AF412721

**Guide to Paediatric Drug Development and
Clinical Research**

# Guide to Paediatric Drug Development and Clinical Research

Editors

**Klaus Rose** Munich

**John N. van den Anker** Washington D.C./Rotterdam

19 figures, and 23 tables, 2010

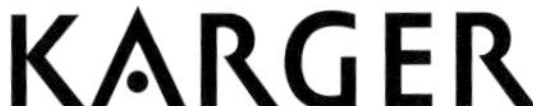

Basel · Freiburg · Paris · London · New York · Bangalore · Bangkok · Shanghai · Singapore · Tokyo · Sydney

**Klaus Rose**
Principal Consultant
Granzer Regulatory Consulting & Services
Zielstattstrasse 44
DE-81379 Munich, Germany

**John N. van den Anker**
Division of Pediatric Clinical Pharmacology
Children's National Medical Center
111 Michigan Avenue, NW
Washington, DC 20010, USA
and
Department of Pediatrics
Erasmus MC – Sophia Children's Hospital
Dr. Molewaterplein 60
NL-3015 GJ Rotterdam, The Netherlands

Library of Congress Cataloging-in-Publication Data

Guide to paediatric drug development and clinical research / editors, Klaus
Rose, John N. van den Anker.
        p. ; cm.
 Includes bibliographical references and indexes.
 ISBN 978-3-8055-9362-5 (hard cover : alk. paper)
 1.  Pediatric pharmacology. 2.  Drug development.  I. Rose, Klaus, 1953-
II. Van den Anker, John N.
 [DNLM: 1.  Drug Evaluation. 2.  Child. 3.  Clinical Trials as Topic. 4.
Infant.  QV 771 G9463 2010]
 RJ560 .G85 2010
 615'.190083--dc22
                                          2010001239



© Copyright 2010 by S. Karger AG, P.O. Box, CH-4009 Basel (Switzerland)
www.karger.com
Printed in Switzerland on acid-free and non-aging paper (ISO 9706) by Reinhardt Druck, Basel
ISBN 978-3-8055-9362-5
e-ISBN 978-3-8055-9363-2

# Contents

# Introduction

Children in the developed world have never enjoyed better medical care. Life expectancy is increasing, and child mortality is improving in most countries. However, the more we can do, the more we also see what could be done better. Every week five new genetically based rare diseases are described – for most of them there is no effective treatment and children with these diseases die early. Cancer in children is no longer untreatable. With the use of chemotherapy, radiation and surgery around 75% of the children survive. However, there are still several cancers in children where treatment is unsatisfactory, and the quality of life of many surviving children is seriously affected. The survival of children with cancer is one of the greatest success stories of medical research in the 20th century. It was not achieved by revolutionary break-through medication, but by combining the chemotherapeutic agents that reached the market in the 1940s and 1950s in new ways and new doses. From 1970 on, with each decade of diagnosis the survival of children with, e.g., acute lymphatic leukemia increased by 10–15% and is today around 90%. But in hindsight, many lives could have been saved earlier had we known how to use the existing medication. This gap was closed by systemic testing and is probably the best argument to show the value of clinical research in and with children. There are other success stories, including the advances in vaccines, surgery, nutrition, and many more.

The rapid advancement of scientific understanding of even more details of the human body combined with the availability of a large group of new genetically engineered medications has increased the desire to make these new treatment options available to children as soon as possible. This is the aim of the EU Paediatric Regulation, in force since January 2007, that has resulted in the formation of the Paediatric Committee, the strengthening of the paediatric department in the European Medicines Agency, and the submission of hundreds of Paediatric Investigation Plans by the pharmaceutical industry.

On the other hand, there are the children in developing countries that are exposed to diseases that in the majority of cases could be easily treated using existing medicines. In the days of modern communication technology, the visibility of these children and the theoretical possibility to help them with access to existing medication have increased the expectations that these children should receive more attention in general and specifically should receive better health care.

The public discussion about medicines for children and the health of children in the developed as well as in the developing world has in the past years reached an unprecedented intensity. One main driver has been the introduction of the EU paediatric regulation, in force now since January 2007, which has exposed pharmaceutical industry to an unprecedented need to include children into the drug development process. An additional driver has been the launch of the WHO campaign 'make medicines child size', which is drawing increased attention to the health of children in the developing world. Further drivers are the increased collaboration between the regulatory authorities of the USA, EU, Japan and other countries and regions in their effort to bundle forces to promote better medicines for children.

On a different level, and less visible for the general public, there have been multiple developments at the clinical, scientific, academic and educational levels. Paediatric clinical pharmacology has established itself as an academic discipline in its own right, represented by the two large international organizations PPAG and ESDP. But what is paediatric clinical pharmacology?

Firstly, paediatric clinical pharmacology is the work of clinical pharmacologists in hospital pharmacies. They advise paediatricians and people in other medical disciplines that take care of ill children on the appropriate dosing of a given medication. They provide the appropriate, mostly extemporaneously prepared, formulation of medications where a child-friendly and age-appropriate formulation is not provided by the manufacturer.

Secondly, paediatric clinical pharmacology is the research undertaken by academic clinical pharmacologists that measure the absorption, distribution, metabolism, and excretion of medicines in children. It was due to their work that a common understanding evolved on how all body functions of the child mature at a different pace. This paediatric clinical pharmacology has, among others, elucidated that a much higher variability in ADME exists in children and that the degree of this high variability further increases if the child or infant has additional issues such as fever, stress, malnutrition or obesity, or is receiving multiple medications.

Thirdly, clinical pharmacology is the discipline in the pharmaceutical industry that tries to predict the dose of a given new medication when administered to children for the first time. Part of this work is modeling and simulation (M&S). M&S allows estimating the first dose of a given medication in a child. This assumed first dose has to be verified against the predicted serum concentration of the medication. If necessary, the prescribed dose has to be adapted based on the observed factual serum concentrations, and, in consequence, the underlying M&S assumptions have to be corrected. It would be unethical to expose children to a drug where basic safety and efficacy data have not yet been established in adults. Consequently, phase 1 clinical trials in healthy volunteers that are routine in adult drug development are not allowed in children. Therefore, clinical pharmacology data in children can only be generated in a setting where a child should benefit from the therapeutic potential of the drug in discussion. As a consequence, paediatric clinical pharmacology in the drug development process can by definition only happen in the framework of phase 2 or phase 3 clinical trials.

Clinical pharmacology is also the discipline in pharmaceutical industry that is part of the multidisciplinary development team that brings a drug through the development process from initial discovery through preclinical and clinical testing to the registration as a medicine. The roles of the clinical pharmacologists in this process include advising on the doses to choose for clinical trials, time point of first exposure of a given drug in adult healthy volunteers, advice on the appropriate time point of a first paediatric exposure, advice on dose adaption in case of renal, hepatic or other impairments, and many more.

The two first types of clinical pharmacology concern drugs that are already existing. Modern drugs have evolved with industrialization and the ability of chemical engineering. Increasingly, biological engineering plays an important role in drug development. When we talk about off-label use of drugs in children we should not forget that modern labels have only evolved since the Kefauver-Harris acts in the USA in 1962 and that drugs in the modern sense of the word only exist for just over 100 years. On the background of this evolution, paediatric clinical pharmacology has been a logical consequence of this development. As always, it only seems to be a logical consequence in hindsight. If we look at the time axis, we see that paediatric clinical pharmacology is only at its early stages.

The level of clinical pharmacology service in hospitals and the level of collaboration with the discipline of paediatrics varies considerably. 'Advanced' hospitals have an own department of paediatric clinical pharmacology. 'Less advanced' hospitals just have a department of clinical pharmacology which may or may not include one paediatric clinical pharmacologist who talks with the paediatricians. And let us not forget those hospitals in less-developed countries that may have only one pharmacologist for the entire hospital. How paediatricians and clinical pharmacologists interact varies from country to country and from hospital to hospital. The collaboration is driven partially by science and partially by tradition.

Research in children is less developed than research in adults. Not all publications on research in children have the methodological scrutiny that has become standard in adult publications. That there is room for improvement is perceived by the most advanced representatives of the professional learned societies of paediatrics, pharmacology, clinical pharmacology and paediatric clinical pharmacology. On the other hand, most paediatricians are rather conservative. They have learned their profession, are proud of their profession, and are not very exposed to paediatric research in their daily clinical work. Speaking of better medicines for children must take into account the different levels of awareness that exists. Conferences on clinical pharmacology and paediatric clinical pharmacology have in recent years had sessions that were specifically dedicated to the new paediatric legislation in the USA and EU as well as to the WHO campaign 'make medicines child size'. Interestingly, the interest of paediatric practitioners has been rather limited. The call for better medicines for children is a movement that is represented and driven forward by a relatively small group within the professional bodies of paediatric pharmacology and clinical pharmacology. It is a movement that still is not strongly represented in the mindset of practicing paediatricians.

Key organizations to promote academic paediatric clinical pharmacology are the IUPHAR and the ESDP. Their key representatives have, together with key representatives from the International Pediatric Association (IPA), established a movement that culminated in the foundation of the IA: International Alliance for Better Medicines for Children. The journal *Pediatric Drugs* is now the official journal of this alliance.

The ethics of research in children is another area. Several issues are at its core. Basic dilemmas are the interest of the child, its inability in young years to represent its interests on its own, and the need of parents to decide in the best interest of their children, in short, their legal status. All involved institutions must balance the potential benefit of a new medication with the potential risk it may carry. But risks are not fully predictable. In consequence, the degree to which potential risks are accepted varies considerably over time depending of tragedies that happen, serious threats like a pandemic that has the potential to change the perception of need risk taking, and many, many more factors.

Ethics committees/IRBs have the institutional obligation to systematically evaluate paediatric research projects. Ethics committees need paediatric expertise. With the number of paediatric research projects increasing, the number of ethics committees that are exposed to paediatric research is increasing as well. The debate of ethics in paediatric research has therefore several elements. One is the question of right and wrong. Another one is the operational organization of decision processes by ethics committees. The literature on ethics in paediatric research is immense and growing. Dilemmas in daily clinical work exist and can by definition not be resolved. They must be handled operationally.

On the other side, the forced exposure of pharmaceutical and medical device industry to paediatric research and an increased academic discussion about paediatric research will also open new dimensions of ethical challenges. Large companies have own departments of quality assurance and are used to scrutiny by the public. Smaller companies have to now deal with paediatric development as well – and they do not have a dedicated paediatric infrastructure. They will be the tempted to find quick solutions. Hopefully this will just remain a temptation. We all know that human nature is immune to temptations. Another temptation will be academicians without proper background and experience who will nevertheless try to get research funds for paediatric projects. For an ethics committee, it is easier to reject a research project from a pharmaceutical company than from a fellow academic. We will over the next years and decades see a lot of movement.

Drug development in general is multidisciplinary. Paediatric drug development reflects as a microcosm the complexity of drug development, narrowed to the specific focus of children. The main disciplines that come in, apart from paediatricians, clinical pharmacologists, ethics, ethics committees and parents and patients, are the departments dedicated to the development of paediatric formulations; the departments that have to run the preclinical pharmacology, safety and toxicology in vitro and in vivo with animals; the clinical development departments, and the departments that are responsible for trial methodology.

This planet is not a perfect place. There is no planet's government. There is war, and there is peace, there are regions with some order and other regions with a lot of corruption. Even in the richest countries children's pharmaceutical and medical treatment was not as perfect as professionals thought long time it was. Diseases that were believed to be near extinction have re-emerged, there are new diseases and new health challenges, and a lot of more challenges. Different institutions address different dimensions. The WHO is focusing on frequent diseases in low income countries, predominantly tuberculosis, malaria and HIV/AIDS. There are other areas that are less visible to the general public. We have included one chapter on paediatric oncology in Europe, and a second one on paediatric oncology in Africa. For any child in Europe the diagnosis of leukemia was a death sentence 60 years ago. It is no longer today. But also a child in Africa has better survival chances today than decades ago. European and US paediatric oncologists support their African colleagues. Paediatricians from rich countries try to support their counterparts in less-rich countries. Where should funds be allocated? Who should allocate them? The development of new drugs for neglected diseases is today done more by private public partnerships than by the pharmaceutical industry. The funding often comes from philanthropic organizations such as the Gates or the Clinton foundation. It is almost impossible to keep an overview over the multitude of initiatives currently going on.

In this edition, we have tried to find suitable representatives of the various disciplines, voices and positions involved. Some key stake holders are heavily involved in operational activities such as the regulatory authorities. Others have a more strategic role, e.g. the World Medical Association. The processes are complex and the different partners are sometimes on different sides. Although we have tried to keep the chapters to a high level, the final composition of this book's faculty can by definition not be perfect. However, we have tried to elucidate the multitude of facets this movement has. The content of this book should give anybody with an interest in paediatric clinical trials and drug development sufficient material to see how complex the matter is and how many completely different disciplines have to work together. We simply tried our best. Many, many thanks to all the authors that have contributed. We hope that you will enjoy the reading.

*John N. van den Anker*
*Klaus Rose*

# The Editors

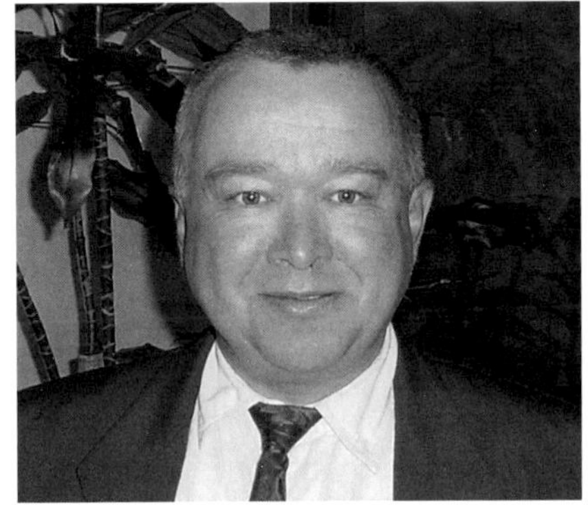

*Dr. Klaus Rose* was born in Heidelberg, Germany. He qualified in medicine in Berlin after initial studies in Romance languages and psychology leading to an MS in psychology. He completed his post-graduate clinical training in General Medicine in Germany and England before joining the pharmaceutical industry in 1991. Since then, he has held various positions in clinical development of progressively increasing responsibility culminating in 2002 in the position of Global Head Paediatrics, Novartis, Basel, Switzerland. In 2005, he joined Roche as Global Head Paediatrics and established a focus for excellence in paediatric drug development. Since 2010, he is Principal Consultant at Granzer Regulatory Consulting in Munich, Germany.

Dr. Rose is a frequent speaker on national and international conferences on paediatric drug development including academic conferences, the EFGCP (European Forum for Good Clinical Practice), the DIA (Drug Information Association), the ECPM (European Course of Pharmaceutical Medicines) and others. He was chairman of the IFPMA paediatric task force from 2008 to 2009 and is chairman of the EFGCP children's medicines working party since its foundation in 2003.

He is married with two daughters. His private interests include Mediterranean-style cooking, good wine, gardening, Latin languages, and classical guitar.

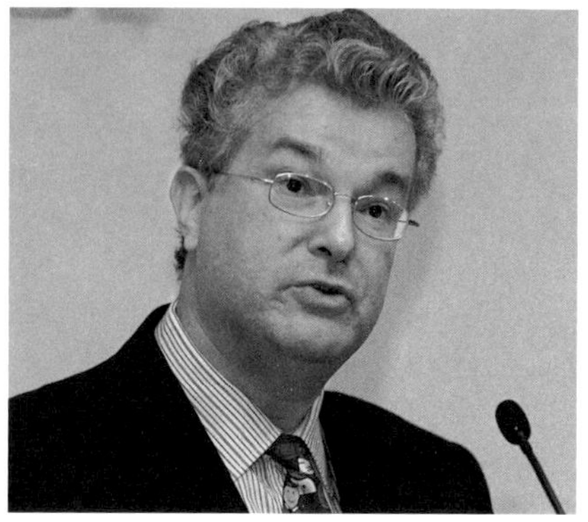

*Prof. Dr. John van den Anker* was born in the Netherlands. He qualified in medicine in Rotterdam in 1983 and completed his post-graduate clinical training in General Paediatrics and Neonatal-Perinatal Medicine in 1991. In 1995, he successfully defended his PhD thesis in Clinical Pharmacology and in 1997 he became the Division Chief of Neonatology at Erasmus MC-Sophia Children's Hospital in Rotterdam. In 2001, he moved to the USA to direct one of the 13 NIH-funded Pediatric Pharmacology Research Units but stayed strongly connected with Erasmus MC-Sophia Children's Hospital. Currently, he is Vice Chair of Paediatrics for Experimental Therapeutics at Children's National Medical Center in Washington, D.C. and holds the Evan and Cindy Jones Chair in Paediatric Clinical Pharmacology. In addition, he is Professor of Paediatrics, Pharmacology and Physiology at the George Washington University.

Prof. Dr. van den Anker is currently 100% funded by the NIH for his clinical and translational research and is a frequently invited speaker on national and international conferences on paediatric clinical pharmacology. He was the President of the European Society for Developmental, Perinatal and Paediatric Pharmacology from 2006 to 2008 and a member of the Board of Directors of the American Society for Clinical Pharmacology and Therapeutics from 2005 to 2008. In 2008, he received the Distinguished Investigator Award from the American College of Clinical Pharmacology and is a member of the editorial board of the major clinical pharmacology journals. Finally, he has been a longstanding member of the Paediatric Working Party of the EMA representing the Netherlands.



The Editors

# Authors' Addresses

**William J. Appleyard, MD, FRCP**
Thimble Hall
108 Blean Common
Blean
Canterbury, Kent CT2 9JJ (UK)
Tel./Fax +44 1227 781771
E-Mail Jimappleyard2510@aol.com

**Hans J. Avis, MD**
Departments of Vascular Medicine, and Pediatrics
Academic Medical Centre
Meibergdreef 9
NL-1105 AZ Amsterdam (The Netherlands)
Tel. +31 20 566 6612, Fax +31 20 566 9343
E-Mail h.j.avis@amc.uva.nl

**Daniel Bar-Shalom**
Associate professor, Department of Pharmaceutics
and Analytical Chemistry
Faculty of Pharmaceutical Sciences
University of Copenhagen
Universitetsparken 2
DK-2100 Copenhagen Ø (Denmark)
Tel. +45 35336351, Fax +45 35 33 60 01
E-Mail dbs@farma.ku.dk

**Daniel K. Benjamin, Jr. MD, PhD**
Department of Pediatrics and
Duke Clinical Research Institute
2400 Pratt Street, #7582
Durham, NC 27715 (USA)
Tel. +1 919 668 7081, Fax +1 919 681 9457

**Claus Bolte, MD, MBA**
Pharmaceuticals Division: Global Medical Director
(Immunology)
F. Hoffmann-La Roche Ltd. - Pharmaceuticals Division
Grenzacherstr. 74, bldg 74/4 Ost/106
CH-4070 Basel (Switzerland)
Tel. +41 414101426
E-Mail clausmannyc@netscape.net

**Jörg Breitkreutz**
Professor for Pharmaceutical Technology
Heinrich-Heine-University Düsseldorf
Institute of Pharmaceutics and Biopharmaceutics
Universitätsstrasse 1
DE-40225 Düsseldorf (Germany)
Tel. +49 211 8110678, Fax +49 211 8114251
E-Mail joerg.breitkreutz@uni-duesseldorf.de

**Francesca Ceddia, MD**
Vice President and Head
Global Clinical Development
GlaxoSmithKline Biologicals
Wavre, Belgium
Avenue Fleming, 20 (W23)
BE-1300 Wavre (Belgium)
Tel. +32 10 85 94 10, Fax +32 10 85 33 63
E-Mail francesca.x.ceddia@gskbio.com

**Dr. Simon Day**
Roche Products Ltd.
Hexagon Place
Shire Park
Welwyn Garden City
Hertfordshire AL7 1TW (UK)
Tel. +44 1707 366409, Fax +44 1707 383145
E-Mail simon.day@Roche.com

**Luc M. De Schaepdrijver, DVM, PhD, MSc**
Global Preclinical Development
Johnson & Johnson Pharmaceutical Research &
Development
Turnhoutseweg 30
BE-2340 Beerse (Belgium)
Tel. +32 14605062, Fax +32 14606138
E-Mail ldschaep@its.jnj.com

**Dr. Oscar E. Della Pasqua, MD, PhD**
Clinical Pharmacology & Discovery Medicine
GlaxoSmithKline
Stockley Park West
Uxbridge UB11 1BT (UK)
Tel. +44  20 8990 3646, Fax +44 20 8990 4654
E-Mail odp72514@gsk.com
and
Associate Professor
Division of Pharmacology
Leiden/Amsterdam Center for Drug Research
POBox 9502
NL-2300 RA Leiden (The Netherlands)

**Patricia Fowler**
Danemount Consulting
Hertford (UK)
E-Mail danemount@live.co.uk

**Ian Friedland, MD**
Cubist Pharmaceuticals, Inc.
65 Hayden Avenue
Lexington, MA 02421 (USA)
Tel. +1 781 860 8421, Fax +1 781 863 1331
E-Mail ian.friedland@cubist.com

**Dr. Sabine Fuerst-Recktenwald, MD**
Pediatrician
Translational Medicine Leader, Metabolism
F. Hoffmann-La Roche Ltd.
Building 682 / 222, Steinentorberg 8/12
CH-4070 Basel (Switzerland)
Tel. +41 61 688 41 04, Fax +41 61 688 03 55
E-Mail sabine.fuerst-recktenwald@roche.com

**Prof. Steffen Gay, MD**
Director, WHO Collaborating Center for Molecular
Biology and Novel Therapeutic Strategies for
Rheumatic Diseases
Department of Rheumatology
University Hospital Zürich
Gloriastrasse 25
CH-8091 Zurich (Switzerland)
E-Mail Steffen.Gay@usz.ch

**Brahm Goldstein, MD, MCR**
Senior Director, Translational Science
Ikaria, Inc., Clinton, NJ
Professor of Pediatrics
University of Medicine and Dentistry of New Jersey
Robert Wood Johnson Medical School
Clinton, NJ 08801 (USA)
Tel. +1 908 399 8346, Fax +1 908 219 2448
E-Mail brahm.goldstein@ikaria.com

**Dr. Ulrich Granzer**
Granzer Regulatory Consulting & Services
Zielstattstr. 44
DE-81379 Munich (Germany)
Tel. +49 89 780 68 98 0, Fax +49 89 780 68 98 15
E-Mail granzer@granzer.biz
www.granzer.biz

**Vincent Grek, MD**
Only for Children Pharmaceuticals
35b rue Henri Barbusse
FR-75005 Paris (France)
Tel. + 33 1 57 27 86 86
Fax + 33 1 57 27 86 80
E-Mail vincent.grek@o4cp.com

**Dr. Daniel B. Hawcutt**
Clinical Lecturer in Paediatric Pharmacology
University of Liverpool
Alder Hey Hospital
Eaton Road
Liverpool L12 2AP (UK)
Tel. +44 151 282 4730, Fax +44 151 282 4719
E-Mail d.hawcutt@liverpool.ac.uk

**Prof. Johannes Hebebrand, MD**
Department of Child and Adolescent Psychiatry
LVR-Klinikum Essen, University of Duisburg-Essen
Virchowstr. 174
DE-45147 Essen (Germany)
Tel. +49 201 7227465
E-Mail Johannes.Hebebrand@uni-duisburg-essen.de

**Dr. Suzanne Hill, B Med (Hons) PhD, Grad Dip Epi FAFPHM**
Medicines, Access and Rational Use,
Essential Medicines and Pharmaceutical Policies
World Health Organisation
20 avenue Appia
CH-1211 Geneva 27 (Switzerland)
Tel. +41 22 7913522, Fax +41 22 791 4167
E-Mail hills@who.int

**Kalle Hoppu, MD, PhD**
Medical Director
Poison Information Centre,
Helsinki University Central Hospital
P.O. Box 790 (Tukholmankatu 17)
FI-00029 HUS, Helsinki (Finland)
Tel. +358 9 471 74 788, Fax +358 9 471 74 702
E-Mail kalle.hoppu@hus.fi

**Barbara A. Hutten, PhD**
Department of Clinical Epidemiology,
Biostatistics and Bioinformatics
Academic Medical Centre
Meibergdreef 9
NL-1105 AZ Amsterdam (The Netherlands)
E-Mail b.a.hutten@amc.uva.nl

**John J.P. Kastelein, MD, PhD**
Department of Vascular Medicine
Academic Medical Centre
Meibergdreef 9
NL-1105 AZ Amsterdam (The Netherlands)
Tel. +31 20 566 6612, Fax +31 20 566 9343
E-Mail j.j.kastelein@amc.uva.nl

**Alastair Kent**
Director
Genetic Interest Group
4D Leroy House
436 Essex Road
London N1 3QP (UK)
Tel. +44 20 7704 3141, Fax +44 20 7359 1447
E-Mail alastair@gig.org.uk
www.gig.org.uk

**D.M. (Meeike) Kusters, MD**
Departments of Vascular Medicine, and Pediatrics
Academic Medical Centre
Meibergdreef 9
NL-1105 AZ Amsterdam (The Netherlands)
Tel. +31 20 566 6612, Fax +31 20 566 9343
E-Mail D.M.Kusters@amc.uva.nl

**Dr. Birka Lehman**
Bundesinstitut für Arzneimittel und Medizinprodukte
Kurt-Georg-Kiesinger-Allee 3
DE-53175 Bonn (Germany)
Tel. +49 228 993073689, Fax +49 228 2073534
E-Mail blehmann@bfarm.de

**Jennifer S. Li, MD**
Department of Pediatrics and
Duke Clinical Research Institute
Duke University Medical Center
Durham, NC 27710 (USA)
Tel. +1 919 668 8682, Fax +1 919 668 7058
E-Mail jennifer.li@duke.edu

**Xavier Liogier d'Ardhuy, PhD**
Clinical Research and Exploratory
Development & Clinical Pharmacology
F. Hoffmann-La Roche Ltd.
CH-4070 Basel (Switzerland)
Tel. +41 61 688 80 95, Fax +41 61 688 60 07
E-Mail xavier.liogier_dardhuy@roche.com

**Prof. Irja Lutsar, MD**
University of Tartu
Ravila 19
EE-50411 Tartu (Estonia)
Tel. +372 737 4171, Fax +372 737 4172
E-Mail irja.lutsar@ut.ee

**Samuel D. Maldonado, MD**
Vice-President and Head
Pediatric Drug Development Center of Excellence
Johnson & Johnson PRD
920 Route 202 South
Raritan, NJ 08869 (USA)
Tel. +1 908 927 2449
E-Mail SMaldon3@prdus.jnj.com

**Giorgio Massimini, MD**
F. Hoffmann-La Roche Ltd.
Pharmaceuticals Division
Grenzacherstr. 124
CH-4070 Basel (Switzerland)
Tel. +41 61 688 9665, Fax +41 61 688 0501
E-Mail giorgio.massimini@roche.com

**Prof. Dr. Dirk Matthys**
Department of Pediatrics
Ghent University
De Pintelaan 185
BE-9000 Ghent (Belgium)
Tel. +32 9 332 35 84, Fax +32 9 332 38 75
E-Mail Dirk.Matthys@UGent.be

**Dr. med. Dirk Mentzer**
Facharzt für Kinderheilkunde
Referatsleiter Arzneimittelsicherheit
Head of Pharmacovigilance Unit
Paul-Ehrlich-Institut
Paul Ehrlich Str. 51-59
DE-63225 Langen (Germany)
Tel. +49 6103 771011, E-Mail mendi@pei.de

**Simon Nadel, MD, FRCP**
Consultant and Honorary Reader in Paediatric
Intensive Care
Imperial College Health Care NHS Trust
St. Mary's Campus
Prased Street
London W2 1NY (UK)
Tel. +44 2078866077, Fax +44 2078866958
E-Mail s.nadel@imperial.ac.uk

**Hidefumi Nakamura, MD, PhD**
National Center for Child Health and Development
2-10-1 Ookura, Setagaya-ku
Tokyo 157-8535 (Japan)
Tel. +81 3 3416 0181, ext. 7063 or 5373,
Fax +81 3 3417 5691
E-Mail nakamura-hd@ncchd.go.jp

**Robert M. Nelson, MD, PhD**
Pediatric Ethicist, Office of Pediatric Therapeutics
Office of the Commissioner, United States Food and
Drug Administration
Silver Spring, MD 20993 (USA)
Tel. +1 301 827 1522, Fax +1 301 827 1017
E-Mail Robert.Nelson@fda.hhs.gov

**Prof. Tony Nunn**
Clinical Director of Pharmacy and
MCRN Associate Director
Alder Hey Hospital
Eaton Road
Liverpool L12 2AP (UK)
Tel. +44 151 252 5314, Fax +44 151 252 5675
E-Mail Tony.Nunn@alderhey.nhs.uk

**Dr. Cor Oosterwijk**
Vice-President EGAN, Director VSOP
Koninginnelaan 23
NL-3762 DA Soest (The Netherlands)
Tel. +31 35 603 4040, Fax +31 35 602 7440
E-Mail c.oosterwijk@vsop.nl
www.egan.eu, www.vsop.nl

**Masahiro Ozaki**
Associate Director, Regulatory Affairs
UCB Japan Co., Ltd.
2-2 Kanda-Surugadai, Chiyoda-ku
Tokyo 101-0062 (Japan)
Tel. +81 3 5283 1733, Fax +81 3 5283 1890
E-Mail masahiro.ozaki@ucb.com
www.ucb.com

**Audino Podda, MD**
Novartis Vaccines Institute for Global Health
Clinical Development & Regulatory
Via Fiorentina, 1
IT-53100 Siena (Italy)
Tel. +39 0577 243496, Fax +39 0577 243540
E-Mail audino.podda@novartis.com

**Ysbrand Poortman**
Vice-President World Alliance of Organizations for
Prevention and Treatment of Genetic and Congenital
Conditions (WAO)
Helios 130, Gerstkamp
NL-2592 CV The Hague (The Netherlands)
Tel. +31 35 683 1920, Fax +31 35 602 7440
E-Mail y.poortman@vsop.nl

**Ronald J. Portman, MD**
Group Director
Pediatric Drug Development Program/CV-metabolics
Bristol Myers Squibb
Rte 206 and Provinceline Road
Princeton, NJ 08543 (USA)
Tel. +1 6092525758, Fax +1 6092526701
E-Mail Ronald.Portman@bms.com

**Prof. Kathy Pritchard-Jones, MD**
The Institute of Cancer Research and
The Royal Mardsen Hospital
Downs Road
Sutton
Surrey SM2 5PT (UK)
Tel. +44 20 8661 3498, Fax +44 20 8661 3617
E-Mail kathy.pritchard-jones@icr.ac.uk

**Prof. José Ramet, MD**
Chairman Department of Pediatrics
University Hospital of Antwerp (UZA)
Wilrijkstraat 10
BE-2650 Edegem (Belgium)
Tel. +32 3 821 4015, Fax +32 3 829 1194
E-Mail Jose.Ramet@uza.be

**Bruno Reigner, PharmD, PhD**
Clinical Research and Exploratory
Development & Clinical Pharmacology
F. Hoffmann-La Roche Ltd.
CH-4070 Basel (Switzerland)
Tel. +41 61 688 4507, Fax +41 61 688 0415
E-Mail bruno.reigner@roche.com

**Prof. Lorna A. Renner, MD**
Consultant Paediatric Oncologist
University of Ghana Medical School
Korle Bu Teaching Hospital
P.O. Box 4236
Accra (Ghana)
Tel. +233 21 665405, Fax +233 21 681080
E-Mail lornarenner@gmail.com

**Benedicte Ricci, PharmD, PhD**
Clinical Research and Exploratory
Development & Clinical Pharmacology
F. Hoffmann-La Roche Ltd.
CH-4070 Basel (Switzerland)
Tel. +41 61 688 5067, Fax +41 61 688 6007
E-Mail benedicte.ricci@roche.com

**William Rodriguez, MD, PhD**
Office of Pediatric Therapeutics
Office of the Commissioner FDA
Rockville, MD 20857 (USA)
Tel. +1 301 827 1996, Fax +1 301 827 1017
E-Mail William.Rodriguez@fda.hhs.gov

**Dr. Andrew C. Rose**
MCRN Industry Liaison Manager
University of Liverpool
Alder Hey Hospital
Eaton Road
Liverpool L12 2AP (UK)
Tel. +44 151 252 5435, Fax +44 151 282 4719
E-Mail andrew.rose@liverpool.ac.uk

**Klaus Rose, MD, MS**
Principal Consultant
Granzer Regulatory Consulting & Services
Zielstattstrasse 44
DE-81379 Munich (Germany)
Tel. +49 89 780 68 98 29, Fax +49 89 780 68 98 15
E-Mail rose@granzer.biz

**Ladislav Šenolt, MD, PhD**
Institute of Rheumatology and
Connective Tissue Research Laboratory
Department of Rheumatology of the First
Faculty of Medicine
Charles University in Prague, Czech Republic
Na Slupi 4
CZ-128 50 Prague 2 (Czech Republic)
Tel. + 420 234 075 232, Fax +420 224 914 451
E-Mail seno@revma.cz or lsenolt@yahoo.com

**Thomas Severin, MD**
Novartis Pharma AG
Novartis Campus
CH-4002 Basel (Switzerland)
Tel. +41 61 324 5424, Fax +41 61 324 2130
E-Mail thomas.severin@novartis.com

**Renee Simar, PhD**
Principal Strategist, Pediatrics
INC Research
3321 Bee Caves Road
Austin, TX 78746 (USA)
Tel./Fax +1 512 858 4928
E-Mail rsimar@incresearch.com

**Dr. Despina Solomonidou**
Global Technical R&D Project Management - Franchise
Head Oncology
Novartis Pharma AG
Fabrikstrasse 12-4.03C.8
Novartis Pharma AG
Novartis Campus
CH-4056 Basel (Switzerland)
E-Mail despina.solomonidou@novartis.com

**Dr. Catherine Tuleu**
Senior Lecturer in Pharmaceutics
Deputy Director Centre for Paediatric Pharmacy
Research
The School of Pharmacy
University of London
29-39 Brunswick Square
London WC1N 1AX (UK)
Tel. +44 2077535857, Fax +44 2077535942
E-Mail catherine.tuleu@pharmacy.ac.uk

**Dr. Mark A. Turner**
Senior Lecturer/Consultant in Neonatology
Neonatal Unit
Liverpool Women's Hospital
Crown Street
Liverpool L8 7SS (UK)
Tel. +44 151 702 4118, Fax +44 151 702 4202
E-Mail mark.turner@liverpool.ac.uk

**Prof. John N. van den Anker, MD, PhD**
Division of Pediatric Clinical Pharmacology
Children's National Medical Center
111 Michigan Avenue, NW
Washington, DC 20010 (USA)
E-Mail jvandena@cnmc.org
and
Department of Pediatrics
Erasmus MC – Sophia Children's Hospital
Dr. Molewaterplein 60
NL-3015 GJ Rotterdam (The Netherlands)

**Prof. Gilles Vassal, MD**
Institut Gustave Roussy
FR-94805 Villejuif Cedex (France)
Tel. +33 1 42 11 65 30, Fax +33 1 42 11 53 08
E-Mail gvassal@igr.fr

**Prof. Timo Vesikari**
Vaccine Research Center
University of Tampere
Biokatu 10
FI-33520 Tampere (Finland)
Tel. +358 3 3551 8444, Fax +358 3 3551 8450
E-Mail timo.vesikari@uta.fi

**Maud N. Vissers, PhD**
Department of Vascular Medicine
Academic Medical Centre
Meibergdreef 9
NL-1105 AZ Amsterdam (The Netherlands)
Tel. +31 20 566 6612, Fax +31 20 566 9343
E-Mail m.n.vissers@amc.uva.nl

**Albert Wiegman, MD, PhD**
Academic Medical Centre
Department of Pediatrics
Meibergdreef 9
NL-1105 AZ Amsterdam (The Netherlands)
Tel. +31 20 566 3468, Fax +31 20 691 9854
E-Mail a.wiegman@amc.uva.nl

**Dr. ElisabethAnn Wright**
Hogan & Hartson
Brussels
rue de l'Industrie 26
BE-1040 Brussels (Belgium)
Tel. +32 2 505 0911, Fax +32 2 505 0996
E-Mail ewright@hhlaw.com

**Prof. Lothar-Bernd Zimmerhackl, MD**
Department of Pediatrics I
Medical University Innsbruck
Anichstrasse 35
AT-6020 Innsbruck (Austria)
Tel. +43 512 504 23501, Fax +43 512 504 25450
E-Mail lothar-bernd.zimmerhackl@uki.at

Rose K, van den Anker JN (eds): Guide to Paediatric Drug Development and Clinical Research.
Basel, Karger, 2010, pp 1–5

# Europe and the Path to Better Medicines for Children

José Ramet[a] · Birka Lehman[b] · Klaus Rose[c]

[a]Department of Paediatrics, University Hospital Antwerp (UZA), Edegem, Belgium, [b]Bundesinstitut für Arzneimittel und Medizinprodukte, Bonn, Germany and [c]F. Hoffmann-La Roche Ltd., Pharmaceuticals Division, Basel, Switzerland

There is increasing awareness worldwide that the pharmaceutical treatment of children is not as scientific in comparison to the scientific and regulatory framework that defines today's drugs for adults. Off-label use of medicines in children is widespread, and the awareness of adverse drug reactions in children does not get as much attention as would be desirable and for many older drugs no evidence-based dosing recommendations are available or differ between countries or even between regions or cities within the same country. This and much more is documented in detail in numerous publications [1–5].

It is helpful to look at child treatment within the framework of a rapidly evolving world, where the position of Europe is not static. Europe's scientific and material superiority compared to other countries and regions cannot be taken for granted. The EU Lisbon strategy set out in March 2000 aims at making 'the most dynamic and competitive knowledge-based economy in the world capable of sustainable economic growth with more and better jobs and greater social cohesion, and respect for the environment by 2010' [6, 7]. What does this mean for children?

We see today how many assumptions that constituted the fundaments of pharmacotherapy of children in the past have had to be corrected. It was, e.g., assumed over the last decades that during the first month of a neonate's life absorption, distribution, metabolization and excretion remain stable. Today, we know that we are confronted with a rapid, nearly daily development especially over the first weeks and months of life and therefore we need to adapt our treatment recommendations and tools more precisely. Our general understanding of the growing child's organ systems, metabolic pathways as well as their neuronal development is exploding [8]. In other words, we have just started. The majority of children in the developed world profit from a health care system that could not even have been dreamed about centuries ago. We just have started to see what is possible, and we might have glimpses of what can be reached in the future. Every day symptoms and diseases and the relationship to each other are being discovered. Many children still die or have a low quality of life because of cancer, genetic disorders, or many other diseases.

Children deserve the brightest minds to be attracted to and retained in paediatric clinical care and research. The active participation of the top representatives of the paediatrics community can ensure that sick children have access to the most advanced treatment options and that parents of a sick child find motivated, interested partners as their medical counterparts when they consider options what to do for their sick child. This is not a task for the single person. It is within the responsibility of society to set frames for current and future child treatment. If research with children is not honoured by society, young people with good prospects will find their careers in other areas. Top quality scientific research with children is part of the competitiveness of any country and region.

An example: Following the evolvement of chemotherapeutic agents for treatment of adult cancer, clinical research in children has led to an impressive reduction of mortality in this area. Not all children with cancer survive, and those that do survive do not all have a quality of life comparable with healthy children. There is still a long way to go, improvements on many levels will be needed and will have to be pushed through against a multitude of barriers. We have started this way, but we are not yet there.

There are hundreds of disease-specific national, regional and global professional paediatric associations and organisations. With Europe growing from a conglomerate of national states into a regional entity, Europe's paediatricians will have to adapt to this new challenge to adequately represent the voice of child health care in Europe. It will also be necessary to work more closely with other professions, including nurses and child nurses. Training schemes and career development in health care will have to adapt and evolve.

Due to the EU Paediatric Regulation [9], in force since January 2007, drug development in Europe is no longer possible without considering the future use of the drug in children. The regulation's main focus is on improving children's pharmaceutical treatment by ensuring that the specific aspects of the growing child's body and mind are considered when companies want to expand the use of medications already available ('today's drugs') as long as they

are patent protected, as well as for medications in earlier development stages ('drugs of the future'). Additional foci are strengthening research on drugs that are no longer patent protected ('mature drugs') and strengthening the European paediatric research infrastructure and competitiveness. As per European infrastructure and organisation, only pharmaceuticals are in the scope of this legislation whereas the US paediatric paediatric legislation which was re-authorized in 2007 [10] includes a paediatric chapter on medical devices. Inclusion of children into the drug development process is mandatory. It is also rewarded with a 6 months' Supplementary Patent Certificate prolongation.

Over the last decades, paediatric clinical pharmacology has evolved as a discipline in its own right. Several chapters in this book describe the operational role of clinical pharmacologists in the daily practice in hospital clinical care, i.e. the research in academic clinical pharmacology that has enormously increased our understanding of the evolving child's body [8]. Less visible to the outside world, paediatric clinical pharmacology has been the second major force that has pushed for paediatric legislation both in the USA and in Europe.

The EU Paediatric Committee (PDCO) [11] was established July 2007. It is comprised by up to 27 representatives of EU member states, including 5 members of the Committee for Medicinal products for Human Use (CHMP) [12], three representatives of patient organisations, and three representatives of the paediatric profession. The PDCO handles paediatric investigation plans (PIPs) submitted by pharmaceutical companies. This includes negotiating with the respective submitting company on proposed development measures, including clinical trials, non-clinical trials, child-adapted galenic formulations, clinical safety, post-marketing commitments, and more. If the negotiations succeed, they could result in a final opinion that includes the agreed measures, deferrals (measures will be considered or started later but the content has to be agreed by the PDCO and included in the opinion) for one or several age groups, or waivers (no development in children). The essentials of the decisions are published at the EMA website [13] after removal of confidential and sensitive information. If the negotiations do not succeed, the final opinion is negative and the PIP is not approved. Further responsibilities of the PDCO include the tracking of submitted PIPs – the respective company has to submit a progress report once per year, and decision about companies' compliance with their PIP towards the end of the patent life.

PIPs are requested for two major reasons. Firstly, a PIP is requested for any new indication, new formulation or new route of administration of any patent-protected medication already on the market. Secondly, a PIP is requested for drugs in development ('drugs of the future') at the end of adult human pharmacokinetic studies. Although there is no precise definition as to when the end of adult human pharmacokinetic studies occur, it is in every developing company's own interest to submit a PIP not too late. Marketing Authorisation Applications (MAAs, the European wording for submitting a request for licensing a new drug) will not be validated by the EMA without an approved PIP.

The PDCO is an entity that is supported by the EMA, the European Medicines Agency. A PIP is not submitted directly to the PDCO, but to the EMA, which produces a PIP summary report that is forwarded to the PDCO, which appoints a rapporteur and a co-rapporteur from two different member states. In the case of the PIPs, the EMA is the body that has the power of enforcement. No new medication can be submitted for licensing in the EU anymore without an agreed PIP. Neither the EMA nor a member state will validate such a submission. As a consequence, drug development is no longer possible in Europe without taking children's needs into consideration. This consideration can start by finding the targeted adult indication on the

EMA list of class waivers [14]. In this case, no formal PIP procedure needs to be undertaken; instead, a letter to the EMA referring to the list of class waivers should be enough and must be presented to the PDCO for information and agreement. If no waiver is granted, an extensive and expensive paediatric investigation plan should be made consisting of several clinical, technical, non-clinical and other measures that all will be scrutinised by the EMA and PDCO towards the end of the time period agreed upon.

The EMA paediatric website [15] is an excellent repository of information. Numerous statistics on the number of PIPs received, accepted or rejected are available.

Regarding the resource for more inclusion of children into the drug development process there are at least two categories. The EMA has scientific administrators that evaluate PIPs submitted by pharmaceutical companies and eventually evaluate data generated on the base of these PIPs. The EU Member States are contributing through their PDCO representatives that act as rapporteur or peer reviewer. Data from the pharmaceutical industry on the resources required to handle the EU paediatric regulation do not exist at present. Industry will in the future have to develop ways to assess these resources.

The degree to which daily healthcare of children has changed with the US legislation is very difficult to assess. The report to congress in 2001 [16] tentatively lists the number of hospital days reduced by better medication of children, or the reduced number of working days lost by parents due to better pharmaceutical treatment of their children. No such data have been published since then. A surrogate parameter might be the percentage of specific paediatric information given in the patient information of drugs on the market. Here things have certainly progressed over the last decade. For such an assessment of the EU regulation more years will be needed.

What is the attitude of paediatricians, parents and the public towards research with children?

Paediatricians are acting in a more conservative way, and not all representatives accept that a continuous critical evaluation of current practices is required.

Is the general European climate facilitating clinical research both in general and in children? The European clinical trials directive has attempted to improve the conditions of clinical research, but this has led to different interpretations of many details in the different EU member states. Of course, the opinions of the different stakeholders about this directive are divided. However, there is probably agreement among all the stakeholders that the attractiveness of Europe for clinical research as compared to other regions of this world has improved over the last decade, but not drastically.

Paediatric research networks in Europe are evolving. We observe the establishment of many national paediatric research networks, including the UK, Germany, France, Austria, Finland, the Netherlands and Belgium. Other networks are disease specific (almost all of them international) and are already exposed to many years of collaboration with the pharmaceutical industry. One of the objectives of the EU paediatric legislation is the creation of a network of networks of paediatric research [17]. In 2010, many questions regarding these networks remain open.

It is the will of the EU legislators to seriously improve child health in Europe and worldwide. Considering the economic position of Europe on a global scale and that drug development today is a global process, this will have a major impact on the global development of medicines. The awareness of this impact is still limited among the parties involved in adult and children's health care. As the dimensions of this impact are certainly enormous, the debate can be expected to gain momentum over the years to come.

There is a high-level agreement between regulators, academics and the pharmaceutical industry that the consciousness of more and better research with children is necessary. Of course, at the detail level there are many areas of diverging opinions. All sides are undergoing a learning curve. It is essential when addressing child health and child research in Europe to keep an open view on the evolving world and Europe's place in this world. Europe's children deserve the best medical care and research. Many barriers remain to be removed. An open constructive dialogue will be essential to move forward.

## References

1 Caldwell PH, Butow PN, Craig JC: Pediatricians' attitude toward randomized controlled trials involving children. J Pediatr 2002;141:798–803.
2 Caldwell PH, Butow PN, Craig JC: Parents' attitude to children's participation in randomized control studies. J Pediatr 2003;142:554–559.
3 Campbell H, et al: A review of randomised controlled trials published in *Archives of Disease in Childhood* from 1982–1996. Arch Dis Child 1998;79: 192–197.
4 Clark RH, Bloom BT, Spitzer AR, Gerstmann DR: Reported medication use in the neonatal intensive care unit: data from a large national data set. Pediatrics 2006;117:1979–1987.
5 Evans JR, Short BL, Van Meurs K, Sachs HC: Cardiovascular support in preterm infants. Clin Ther 2006;28:1366–1384.
6 http://en.wikipedia.org/wiki/Lisbon_Strategy
7 European Commission, Directorate-General for Research: 'Towards a European Research', Area Science, Technology and Innovation. 2003, key figures, 43–44. http://ec.europa.eu/research/era/pdf/indicators/benchmarking2003_en.pdf
8 Kearns GL, et al: Developmental pharmacology – drug disposition, action, and therapy in infants and children. NEJM 2003;349:1157–1167.
9 http://www.ema.europa.eu/htms/human/paediatrics/regulation.htm
10 http://www.fda.gov/RegulatoryInformation/Legislation/FederalFoodDrugandCosmeticActFDCAct/SignificantAmendmentstotheFDCAct/FoodandDrugAdministrationAmendmentsActof2007/default.htm
11 http://www.ema.europa.eu/htms/human/paediatrics/pdco.htm

12  http://www.ema.europa.eu/htms/general/contacts/CHMP/CHMP.html

13  http://www.ema.europa.eu/htms/human/paediatrics/decisions.htm

14  http://www.ema.europa.eu/htms/human/paediatrics/classwaivers.htm

15  http://www.ema.europa.eu/htms/human/paediatrics/introduction.htm

16  http://www.fda.gov/downloads/Drugs/DevelopmentApprovalProcess/DevelopmentResources/UCM049915.pdf

17  http://www.ema.europa.eu/htms/human/paediatrics/network.htm

Klaus Rose, MD, MS
Principal Consultant
Granzer Regulatory Consulting & Services, Zielstattstrasse 44
DE–81379 Munich (Germany)
Tel. +49 89 780 68 98 29, Fax +49 89 780 68 98 15, E-Mail rose@granzer.biz

Rose K, van den Anker JN (eds): Guide to Paediatric Drug Development and Clinical Research.
Basel, Karger, 2010, pp 6–11

# European Union Paediatric Regulation: Theory and Practice

ElisabethAnn Wright[a]  ·  Klaus Rose[b]

[a]Hogan & Hartson, Brussels, Belgium and [b]F. Hoffmann-La Roche Ltd., Pharmaceuticals Division, Basel, Switzerland

This chapter examines the legal framework established by the EU Paediatric Regulation[1]. It also examines the role of the European Medicines Agency (EMA) Paediatric Committee (PDCO). Practical experience thus far of the application of the regime for which the regulation is assessed and possible improvements are also discussed.

## Background

The statistics, well known and often repeated, that although almost 20% of the population of the EU is aged under 16 years and that an estimated 50–90% of medicinal products for human use are not designed, developed, tested or evaluated for use in the paediatric population were an important influencing factor in the adoption of the EU Paediatric Regulation.

It was concluded that any adequate solution to the existing limited sources of medicinal products specifically developed for the paediatric population should have a number of basic elements. These elements included steps to improve the health of the children through stimulation of ethical and high quality research in the field of paediatric indications, an increase in the number of available products with paediatric indications and means to channel the appropriate information to healthcare professionals treating children. At the same time, it was necessary that this objective be achieved while avoiding unnecessary clinical investigations involving children and that it should not prejudice development and access to innovative treatment available to the general population.

A key element of the EU Paediatric Regulation was the introduction of a new element to the EU marketing authorisation procedure for medicinal products requiring applicants to include information relating to potential paediatric use of the product. The philosophy of the regulation was to establish a system of obligation and awards for the companies researching and developing medicinal products to include paediatric indications.

The EU Paediatric Regulation was adopted on December 12, 2006 and entered in force as of January 26, 2007. All of the transitional periods provided for the regulation expired as of January 26, 2009.

---

[1] Regulation (EC) No. 1901/2006 of the European Parliament and of the Council of December 12, 2006 on medicinal products for paediatric use.

## The EMA Paediatrics Committee

On July 26, 2007, the Paediatric Committee (PDCO) was established. It is composed of the representatives of the EU member states, works in close collaboration with the EMA, but is not part of the EMA. The PDCO is responsible for providing scientific assessment of the paediatric investigation plans (PIPs) required by the EU Paediatric Regulation. Its main responsibility is to assess the content of PIPs and adopt opinions on these in accordance with the provisions of the regulation. This includes the assessment of applications for a full or partial waiver of PIPs and assessment of applications for deferrals. The PDCO does not, however, provide opinions on applications for marketing authorisation for medicinal products for paediatric use. This remains entirely within the remit of the EMA's Committee for Medicinal Products for Human Use (CHMP).

*The Obligations*

Following entry into force of the EU Paediatric Regulation, all applications for marketing authorisation of products that were not yet authorised by July 26, 2008 must include the results of studies conducted according to a Paediatric Investigation Plan (PIP) previously approved by the PDCO. The PIP includes information concerning the timing and measures proposed to obtain a paediatric indication, with an age-appropriate formulation, in all paediatric subsets affected by the condition. Applications for a PIP, including applications for deferral or for a waiver, should generally be submitted at the completion of human pharmaco-kinetic studies of the product in adults. Once agreed by the PDCO, the PIP is binding for the company. Within the submitted PIP, the company can request partial of complete waiver(s) or deferral(s). All these requests must be well justified.

The obligation to submit a PIP extends to applications for new indications, pharmaceutical forms and/or ways of administration of already authorised medicinal products that are still protected by a supplementary protection certificate (SPC), or by a patent eligible for a SPC. In such cases, the PIP must cover not only the new indications, but also the already authorised, existing indications.

The PIP is an evolving document. When new information and clinical data become available in the course of the development of a medicinal product the company may submit an application for modification of the PIP to the PDCO.

When assessing a PIP, the PDCO also takes into consideration the 'interest of the children'. An indication as to what falls within the concept of the 'interest of the children' can be found in several lists identifying needs in major therapeutic areas. Those lists are published on the EMA website.

Finally, some medicinal products are exempt from the obligation to submit a PIP. The list includes the generic medicinal products, hybrid medicinal products, biosimilars and medicinal products containing one or more active substances of well-established medicinal use, as well as the homeopathic and (traditional) herbal medicinal products.

*Class Waivers*

Soon after the implementation of the EU Paediatric Regulation the PDCO initiated to publish class waivers, i.e. lists of diseases that do not exist in children. A company that plans to develop a drug in on of these diseases does not need to submit a PIP but can get an exemption form a PIP through a letter to the EMA referring to the list of class waivers. EMA will confirm this in written.

In the meantime, the list of class waivers has been consolidated into one list. Furthermore, a first disease has been removed from the status of adult-only disease: melanoma. Melanoma is now considered to occur frequently enough in adolescents (12–18 years) to be considered as a paediatric disease. As the decision to revoke the class waiver status was published officially on July 14, 2008, companies that plan to submit a marketing authorisation application for a melanoma drug could do so without the obligation to submit a PIP until the July 13, 2011.

*The Benefits*

The EU Paediatric Regulation includes incentives and awards for compliance with PIPs by applicants for marketing authorisation.

When a manufacturer submits trial results that comply with the agreed PIP with its application for marketing authorisation for a new product, or new indication or formulation of an existing product the related SPC for the product will be extended by 6 months.

This award is, however, conditional to a number of provisos. The medicinal product must be protected by an SPC or by an eligible basic patent. The SPC must include the information relevant to any paediatric indication. Furthermore, the product must be authorised in all EU Member States. Finally, if the paediatric indication was used to apply for and benefit from an additional year of data exclusivity as an innovative indication, the product cannot benefit from the additional six months SPC period related to the PIP.

It is also possible for products that have been designated as orphan medicinal products to benefit from a 10-year period of market exclusivity. Such products are not commonly protected by patent. As a result, the reward of an extension of the related SPC is not available. Consequently, rather than an extension of the SPC supplementary protection certificate, for orphan medicinal products the 10-year period of orphan market exclusivity is extended to 12 years if the requirement for data on use in the paediatric population is fully met.

The EU Paediatric Regulation also provides incentives for medicinal products that have been on the market in EU Member States for some time and are, therefore, no longer covered by patent or SPC protection. The Paediatric Use Marketing Authorisation (PUMA) procedure permits application for authorisation of a paediatric indication for an existing medicinal product. A successful application results in a grant of 10 years' data exclusivity. This period is independent of the product's patent or SPC status.

There is an important distinction to be underlined concerning the benefits available on the basis of the EU Paediatric Regulation. The additional 6-month SPC period award for new and patented medicinal products is granted even the marketing authorisation for the product does not include the paediatric indication(s). This is also the case for the additional 2 years market exclusivity period granted to orphan medicinal products. However, the 10 year data exclusivity period granted on the basis of the PUMA will be available only if a marketing authorisation for this indication is granted.

**The EU Paediatric Regulation in Practice**

The EU Paediatric Regulation is still relatively new, with the transitional periods for which it provides having expired only in January 2009. It is, therefore, still difficult to fully assess the impact that the regulation has had and even less the success (or failure) of the established framework. The extent to which the basic aim of the Regulation has been achieved (i.e. increase in the research in the field of paediatric indications and an increase the number of available products with paediatric indications) is unlikely to be evident for some time.

Nevertheless, some quantitative and qualitative experience has been acquired and a number of difficulties and shortcomings have been identified, essentially concerning the implementation of the theoretical framework in practice.

Between its entry into force in late July 2007 and May 2009, the PDCO had validated 459 PIPs and/or waiver applications. These included:
- 292 of applications concerned new product;
- 18 PUMA applications;
- 742 waiver applications.
  The results of these consultations were:
- 85 positive opinions on full waiver;
- 143 positive opinions on PIP (including deferrals);
- 12 negative opinions;
- 7 positive opinions on compliance with PIPs, and
- 16 positive opinions on modification of a PIP.

Although it is difficult to draw any qualitative conclusion out of those numbers, it appears that the system is functioning and that the industry is adapting to the system which the EU Paediatric Regulation has introduced. However, a number of issues associated with the application of the provisions of the in practice have emerged.


*What Is the Extent of the Relative Discretion of the PDCO and of the CHMP?*

The point at which the role of the PDCO ends and that of the CHMP begins is currently unclear. Experience suggests that a delineation between the roles of the two committees could usefully be established.

Moreover, it is emerging that EMA and PDCO consider the EU Paediatric Regulation to have attributed to them an important margin of appreciation and discretion to modify the submitted PIP as they consider appropriate. According to their current interpretation of their powers, these include imposition of additional elements in the PIP which can, on occasion, be extended to including new indications not foreseen by the applicant but considered necessary by the PDCO and EMA. While the power of the PDCO and EMA to approve a PIP while imposing modifications is not disputed, the power to require modifications that essentially lead to a significantly different PIP and the criteria on which this power is based could usefully be addressed.

The confusion as to the extent of the EMA power in this area has already led to conflict and an action before the European Court of First Instance (CFI). Nycomed Danmark ApS has challenged a decision by the EMA to refuse to accept its application for a waiver of its PIP obligations in relation to a new in vivo diagnostic product, claiming that the EMA has misinterpreted the concept of 'a disease or condition for which the medicinal product is intended'. The company further argues that the EMA abused its power in refusing to accept its request for a waiver.

The case arose following the developments by Nycomed of an ultrasound echocardiography imaging agent for which the company intended to apply for marketing authorisation through the centralised authorisation procedure. The company's intended indication for the product was diagnosing coronary artery disease in patients with chest pain being evaluated for inducible ischemia. Having conducted clinical trials in adults with coronary artery disease (CAD), the company submitted an application for a PIP waiver on the ground that the product was intended as a diagnostic agent for CAD, which occurs only in the adult population.

Endorsing a negative opinion by the PDCO the EMA rejected Nycomed's application for a waiver. It concluded that the diagnostic agent was used to reveal myocardial perfusion abnormalities which can be various heart diseases occurring both in children and adults. The EMA concluded that the product was, therefore, likely to be applied in children sooner or later irrespective of the fact that Nycomed had selected an indication occurring only in the adult population.

On April 24, 2009, the CFI refused an application by Nycomed for interim measures suspending the decision of the EMA. However, the main dispute between the parties will now be addressed. This is essentially how much discretion the PDCO and EMA have under the EU Paediatric Regulation and the extent to which they may refuse a product-specific waiver or impose requirements that go beyond the therapeutic indication which the applicant intends to include in the application for marketing authorisation.

*Some Practical Shortcomings of the Award System*

One of the requirements that must be fulfilled if a patented product is to benefit from 6 months extension of the SPC protection is that the product is authorised in all EU member states. When applied to medicinal products that have been authorised through the EU centralised marketing authorisation procedure this obligation does not pose any great problem. The result of a centralised authorisation is that the product is automatically authorised in all 27 EU member states.

However, at the present time, and partially due to the criteria governing authorisation through the centralised procedure, a significant number of medicinal products are currently authorised in the EU through the decentralised marketing authorisation procedure. Application in practice of the obligation to have a medicinal product authorised in all EU member states in order to benefit from the six months extension to the SPC means that, where the medicinal product is authorised in accordance with the decentralised or mutual recognition procedures, the authorisation holder must seek marketing authorisation in all 27 EU member states.

For various reasons, not all medicinal products are authorised in all EU member states. An intended incentive to research and development of paediatric indications may be discouraged due to the fact that, even if medicinal products fulfil all the requirements for which the EU Paediatric Regulation provides, they are excluded from benefitting from the 6-month SPC extension because the product is not authorised in all member states.

Moreover, the competent authorities of EU Member States can take several months, or on occasion years, to update marketing authorisation dossiers. This can create the risk of missed deadlines for the SPC application and losing the benefit provided for by the EU Paediatric Regulation.

One solution to this difficulty could be found in a flexible interpretation of the provisions of the EU Paediatric Regulation. The requirement for a 'product' to be authorised in all member states could possibly be interpreted in practice as referring to the active substance of the original product being authorised in all member states, independently of consecutive product variations and line extensions. The European Commission currently adopts a strict interpretation of the obligation which may exclude this interpretation. However, evidence that it is limiting application of the Regulation may encourage some flexibility.

*One PIP or Several PIPs*

The development of medicinal products is a complex process that on one side can be planned, but on the other side often is facing complex challenges. Companies may develop a product initially in the two indications A and B and later decide to drop indication B or to investigate a new indication C, or D, or E. If the decision to seriously develop the new indication C, D, or E is made with a sufficient time gap from the initial PIP submitted, it may be more practical for the company to submit an entirely new PIP, especially if the originally submitted PIP has already been accepted by the PDCO and published on the EMA website. A year later a next PIP may be submitted for yet another new indication. While this appears to seem a mere formality to an outsider, it can carry considerable weight for the company. Once the measures in the first PIP are fulfilled, the company is entitled to the reward in the form of the SPC extension. Would, however, the EMA only accept requests for modifications of the original PIP, the company might find itself in a situation where due to additional new modifications compliance with the PIP might not be possible before the expiry of the patent or the existing SPC. In many cases, it may be more practical for the company to submit different PIPs, and again time will show to what degree of practicality EMA and PDCO will handle companies' requests.

## Conclusion

Quantitative data suggests that the pharmaceutical industry is adopting to the new system introduced by the EU Paediatric Regulation. However, the implementation of the Regulation in practice is raising issues which will need to be addressed if the system is to work and the industry is to have faith in the authorities that are applying it. Both sides are here on a learning curve.

Klaus Rose, MD, MS
Principal Consultant
Granzer Regulatory Consulting & Services, Zielstattstrasse 44
DE–81379 Munich (Germany)
Tel. +49 89 780 68 98 29, Fax +49 89 780 68 98 15, E-Mail rose@granzer.biz

Rose K, van den Anker JN (eds): Guide to Paediatric Drug Development and Clinical Research.
Basel, Karger, 2010, pp 12–14

# United States Paediatric Legislation Impact on Paediatric Drug Studies

William Rodriguez[a], * · Samuel Maldonado[b]

[a]Office of Paediatric Therapeutics, Office of the Commissioner FDA, Rockville, Md., and [b]Paediatric Drug Development Center of
Excellence, Johnson & Johnson PRD, Raritan, N.J., USA

The paucity of information about the use of drugs in paediatric patients and the off-label use of drugs in children with little or no scientific support led to important regulatory changes in an effort to improve and modernize the study of drugs in children. In 1994 to increase paediatric information in labeling, a final rule amended regulations on the 'Paediatric Use' subsection of drug labeling. One aspect of this regulation stated that information derived from studies in adult could be extrapolated for conditions where the pathophysiology of the condition as well as the response to the therapy in children paralleled that of the adult. However, safety and pharmacologic studies would be required in the paediatric population to support the use [1]. The 1994 final rule did not substantively increase the number of products with adequate paediatric labeling. In 1997, given the lack of results of the previous approach and the belief that a more focused legislative approach would encourage paediatric drug development, the Food and Drug Administration Modernization Act (FDAMA) was passed which contained an exclusivity incentive to encourage paediatric drug development [2]. The exclusivity incentive was reauthorized with the

Best Pharmaceuticals for Children Act (BPCA) in 2002 [3]. The paediatric exclusivity incentive provided for the granting of 6 months of market exclusivity to companies who reasonably conducted the requested paediatric studies as outlined in a written request (WR) issued by the FDA and submitted the studies in the agreed time to the agency. The WR is an instrument that defines the quality and type of clinical trial work. It is a legal document and not a protocol. It is a document issued by the FDA to sponsors requesting needed studies in the paediatric population. The sponsor may or may not accept the request. In order to prospectively promote and require studies in the paediatric population, the Food and Drug Administration passed the Paediatric Rule in 1998 [4]. This rule allowed FDA to require studies of products for which the sponsor had submitted an application to the Agency for a condition in adults which also occurred in children. The rule was enjoined in 2002. However in 2003, the Paediatric Research Equity Act (PREA) was passed by Congress essentially reestablishing the mandate of the paediatric rule [5]. Although the WR permitted FDA to request indications not existing in the adult population or authorized in

---

* The views expressed are those of the author. No official support or endorsements by the US FDA are provided or should be inferred. No commercial interest or other conflict of interest exists between the author and the pharmaceutical companies.

adults, PREA's requirement was subject to the adult indication(s) sought by the sponsor.

The success of the paediatric incentive (FDAMA/BPCA) and PREA was contributory to Congress passing the Food and Drug Administration Amendments Act (FDAAA) in 2007. The act (FDAAA) reauthorized both BPCA and PREA. The Paediatric Medical Devices Safety and Improvement Act also added and contained the legislation intended to foster medical devices with potential use and benefit for children [6].

FDAAA required paediatric studies of certain drugs and biological products; reauthorized the Paediatric Advisory Committee; as well as required the formation of an internal committee of the FDA with the responsibility of assessing quality and consistency in paediatric information contained in a paediatric plan, assessments, waivers and deferrals as well as the WRs. The committee has been named the Paediatric Review Committee (PeRC) by the FDA. This internal multidisciplinary committee makes recommendations and provides consultation to the review divisions on all paediatric plans and assessments prior to approval of an application of a supplement for which paediatric assessment is required, or the granting of a deferral or a waiver. These recommendations are not mandatory.

In an effort to improve the dissemination of paediatric information, FDAAA requires FDA to make available to the public, the medical, statistical and clinical pharmacology reviews no later than 210 days after studies submission. The law also mandates that the sponsor disseminates information on labeling changes to physicians and health care providers.

Both positive and negative results of the studies are included in the labeling. If a waiver is granted on the basis of a safety concern, that information must also go in the labeling.

Unlike adult studies where failed studies in a submission do not become public and the FDA is not permitted to reveal the results of those studies, this legislation has had profound impact. It has enhanced our knowledge of paediatric therapeutics by making the information available to the public about these studies even when they failed or were unable to prove efficacy. This has been particularly important for children where studies are small or few in numbers.

The process for PREA is rather straight forward. The sponsor submits an application (IND/NDA/BLA) at phase 2/3 for the adult indication(s). The division then presents recommendations for waivers, deferrals and proposed studies to PeRC which advises concerning such paediatric studies, deferrals or waivers. For required studies, a timetable in a general outline is decided before action is taken on the application. (This is not a marketing hold.) A request for tracking of outcomes is agreed on. The sponsor presents a paediatric study plan stating date of start, completion and submission.

Once the study is completed and the FDA makes a regulatory decision, the product labeling is updated to include new paediatric information. FDAAA requires a safety review be presented to the Paediatric Advisory Committee one year after the labeling change for drugs, biologicals and certain devices.

The paediatric exclusivity incentive created in FDAMA and reauthorized in BPCA is a major driver of paediatric studies. However, the exclusivity incentive applies to drugs and not to biologics approved under the Public Health Services Act. The language matched PREA's mandate for transparency and interaction with the PeRC.

The success of both processes has been dramatic. As of July 31, 2009, the FDA has issued 376 WRs and received submissions for over 180 products. Of these 167 have been granted exclusivity and 171 products have had labeling changes to incorporate new paediatric information (please see below for labeling changes under PREA). We have learned a lot from this process such as new dosing information, lack of effectiveness for some, or detected new paediatric safety issues [7]. Some of the safety issues were recognized in the mandated 1 year post-exclusivity (now labeling/approval) report to the PAC [8]. This committee provides recommendations for any safety issue presented to them on those products.

We have also realized that long term safety effects on growth, learning and behavior continue to be understudied and that neonates is the group most understudied in the area of safety and efficacy of the therapies being used to treat them.

We also found that in an analysis of 99 drugs studied under BPCA between 2002 and 2007, the distribution of sites and patients reflected a global approach. The USA provided 60% of the patients. Fifty-four percent of the studies were international. Hence, paediatric studies conducted under BPCA have resulted in a globalization in paediatric drug development.

We have also learned a lot from the PREA effect on paediatric drug development. As of July 31, 2009, there have been 110 new labeling changes associated with PREA. PREA has made the sponsor think of how the product will be used in the paediatric population early in the drug development process.

The most recent 'kid in the block' in the paediatric regulatory aspect of drug development is the EMA which passed in 2007 EEC/EMA request for sponsors of drug development to submit a Paediatric Investigational Plan (PIP) earlier in the process (end of phase 1) than the USA legislation. Collaboration of the two regulatory agencies (FDA and EMA) has developed dramatically leading to personnel exchanges for educational purpose, regular teleconferences. The confidential and secure electronic exchanges of information have the purpose to facilitate harmonization and protect our children during paediatric drug development, promote ethical considerations of paediatric patients in trials such as avoidance of duplication of studies for the same condition. Although technical experts may have different approaches there is mutual respect for differences such as those extant in differences in standard of care.

Thus, global development in paediatric drug development and regulatory approaches offer many opportunities and challenges. The most important result is that it provides an opportunity for regulatory agencies and industry to apply knowledge learned to benefit children around the world by working together.

## References


1 Food and Drug Administration: Specific requirements on content and format of labeling of human prescription drugs: revision of 'paediatric use' subsection in the labeling. Fed Regist 1994;59:64240–64250.
2 Food and Drug Administration Modernization Act of 1997. 111 Stat 2296, vol 105. 105th Congress ed, 1997, pp 107–109.
3 Best Pharmaceuticals for Children Act. Pub L No. 107–109, 115 Stat 1408 (2002). Available at:http://www.fda.gov/Drugs/DevelopmentApprovalProcess/DevelopmentResources/ucm049876.htm
4 Food and Drug Administration: Regulation requiring manufacturers to assess the safety and effectiveness of new drugs and biological products in paediatric patients: final rule. Fed Regist 1998;63:66631–66672.
5 Paediatric Research Equity Act of 2003, S 650, 108th Congress. Available at: http://frwebgate.access.gpo.gov/cgi-bin/getdoc.cgi?dbname_108_cong_bills&docid_f:s650enr.txt
6 The Food and Drug Administration Amendments Act of 2007 (FDAAA) (Public Law 110–85) September 27, 2007. 110th Congress Public Law 110–85.
7 Rodriguez W, Selen A, Avant A, et al: Improving paediatric dosing through paediatric initiatives: what we have learned. Paediatrics 2008;121:530–539.
8 Smith PB, Benjamin DK Jr, Murphy MD, et al: Safety monitoring of drugs receiving paediatric marketing exclusivity. Paediatrics 2008;122:e628–e633.



William Rodriguez, MD, PhD
Office of Paediatric Therapeutics, Office of the Commissioner FDA
Rockville MD 20857 (USA)
Tel. +1 301 827 1996, Fax +1 301 827 1017, E-Mail William.Rodriguez@fda.hhs.gov

Rose K, van den Anker JN (eds): Guide to Paediatric Drug Development and Clinical Research.
Basel, Karger, 2010, pp 15–22

# Facilitation of Paediatric Research in Japan

Hidefumi Nakamura[a] · Masahiro Ozaki[b]

[a]Division for Clinical Trials, Clinical Research Center, National Center for Child Health and Development, and
[b]Regulatory Affair Division, UCB Japan Co., Ltd., Tokyo, Japan

## Japan and the Rest of the World

One fundamental difference between pharmaceutical treatment in Japan and US/EU is the low penetration rate of generics. Essentially, the voluntary part of US and EU paediatric legislation is an incentive towards research-based pharmaceutical industries. In exchange for paediatric drug development, generic competition is delayed for 6 months. Without a strong generic competition, this path may not be an effective option for the Japanese legislator. The first attempt as an incentive was postponement of the re-examination period, which is discussed below and was not very successful. At present, higher prices for paediatric medicines are considered as the way forward, and it remains to be seen if this will work.

Another fundamental difference is that many modern drugs are approved in Japan late in comparison to the US and EU. Today, the lag in introducing modern medication in Japan is perceived especially serious in cancer therapy and has become a national concern that has triggered several Ministry of Health, Labour and Welfare (MHLW) activities.

In the following, various aspects of paediatric drug development in Japan are discussed from different view points, i.e. from the view of a clinician, of the pharmaceutical industry, from government, and from paediatric clinical trial advocates.

## Current Status of Extemporaneous, Off-Label and Unlicensed Use of Drugs in Japanese Children

Extemporaneous, off-label and unlicensed use of medicines in children is as common in Japan as in the rest of the world. In 2005, Kato et al. [1] described the incidences of dosage form changes at 32 institutions in 1 month. On 1,227 occasions, age appropriate powders were made either by crushing tablets and/or adding sucrose. The top 5 drugs for dosage form changes on prescription number basis were warfarin potassium, methyl digoxin, enalapril maleate, dantrolene sodium and lisinopril. Morita [2] described the off-label status of paediatric drugs prescribed in 5 hospitals during 1997 and 1998. 2,032 drugs were prescribed on 531,137 occasions in 1 year. Among these, only 24.4% had sufficient information for paediatric dosage on the package inserts. Approximately 40% had the description 'Safety is not established in children', and approximately 2% were either 'contraindicated' or 'not recommended' for certain age groups.

'Raw' chemical compounds including sodium benzoate, betaine, cysteamine and glycine are dispensed for certain orphan diseases. Among these, betaine and cysteamine are already approved in other countries. It appears to be difficult for the MHLW to find companies to provide betaine and some other drugs to the Japanese market.

## Guidance and Notifications for Paediatric Drug Developments

*Impact of ICH E11*

The primary law governing drug development in Japan is the Pharmaceutical Affairs Law (PAL) [3]. There is no regulation equivalent to the EU Paediatric Regulation, and the ICH E11 guideline is the only official guideline for paediatric drug development. However, ICH E11 is not a binding legal document. There is an agreement in paediatric academia that more clinical trials in children are necessary, but the actual number of paediatric clinical trials seems to have increased only moderately in the last decade.

The paediatric task force team of the Japan Pharmaceutical Manufacturers Association (JPMA) reviewed the evaluation reports issued by the Pharmaceuticals and Medical Devices Agency (PMDA) from April, 2001 to January, 2006 to investigate what types of drug development were performed. 50 drugs were approved. Among these, paediatric clinical trials were performed for 31. For the remaining, 12 were approved based on Notification No. 104 which is described later, 2 were emergently approved as an antiterrorism measure and 5 were based on overseas data and post-marketing study results. For the drugs with paediatric clinical trials, 17 (54.8%) were with a single paediatric trial. Among 56 clinical trials for 31 drugs, approximately 7 tenths (69.6%; 39/56) were open-label, uncontrolled trials. Double-blind studies were carried out in 26.8% (15/56) of which 2 were placebo-controlled studies. Pharmacokinetic studies were performed for 16 drugs (51.6%), of which all but one were performed during open-label studies.

*The Official Notification on Procedures for Approval of Off-Label Drugs (Notification No. 104)*

This ordinance is classified as Kacho-tsuchi, sub-ministerial Division notification that is sometimes translated as 'guideline' [4]. This notification was issued jointly by the Evaluation and Licensing Division (ELD) of the Pharmaceutical and Medical Safety Bureau and the Research and Development Division (RDD) of the Health Policy Bureau, MHLW, in 1999.

According to this notification, RDD will encourage a company to consider a clinical development for expansion of the already approved indication(s), in cases where there are both a formal petition from the academic society *and* a recognized medical necessity for the indication. When conditions are met, this notification allows off-label indications to be approved with a literature-based application, waiving some or all domestic registration-directed clinical trials (Chiken). Consultation with the ELD prior to the application submission is recommended. The following are the three situations when domestic Chiken may be waived.

1  The proposed indication has already been approved in a foreign country which has an equivalent drug approval system to Japan (e.g. the US and EU), and there is a sizable body of data accumulated from clinical practice. If this is the situation, and the material submitted to the overseas approving authority can be submitted according to the Japanese requirement, domestic Chiken may be waived.

2  In cases when the indication has been approved according to the conditions stipulated above, a sizable body of data from use in clinical practice has been accumulated *and* reliable results are published in internationally recognized journals. To meet this standard, the data should be of high scientific quality.

3 In cases when scientifically reliable data exists from studies conducted under the auspices of a publicly sponsored organization such as the MHLW. To meet this standard, such studies must have been conducted in accordance with currently accepted international ethical and scientific standards.

*Extension of the Reexamination Period*

Extension of the reexamination period was introduced in December 2000. The reexamination period is applied to all newly approved indications. Standard reexamination period was 6 years before April 2007 and was then extended to 8 years. Data protection is applied during the re-examination period. When a company conducts clinical trials for a paediatric indication during the reexamination period, the period may be extended up to 10 years. This extension is intended to cover the clinical trial period. Ironically, this extension which should be an incentive for companies, has been delaying the paediatric drug development process. Based on the examination of recent evaluation reports, many companies wait to start post-marketing paediatric clinical trials until the last moment before reexamination period expires to get maximum extension.

*Basic Principles on Global Clinical Trials*

The PMDA considers inclusion of Japanese patients into global studies as a key factor to resolve the approval lag of modern drugs in Japan. It has issued 'basic principles on global clinical trials' jointly with the ELD of the MHLW (Notification No. 928010) on September 28, 2007, encouraging companies to consider active involvement of Japan in global studies [5]. The PMDA also has been offering preferential arrangement of in-person consultation on global studies since 2008.

This notification has been made based on past review/consultation experience by PMDA and summarizes the basic idea for planning and conducting global studies. A reference flow chart for developmental strategies utilizing global trials is shown in figure 1. As there has been limited experience in paediatric global trials in Japan, this notification has to be interpreted with caution when applying to paediatric clinical trials. For each individual case, early consultation with the PMDA is strongly recommended.

As of January 2007, the PMDA has conducted 52 trial consultations concerning global studies, and approved following 3 drugs for adult indications by accepting results from global studies: Gefitinib for inoperable or recurrent non-small cell lung cancer, Tolterodine tartrate for overactive bladder, and Losartan for diabetic nephropathy. As of November 2008, 24 companies were conducting a total of 90 global studies.

## Recent Government Efforts to Facilitate Drug Development in Japan

Lack of domestic approvals in a significant number of drugs in children has become a national concern, and there are ongoing MHLW activities to resolve the off-label and unlicensed use of drugs in children.

*Expert Panel on Unapproved Drugs (MHLW, January, 2005–October, 2009)*

This expert panel started in January 2005 to oversee the situation of approval lag, to evaluate the need to introduce unapproved drugs in Japan, and to lead them to the clinical development stage. 22 formal meetings were held, and development and approval strategies for 44 drugs were discussed. Of these 44 drugs, 23 are oncology drugs and 15 are paediatric drugs. The MHLW reported that 20 of 44 drugs have been approved as of February, 2009,

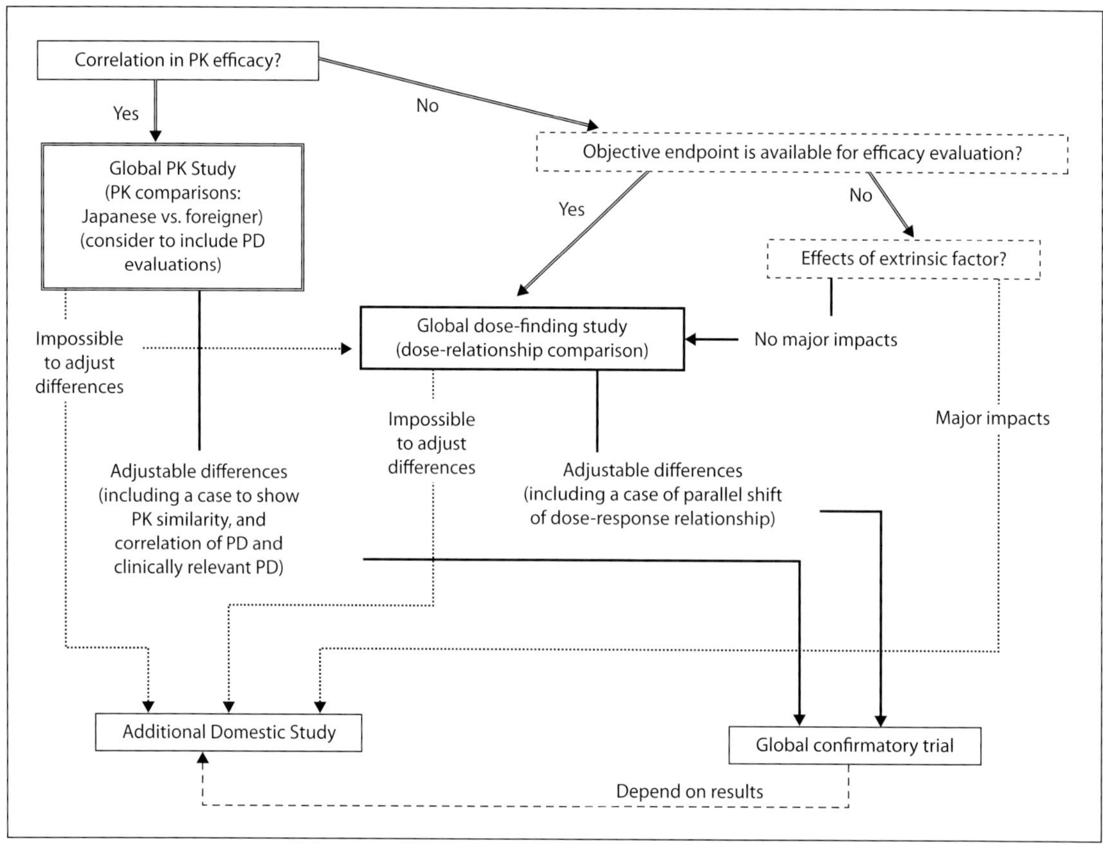

**Fig. 1.** A reference flow chart for developmental strategies utilizing global trials (Notification #928010).

including 5 paediatric indications. Developments of the most of the other paediatric drugs evaluated have been initiated.

In June, 2009, the MHLW decided to reorganize the Expert Panel on Unapproved Drugs, the Expert Panel on Paediatric Drug Therapy and other activities related to off-label and unlicensed drugs to form a new 'Expert Panel on Unlicensed and Off-Label Drugs'. The government has decided to spend 10 billion yen for the development of unlicensed drugs and 4.2 billion Yen to fasten PMDA review process over the 2009–2011 period. The first meeting of this new 'Expert Panel' was held in February, 2010. Under the panel, there are 6 working groups by therapeutic category such as cardiovascular medicine and psychiatry/neurology, and a paediatric working group which covers all paediatric issues interacting with other 6 working groups. These working groups have started to evaluate 374 drugs/indications (89 unapproved drugs, 285 unapproved indications) listed by medical societies and patient groups for the relevance of the medicines and the development/approval strategies. The development of products requested from the MHLW based on the decision of the new 'Expert Panel' is a condition for granting *'The Premium for the Development of New Drugs and Elimination of Off-label Indications'*, which is explained later.

*Expert Panel on Paediatric Drug Therapy (MHLW, March, 2006–July, 2009)*

The Expert Panel on Paediatric Drug Therapy focuses on a solution of the off-label use of paediatric drugs. A list of 99 drugs chosen from the Japan Paediatric Society's 'priority list' were submitted to the expert panel by paediatric subspecialty societies. The expert panel investigates the approval status and related information in the US, UK, France and/or Germany, the current Japanese situation, and other clinical evidence available in the literature. When the investigation shows that there is 'sufficient evidence' for the indication and/or dosage, the MHLW issues approval based on those investigations. 6 meetings were held and evaluation of acetaminophen, flecainide, methotrexate, botulinum toxin type A and acyclovir were completed.

The necessity of new formulations has been well recognized, but development has not been recommended to the industries due to the lack of incentives and financial support. The new 'expert committee' will evaluate the clinical necessity primarily, but some budget may be also spent for the development of age-appropriate formulations for certain essential drugs. As there are still 94 drugs remaining on the 'priority list', similar activity will be continued by one of the working groups of the new 'expert committee'.

*Paediatric Premium for a Comparator Pricing Method*

At present, a higher drug price for paediatric medication is considered as the most feasible incentive for companies. In 2006, a paediatric premium was newly introduced for a comparator pricing method. The premium was originally 3–10% and only for drugs which have no other pharmacologically comparable drugs in the market. In 2008, the premium was increased to 5–20% and became applicable to all the drugs whose comparators have not received a paediatric premium.

*Premium for the Development of New Drugs and Elimination of Off-Label Indications*

This premium is newly introduced in 2010 and is established for all the drugs pending patent which have no competitors in their classes. In contrast to most of the drugs whose prices are harshly cut every 2 years, the prices will be rather well maintained for these drugs during the patent-pending period, under the condition that the development of the new drugs and off-label indications requested by the MHLW (based on the new 'Expert Panel's' decision) will be initiated in a timely manner.

## Government Efforts to Promote Clinical Trials in Japan

The MHLW and related government agencies have been implementing strategies to facilitate clinical trials in the last few years. At least partially due to these strategies, the total number of clinical trials for all age groups has started to increase gradually after it bottomed in 2003.

*Sponsor-Investigator Trials*

The revision of PAL in 2002 enabled physicians to conduct sponsor-investigator trials in Japan. The Committee on Drugs of the Japan Paediatric Association (JPA) recommends that JPA members to actively involve in sponsor-investigator trials and utilize them to set up a stronger infrastructure for paediatric clinical trials. There have been 9 protocols for 6 drugs in children completed or ongoing as of July, 2009.

*New Five-Year Clinical Trial Promotion Plan
(MHLW and MEXT, 2007–2011)*

In March 2007, the MHLW and Ministry of Education, Culture, Sports, Science and Technology (MEXT) published the 5-year promotion plan that follows the previous three-year plan which was a limited success. The new plan succeeds the previous plan to create several large networks of clinical institutions. The MHLW chose 10 COEs and 30 affiliated major hospitals, based on regional and therapeutic needs as well as their performance in clinical trials. For a clinical trial network for paediatrics, the National Center for Child Health and Development has been chosen as the COE, and the Kanagawa Children's Medical Center, the Osaka Medical Center and Research Institute for Maternal and Child Health, and the Tokyo Metropolitan Children's Medical Center were chosen as affiliated major hospitals. These hospitals have employed staff including, research nurses, pharmacists, biostatisticians and data managers through budgetary supports. Networking with other children's hospitals is ongoing, and a possible collaboration with the JPS to attract global trials is also being discussed.

According to this new 5-year plan, training programs for investigators, research nurses and pharmacists are provided intensively. To attract more industry sponsors, the MHLW has promised to remove administrative red tapes and streamline operations in the networks. Improvement in speed, quality and the price are important components of the objective of this plan.

*Expert Panel on Faster Access to Innovative Drugs
(MHLW, 2006–2007)*

The MHLW convened an expert panel to discuss the bottlenecks to the introduction of new drugs in Japan in October 2006. This Expert Panel focused on the principles of new drug approval, post-marketing safety measures, and enhancement of the PMDA review.

In the final report of this Expert Panel issued in July 2007, it is specified that the government should consider stronger incentives for industry and other regulatory measures to facilitate paediatric drug development. It is in response to the request from the Committee on Drugs of JPA at the public hearing.

*Five-Year Strategy for Developing Innovative
Drugs and Devices (MHLW, MEXT, METI and
Cabinet Office, 2007–2011)*

This strategy was made by 3 ministries, the MHLW, MEXT and the Ministry of Economy, Trade and Industry (METI). The major goals of this strategy is to reinforce clinical research infrastructure to ensure safe and secure patients' access to new drugs and devices, i.e. (1) institutional infrastructure building for clinical research centers' networks, (2) human resource development, and (3) regulatory research promotion and approval system reform. Starting 2007, the PMDA started major reform and has been increasing the number of reviewers to facilitate the review process.

In 2007, MHLW decided to spend 1.8 billion Yen to strengthen translational research infrastructure at National Centers to accelerate R&D and promote new partnership with industries. Receiving 0.4 billion Yen, NCCHD has build a new facility devoted for paediatric drug and device developments in March, 2010.

## Activity of the Japan Paediatric Society in Promoting Paediatric Drug Development

The Members of the Committee on Drugs of the JPS organized a working group to study the approval status of paediatric drugs and make a priority list of off-label drugs in 1998 as part of the

MHLW supported research. As of March, 2010, representatives of 23 associated subspecialty societies joined the working group. The priority list has been utilized for the selection of drugs for the evaluation by the Expert Panel on Paediatric Drug Therapy and the new 'Expert Panel'.

The working group also accumulates information on unlicensed drugs which need to be approved urgently in the country. After the drugs have been evaluated and listed, associated paediatric subspecialty societies submit requests to the MHLW for evaluation by the Expert Panel on Unapproved Drugs and the new 'Expert Panel'.

The committee has also been involved in several activities to facilitate clinical trials, drug development and the approval process. At the public hearing in December 2006, the Committee requested the Expert Panel on Faster Access to Innovative Drugs to consider several issues including the following.

1   To set up certain obligations and incentives similar to the EU/US paediatric regulation.
2   To take appropriate measures to fasten and strengthen the NDA review process for paediatric drugs by the PMDA.

Informal discussion on possible PAL revision and other incentives to promote paediatric clinical trials is ongoing between JPS, JPMA, PMDA and MHLW.

## Pharmaceutical Industry Efforts to Promote Clinical Trials in Japan

The JPMA, a voluntary organization with 69 R&D-oriented pharmaceutical corporate members (as of April, 2009), works on multidimensional projects including solution of common obstacles among pharmaceutical industries and cultivation of philosophy on drug development as well as on international cooperation. Also, special efforts are put toward development of robust corporate structures of the members through strengthening policy proposals, adapting to internationalization, and strengthening public relations.

### *Establishment of 'Development Support Center for Unlicensed Drugs'*

The JPMA established 'Development Support Center for Unlicensed Drugs' on May 29. The purpose of the Center is to assist pharmaceutical companies in obtaining marketing authorization for new drugs and approval of new indications in order to eliminate drug lag in Japan. The decision is being put in motion rather quickly, and the centre will reportedly collaborate with the MHLW to support the development of unlicensed drugs including the three paediatric drugs that no industry so far has agreed for the development.

The centre will also start to offer partial financial support for consultation with and application to the PMDA. It is planning to provide support on the development of 5 drugs per year.

### *The Paediatric Task Force Team to Promote Clinical Trials*

The JPMA has a paediatric task force team inside the Drug Evaluation Committee and has been making efforts to promote paediatric clinical trials in cooperation with the JPS. From September to October in 2008, the team conducted a survey of corporate members on the obstacles and possible solutions to facilitate paediatric drug development. Results are summarized as follows.

Twenty-seven of 45 respondents (60.5%) answered that 'securement of corporate profitability' was an issue.

Difficulty in safety assessment of paediatric trials was one of the obstacles, suggesting that consultation and evaluation system that can properly advice and assess the safety is necessary.

Regarding new rules/regulations, 53.3% answered 'are necessary if corporate incentives exist' and 26.7% answered 'necessary', totaling 80%. The most popular incentive appeared to be 'fast review/approval of drugs when paediatric clinical trials are performed' (78.6%), followed by 'extension of data protection period (re-evaluation period and/ or patent)' (67.9%) and 'drug price raise' (64.3%).

As can be seen by this survey, many believe that new rules/regulations for paediatric drug development (incentives, system enhancement of paediatric trial consultation and evaluation, etc.) have to be developed especially to enhance corporate profitability as in EU and the US.

## Prospect for the Near Future

At present, Japan does not have rules/regulations similar to the EU Paediatric Regulation or US FDAAA. However, discussion for new rules/regulation is ongoing between the relevant parties on a national level. Networks for paediatric clinical trials are being established and discussion with paediatric pharmacologists in other Asian countries including Korea and China has been started. With strong support from the government, we hope that Japan will build up and sustain a robust paediatric clinical trial infrastructure and will increase its international collaboration in this regard on both a regional Asian as well as truly global level.

## References


1   Kato Y, Ishikawa I, Kushida K, Nakamura H: Survey of paediatric dosage form changes in Japan. In preparation.
2   Morita S: Prescription and Package Insert Description Analysis in Paediatric Drug Use (in Japanese); in 1999 MHLW project report for the research on current status of the off-label use of drugs in children and possible solutions (PI: Onishi S), 2000, pp 52–99.
3   Ono S: Ministry of Health, Labour and Welfare (MHLW, Japan); in D'Agostino RB, Sullivan L, Massaro JM (eds): Wiley Encyclopedia of Clinical Trials. Hoboken, Wiley, 2007.
4   Fujiwara Y, Kobayashi K: Oncology drug clinical development and approval in Japan: the role of pharmaceuticals and medical devices evaluation centre (PMDEC). Crit Rev Oncol Hematol 2002;42:145–155.
5   Website for the recent notifications: http://www.pmda.go.jp/english/service/notifications.html



Hidefumi Nakamura, MD, PhD
National Center for Child Health and Development
2–10–1 Ookura, Setagaya-ku
Tokyo 157-8535 (Japan)
Tel. +81 3 3416 0181, ext. 7063 or 5373, Fax +81 3 3417 5691, E-Mail nakamura-hd@ncchd.go.jp

Rose K, van den Anker JN (eds): Guide to Paediatric Drug Development and Clinical Research.
Basel, Karger, 2010, pp 23–31

# Ethical Imperatives in Medical Research on Child Subjects – Reflections of a Past President of the World Medical Association

William J. Appleyard

Canterbury, Kent, UK

## Historical Outline

Significant progress in medicine has been based on research whether it be from a chance observation or the result of painstaking analysis. Essential to the practical application of these new discoveries has been experimentation on human subjects. Key to their involvement has always been the sense of trust for the physicians undertaking research and in the validity of their observations and findings.

Sir William Osler, the doyen of Canadian, American and British Medicine one hundred years ago [4] traced the 'Evolution of Modern Medicine' from the 'primal sympathy of man with man' through the remarkably civilized state on the banks of the Nile in Egypt and in Mesopotamia, modern day Iraq. Knowledge was acquired and skills developed and it was handed down by apprenticeship. Medicine was ancillary to religious belief and rituals and importantly the famous Hammurabi code of laws, civil and religious inscribed in stone around 2,000 BC many of these related to the medical profession. And on to the 'golden age' in Greece with the numerous collections of observations and the acquired wisdom by Hippocrates summed up by the phrase 'Where there is love of humanity, there will be love of the profession'.

The high 'watermark' of professional morality was reached in the 'credo' of the Hippocratic Oath. Out of mysticism, superstition and religious ritual Hippocrates went directly to nature and was the first to grasp that the conception of Medicine as an Art, based on accurate observation, and an integral part of the Science of man. His famous saying in 'The Law' – 'There are in effect two things, to know and to believe one knows; to know is science, to believe one knows is ignorance'. The tension between the acquisition of knowledge against systems of 'belief', be they religious or political, persists until this day. During the ages when 'belief' dominated scientific advances occurred slowly.

With the scientific advances of the 19th century, physicians recognized that both benefit and harm could come from them. Individual codes of practice were developed by leading physician researchers such as Thomas Percival in England, William Beaumont in the USA and Claude Bernard in France.

In 1886, Charles Francis Withington [5] noted the 'possible conflict between the interests of medical science and those of the individual patient'; he sided with the latter's indefensible rights.

William Osler, in 'The Evolution of the Idea of Experiment' [6], required investigators to obtain the consent of the subject: 'For man absolute safety and full consent are the conditions which make such tests allowable. We have no right to use patients entrusted to our care for the purpose of experimentation unless direct benefit to the individual is likely to follow. Once this limit is transgressed, the sacred cord which binds physician and patient snaps instantly'.

During the first two decades of the 20th century, major progress was being made in pathology and medicine in the centres of medical excellence in Germany.

Criticism of unethical human experimentation emerged in the political press and in the German Parliament. In 1931, the Reich government issued detailed 'guidelines for new therapy and human experimentation'. The guidelines clearly distinguished between therapeutic ('new therapy') and non-therapeutic research ('human experimentation') and set out strict precautions [7].

Besides the principles of beneficence and non-malfeasance, the Reich regulations were based on patient autonomy and a legal doctrine of informed consent.

'New therapy may be applied only if consent or proxy consent has been given in a clear and undebatable manner following appropriate information. New therapy may be introduced without consent only if it is urgently required and cannot be postponed because of the need to save life or prevent severe damage to health...' In those cases a written report must clearly outline the preconditions. But non-therapeutic research was 'under no circumstances permissible without consent'. Written documentation and a clear structure of responsibility for each clinical trial were required.

Furthermore 'experimentation involving children or young persons under 18 years of age shall be prohibited if it in any way endangers the child or young person'.

After Hitler and his Nazi Regime came to power 2 years later, there was an increasing discrepancy between the regulatory code and the actual behaviour of the Nazi doctors and the subsequent research practices in German concentration camps. This resulted in the loss of trust in physicians and between physicians and in the medical ethical standards of nations and between nations.

After the end of World War 2, the Nuremburg Code 1947 was formulated. The code restated the essential safeguards spelt out in the 1931 Reich Guidelines [8]
– voluntary and informed consent
– experimentation on humans had to be necessary and yield benefit that overweighed the risk
– right to withdraw without penalty
– subject must be protected against possible injury, disability, or death
– research only conducted by scientifically qualified personnel.

Physicians in over 30 countries including Germany, France, United States and Britain came together in 1946 in London and formed the World Medical Association whose first task was to restore the explicit 'Hippocratic' professional relationship with society through the Declaration of Geneva in 1948 [9]. Germany aimed at re-establishing trust – the Declaration forming the new understanding or 'contract' between the medical profession and society worldwide. This led on to the Declaration of Helsinki on medical research on human subjects.

The first Declaration of Helsinki was issued in 1964, with a major revision in 1975. Since then the Declaration has been recognised throughout the world by physicians and most medical research scientists as the premier medical ethical reference for research on human subjects [10].

Children had been subject to research studies in residential institutions. The most public and controversial research study on children during the second half of the 20th century was the 'Willowbrook Hepatitis Study' started in 1956 at a New York State Institution for mentally defective persons' [11].

Such examples led to the persistence of a predominantly protective approach towards research in children. So much so that with the growing number of medications available to adults in the last half century, children were increasingly being 'left behind'. The market for new drugs amongst children was much smaller and a combination of the inherent protective environment with the increased cost of clinical trials meant that pharmaceutical companies did not undertake the relevant trials in children. Practicing paediatricians faced the dilemma of knowing how effective a new chemical substance had been found in adult studies, feeling 'duty bound' to try them on their child patients 'off label'.

By the 1990s this practice had reached such a proportion of prescriptions for children that paediatricians were pressing for changes in the system.

Recognising these significant risks in the care of their patients, practicing paediatricians, particularly in the USA pressed for changes in the regulation of medicines for children. In 1996, The American Academy of Paediatrics (AAP) reported that only a small fraction of all drugs and biological products marketed in the US at that time had had clinical trials performed in paediatric patients. A majority of marketed drugs were not labeled for use in paediatric patients. The AAP also pointed out that many drugs used in the treatment of both common childhood illnesses and more serious conditions carried little information in the labels about use in paediatric patients [12].

An expert group, bringing together the research community, industry and regulators was set up by the International Conference on the Harmonisation of Technical Requirements for the Registration of Pharmaceuticals for Human use (ICH). Their consolidated 'guidance' on Good Clinical Practice in 1996 was gleaned from their participants [13].

This has provided a uniform standard for the European Union (EU) Japan and the United States for designing, conducting, recording and reporting clinical trials on human subjects (ICH. GCP). In the introduction, the guidance states that 'Compliance with this standard provides public assurance that their rights, safety and well-being of trial subjects are protected. consistent with the principles that have their origin in the Declaration of Helsinki and that the Clinical Data are credible.' Such guidance is very helpful but always must refer to the core ethical principles of the medical profession. Guidelines devoid of underlying ethical principles develop a bureaucratic momentum of their own and the physician researchers experience an inner detachment from the policies and guidelines to which they do not relate professionally.

Paragraph 2 of the Declaration of Helsinki for instance states 'It is the duty of the physician to promote and safeguard the health of the people. The physician's knowledge and conscience are dedicated to the fulfillment of this duty'.

Regulations are important within the legal framework of each country. Medical research is increasingly a global imperative. and the relevant common ethical standards need to be international [15].

Revelations that financial relationships and conflicts of interest had become 'pervasive' and were undermining public trust in the integrity of Science resulted in the call for greater transparency (honesty) within the US regulatory framework. The Office for Human Research Protections (OHRP) was set up in 2000 from the former Office for Protections from Research Risk (OPRR) It reports to the Assistant Secretary of Health and Human.

The National Institutes of Health is by far the largest human research funding agency worldwide. To carry out its research mission, nearly 10,000 universities, hospitals and other Research Institutions in the United States and internationally have formal agreements (assurances) with OHRP to comply with the US regulations related to human subject protection.

The introduction of paediatric exclusivity provision into the Food and Drug Administration

Modernisation Act of 1997 as well as the introduction of the Paediatric Research Equity Act (PREA) in 2003 is discussed in the chapter provided by Rodriguez and Maldonado in this book.

In January 1997 the National Institute of Health, a major 'funder' of clinical research worldwide, developed the policy that children (defined as individuals under the age of 21) must be included in all human subjects research, conducted or supported by the NIH, unless there are scientific and ethical reasons not to include them.

The various aspects of the introduction of the EU paediatric regulation are discussed in several further chapters in this book.


## Current Protection

As the existing protections of human subjects in medical research have taken shape several levels of 'protection' for child subjects have emerged:
- The regulatory oversight available in each country.
- Specific guidance, in the form of 'consensus' guidelines, e.g. ICH Good Clinical Practice without compliance with which, most 'ethical' pharmaceutical companies will not conduct a clinical trial.
- Professional ethical codes of practice such as the Declaration of Helsinki provide the 'external' governance of medical researchers [18].
- The 'conscience' of the medical profession – an essential 'internal' governance based on medical ethics.
- Establishment of local research ethics committees and institutional review boards in the USA which provide essential 'ethical' scrutiny by their professional and 'lay' membership.
- The universal recognition of over-riding importance of the need for the consent of Individual in UN Convention on Human Rights (see Appendix).

## Reluctance to Be Involved

There has been a historical reluctance to include children in medical research, especially in clinical trials. Reasons for this include:
- Because of a child's increased vulnerability, there is an understandable parental reluctance to add any risk to their children's welfare.
- Children have different physiological, psychological and pathogenic features occurring at the different ages and stages of their growth and development from the premature newborn infant through adolescence.
- Risks to child subjects may be increased both in the short and the long term.
- Because of the complexity, high cost and relatively low financial return, pharmaceutical companies are reluctant to invest in this field.

Importantly, outside North America, Europe and Japan there is a lack of universal ethical and regulatory guidance for researchers and sponsors upon which parental trust depends.

Every child and young person under 18 has rights and responsibilities which are protected by the United Nations Convention on the Rights of the Child (UNCRC). The Convention was adopted by the United Nations General Assembly in 1989 and has been ratified by 191 of 193 countries, territories and states, making it a truly global bill of rights. UNICEF uses the UNCRC as a framework for its work for all the world's children.

*Ethical Principles*

The original Declaration of Helsinki in 1964, did not include any reference to the specific needs of children. The Belmont Report [19] in the United States highlighted three ethical principles – respect for persons (autonomy), beneficence and justice. Recent publicity about adverse events in clinical trials has heightened public anxiety and revealed the serious failures related to issues of non-malfeasance, honesty and transparency.

In my view, medical research as an essential part of medical care and professional practice should be underpinned by seven rather than three core 'ethical' principles [20] namely.

## Seven Ethical Pillars of Clinical Research

- Autonomy
- Beneficence
- Non-malfeasance
- Fidelity
- Truthfulness
- Confidentiality
- Justice

## Patient Autonomy

Patients' decisions about their care must be respected. Their consent is a prerequisite for their participation in any research. Their dissent should be abided by

*Beneficence* – Physicians must always aim to do good, look after patients' best interests in any clinical research and recognize circumstances where conflict of interest may compromise professional judgment.

*Non-Malfeasance* – Physicians must endeavour to do no harm – 'primum non nocere' – avoiding unnecessary risks with treatments.

*Fidelity* – Physicians' 'duty of care' is the free acceptance of a commitment to service. This commitment entails being available and responsive when needed, accepting inconvenience to meet the needs of patients, advocating the best possible care within the available resources.

*Truthfulness* – Physician researchers must ensure that patients are completely and honestly informed before consenting to any research and after any clinical trial has started. They must not mislead patients when medical errors or adverse events have occurred. Truthfulness implies keeping one's word and meeting commitments. It also requires the recognition of possible conflicts of interest and avoidance of relationships that allow personal gain to supersede the best interest of the profession.

*Confidentiality* – Confidentiality is one of the foundations on which the trust between patient and physician is based. It may only be breached where there is a real and imminent threat to the patient or to others if this confidentiality were maintained

*Justice* – Physicians must treat all people equally according to their need. Physicians should work actively to eliminate discrimination based on race, gender socio-economic status, religion or ethnicity and promote justice in a health system based on individual and community clinical need.

These 'principles' need to be 'internalized' and become a physician's professional conscience, a compass guiding the journey through the complex and sometimes conflicting scientific dilemmas. The seven principles provide a check list to examine the ethics of any research proposal.

The physician's individual conscience should therefore reflect the 'morality' of the medical profession. It provides the foundation of the 'trust' given by the patient as a research subject to the physician as a clinical researcher The conscientious physician has to earn this trust by children and their families. The profession's 'collective' conscience shapes the essential wider 'contract' between the medical profession and society in general.

The application of our knowledge and skills within the framework of our collective professional 'conscience' to make judgments in the best interests of individuals seeking our advice about clinical research is part of the real 'art' of medicine.

The 'seven' principles or 'ethical pillars' of medical research need to underpin the statements in the medical professional ethical codes and codes of practice.

The recently revised WMA Declaration of Helsinki (http://www.wma.net/e/policy/b3.htm)

encompasses these principles. The Declaration is the only 'universal' guide to medical ethical practice in all the nations of the world. Child subjects, however, need special protections beyond those important general principles which apply to all research subjects. In the revised Declaration, children are included under the safeguards required for 'incompetents' as is illustrated by paragraphs 11, 12, 27 and 28.

*Paragraph 11*

For a potential research subject who is *incompetent*, the physician must seek informed consent from the legally authorized representative. These individuals must not be included in a research study that has no likelihood of benefit for them unless it is intended to promote the health of the population represented by the potential subject, the research cannot instead be performed with competent persons, and the research entails only minimal risk and minimal burden.

*Paragraph 12*

When a potential research subject who is *deemed incompetent* is able to give assent to decisions about participation in research, the physician must seek that assent in addition to the consent of the legally authorized representative. The potential subject's dissent should be respected.

*Paragraph 27*

For a potential research subject who is *incompetent,* the physician must seek informed consent from the legally authorized representative. These individuals must not be included in a research study that has no likelihood of benefit for them unless it is intended to promote the health of the population represented by the potential subject,

the research cannot instead be performed with competent persons, and the research entails only minimal risk and minimal burden.

*Paragraph 28*

When a potential research subject who is *deemed incompetent* is able to give assent to decisions about participation in research, the physician must seek that assent in addition to the consent of the legally authorized representative. The potential subject's dissent should be respected.

The general wording of the Declaration of Helsinki does not reflect the integrity and *relative* autonomy of an 'incompetent' person such as a child. Children are defined as that part of the population aged between birth and 18 years.

But there is a lack of universal ethical guidance. The WMA's current initiative in including Research on Child Subjects as part of their revised Declaration of Ottawa (1998) is setting out to address this. Families with children need to understand the need for clinical research, have confidence in the research process – the research protocols – and trust those who conduct research on their children – experienced paediatric researchers and their teams. There needs to be clear statements on the ethical principles that flow from the fact that 'children involved in research need *special* protection'.

The following is a compilation of self standing statements that are in addition interrelated to the others. The author is aware that further statements might be proposed or added in the ensuing debate.

**Scientific Necessity**

There must be a scientific necessity for *any* research to be undertaken on children, i.e.: Children should not be enrolled in a clinical investigation unless absolutely necessary to answer an important scientific question about the health and welfare of children. Biomedical studies involving children as research subjects should be focused on the knowledge of epidemiology, pathogenesis, diagnosis and treatment of diseases or conditions of childhood. A child should not be involved in research that can be carried out on laboratory models, animal subjects or adult persons.

## Relative Autonomy

Physicians must respect the personhood and relative autonomy of a child.

- *Consent:* The issues of consent, assent and dissent are of key concern in the paediatric age group. Children are 'minors' who have not reached the legal age for self-responsible consent.
- *Informed consent* means the permission of the child's parents or legal representative for the participation of their child in a research study, following sufficient information to enable them to make an informed judgment.
- *Informed assent* means the agreement of the child to participate in the research, following information being provided in a form understandable to his/her age.
- *Dissent* – the refusal to participate in the research by a child, if capable, must be respected.
- Where possible, the consent of both parents should be sought prior to enrolling a child in a biomedical research project.
- There must be no forced or undue influence, financial or otherwise on the child's decision to participate in the research or on the parent's/legal representative's permission.

## Beneficence/Non-Malfeasance

*Assessment of Risk:* The Declaration of Helsinki insists that the risk to any subject who lacks 'competence' is only 'minimal'. Risk is defined as potential harm (real or theoretical) or potential consequence of an action. It may be physical, psychological, or social, and may be immediate or delayed. It may vary according to age groups. Risk should be assessed in terms of probability, magnitude and duration.

Physicians should avoid unnecessary risks, discomfort, stress or potential harm leading to physical, psychological, social, spiritual impairment.

In practice there is a hierarchy of risk for children which needs to be assessed in relation to the seriousness and severity of any clinical condition. Children and their families must be confident that the necessary safeguards related to the 'risk' taken by their child are in place. This underpins the trust in their physician researcher.

There is thus a need to balance the potential direct or indirect benefits to children with the degree of risk involved in the research. For instance in clinical trials on children's medicines, risk assessment includes the evaluation of the risk of the medicinal product tested or the control, the risk of withholding active treatment in some cases, with the risk of the disease itself.

Potential harms include the invasiveness and intrusiveness of the research, the severity as well as seriousness of potential harms, the reversibility of adverse effects and reactions, and their preventability.

- Minimal risk involves routine procedures, questionnaires, observation and measurements. A minor increase over minimal risk may be undertaken when the research is concerned with diagnoses and treatment and the direct and indirect benefits to the child subject outweigh the known or anticipated risks involved.
- A greater than minor increase in risk where:
- the research is likely to yield justifiable generaliseable knowledge of vital importance about the child's disorder or condition, which is of vital importance for the understanding or amelioration of the disorder or condition,
- the research presents a reasonable opportunity to further the understanding,

prevention, or alleviation of a serious problem affecting the health or welfare of children,
–  the research provides the only opportunity to identify, prevent or alleviate a rare disease confined to childhood.

OHRP give guidance on the Department of Health and Human Services Regulations in the USA [21].

## Fidelity – Duty of Care

Study protocols and study designs must be child specific and include the scientific justification for the research.

The performance of a study must be guaranteed to be conducted by experts competent in childhood diseases and disorders, empathetic and truly conversant with children, parents and the legal requirements where the interests of the child are paramount.

## Confidentiality

All personal and health-related information collected and stored about the child subject and the family must remain confidential.

## Beneficence

The interests of the child subject should always be represented on independent research ethics committees by members who are knowledgeable in paediatric, clinical, psychosocial and ethical issues.

These statements should act as reference ethical 'standards' for all children's physicians and children's physician researchers throughout the world, against which their actions will be judged by their peers. Each national medical association can derive from these standards their local culturally sensitive guidelines. With the trust that is earned when medical researchers act in an ethical and transparent manner to prevent the ethical abuses of the past and to plan for the future [21, 22], it is hoped that more parents will recognize the benefits that research on their children can bring to them and all children worldwide.

## Appendix – Note

The 1989 United Nations Convention on the Rights of the Child (CRC) is a comprehensive human rights treaty which enshrines specific children's rights in international law. These rights define universal principles and standards for the status and treatment of children worldwide.

Human rights are founded on respect for the dignity and worth of each individual, regardless of race, gender, language, religion, opinions, wealth or ability and therefore apply to every human being everywhere.

The Convention on the Rights of the Child is presently the most widely ratified international human rights treaty – all UN member states except for the United States and Somalia have ratified the convention.

In addition, the CRC is the only international human rights treaty which includes civil, political, economic, social and cultural rights, and sets out in detail what every child needs to have for a safe, happy and fulfilled childhood. It is the most complete statement of children's rights ever produced and has 41 substantive articles.

## References


1  World Health Organisation: Sixtieth World Health Assembly 'Better medicines for Children', 2007.
2  Child Health Research – A Foundation for Improving Child Health. Geneva, World Health Organisation, 2001.
3  Seyberth HW, Demotes-Mainard J, Wrobel P: Developing a European framework for research on children's medicines. Paediatr Nephrol 2005;20:1537–1540.
4  Osler W: The Evolution of Modern Medicine. New Haven, Yale University Press, 1922.
5  Withington CF: The Relation of Hospitals to Medical Education. Boston, Cupples, Upham & Company, 1886.
6  Osler W: The evolution of the idea of experiment. Trans Cong Am Phys Surg 1907;7:1–8.

7   Sass H-M: Reichsrundschreiben 1931: Pre-Nuremberg German Regulations Concerning New Therapy and Human Experimentation. J Med Phil 1983;8:99–111.

8   Katz J: The Nuremberg Code and the Nuremberg Trial: a reappraisal. JAMA 1996;276:1662–1666.

9   Declaration of Geneva. World Medical Association, 1948.

10  Carlson RV, Boyd KM, Webb D: The revision of the Declaration of Helsinki: past, present and future. J Br J Clin Pharmacology 2004;57:695–713.

11  Krugman S: Experiments at the Willowbrook State School. Lancet 1971;i:966–967.

12  American Academy of Pediatrics Committee on Drugs: Unapproved uses of approved drugs: the physician, the package insert, and the Food and Drug Administration: subject review. Pediatrics 1996;98:143–145.

13  Clinical Investigation of Medicinal Products in the Paediatric Population (E 11), CPMP/ICH/271199. Guideline for Good Clinical Practice (E 6), CPMP/ICH/135/95.

14  Additional Safeguards for Children in Clinical Investigations, section 50.50–56. Food and Drug Administration, 2007.

15  Appleyard WJ: The challenge of building an International Framework for Research on Medicines for Children. The Joseph J Hoet Lecture 2005. Bruxelles, The European Forum for Good Clinical Practice, 2005.

16  Guideline on Ethical Considerations for Clinical Trials Performed in Children within the Scope of the EU Clinical Trials Directive 2001/20/EC. The European Agency for the Evaluation of Medicinal Products (EMA), 2006.

17  Ethical Principles and Operational Guidelines for Good Clinical Practice. Paediatric Research Confederation of European Specialist in Paediatrics, 2002.

18  Ethical Principles and Guidelines for the Protection of Human Subjects of Research. 'The Belmont Report'. US Department of HEW, 1979.

19  Appleyard WJ: Who cares? The Declaration of Helsinki and 'The Conscience of physicians'. Res Ethics Rev 2008;4:106–111.

20  Children Involved as Subjects in Research: Guidance on the HHS 45 CFR 46.407 ('407') Review Process.

21  Choonara I: Regulation of drugs for children in Europe. BMJ 2007;335:1221–1222.

22  Sammons HM, Gray C, Hudson H, et al: Safety in paediatric clinical trials – a 7-year review. Acta Paediatr 2008;97:474–477.



William J. Appleyard, MD, FRCP
Past President World Medical Association (2003–2004), Hon Secretary to the Board of Trustees
International Association of Medical Colleges, Thimble Hall,
108 Blean Common, Blean, Canterbury, Kent CT2 9JJ (UK)
Tel./Fax +44 1227 781771, E-Mail Jimappleyard2510@aol.com

Rose K, van den Anker JN (eds): Guide to Paediatric Drug Development and Clinical Research.
Basel, Karger, 2010, pp 32–39

# Paediatric Clinical Research: The Patients' Perspective

Alastair Kent[a,b] · Cor Oosterwijk[b,c] · Ysbrand Poortman[d]

[a]Genetic Interest Group, London, UK; [b]European Genetic Alliances' Network, Brussels, Belgium; [c]Dutch Genetic Alliance VSOP, Soest, and [d]International Genetic Alliance, The Hague, The Netherlands

For any parents experiencing the arrival of a newborn baby the first question that is asked is 'Is my baby all right?' Fortunately, for most couples the answer to this question is 'yes'. Sadly for some, they cannot be reassured because their baby has a chronic health problem that will potentially limit the quality and possibly the length of life their child can expect.

Even for the parents of a healthy baby, the future may be uncertain, as their child will have to face threats to his or her health ranging from the normal diseases of childhood (which are usually relatively mild but which can sometimes be very severe or even fatal) to more severe destiny for which medical science may not have found a yet is some cases. Paediatric clinical research today still faces the challenges of potentially fatal attacks of violent infections, paralysis, cancer, accidents, etc.

Fortunately, thanks to advances over the last 50 years or so many diseases which were formerly untreatable have become curable as a result of the development of antibiotics and other medicines or preventable by vaccination and other measures to reduce their threat. However, it is still the case today that the vast numerical majority of childhood diseases remain untreatable. Here the doctor only has recourse to palliation of some of the symptoms when offering care and support to the affected child and his or her family. Many, if not most of these intractable conditions are rare. They often have a (partly) genetic origin or are related to periconceptional, prenatal or perinatal circumstances. For the vast majority there is currently little or nothing that can be done to alter their natural course, or change the prognosis for the affected child [1]. Paradoxically, despite the fact that individually these diseases may be rare, because there are many thousands of different conditions (estimates vary, but at least 6,000–8,000 have been described), rare diseases are not uncommon [2] and every doctor will meet some of these during the course of his/her professional life. Other childhood diseases are more common and for these, the need for effective, safe therapies is just as great.

**Research Involving Children**

For children affected by currently untreatable disorders hope for the future rests on the undertaking of high quality biomedical research, and the speedy application of the outputs from that research in the form of safe effective medical products – whether drugs, gene therapy [3], cell or tissue therapies or other forms of innovative intervention targeted at their unmet medical needs.

Involving children in research is a sensitive and a contentious issue. The younger the child the more sensitive the issue becomes, because of their inherent vulnerability and their inability to withhold consent to participation. Understandably, there is a fear that parents, desperate for a cure for their sick child, will be pressured into consenting to research that is neither in the interests of their child, nor of others yet to come who have the same condition. Because of this very natural reticence (and for economic reasons too) research into novel medicines for childhood-onset diseases has been limited. For the same reasons, medicines developed for diseases of adulthood which start in childhood have often not been properly tested on children prior to being given a Marketing Authorisation by the European Medicines Agency (EMA) or National Competent Authorities. This leaves doctors in the unenviable position of having to rely on their expertise when deciding appropriate dosages for their paediatric patients, resulting in ineffective treatment. More importantly it leaves already sick children vulnerable to unexpected adverse events occurring due to difference in their ability to metabolise drugs as they grow and develop.

Properly conducted ethically sound research is essential if children with serious health problems are to be able to hope for novel medicines that will alleviate, prevent or cure their condition. Indeed, it is arguable that not to do such research when you have the opportunity to do so is unethical, because it leaves sick children experiencing the impact of diseases which might have become curable, but which, without research, will remain untreatable.

For many of the rare genetic disease of childhood there is no option but to do research on children because, sadly, they do not live long enough to reach adulthood.

The need for high quality research into medicines for childhood diseases is immense. The opportunity to do this research, in a properly regulated, ethical manner that prospects the interests of the child and safeguards against exploitation is growing. This is a result of the coming together of a number of circumstances which are detailed below.

## Increased Awareness of Childhood Diseases and Paediatric Research

Largely as a result of recent advances in genetics, it has become increasingly possible to provide a definitive diagnosis for growing numbers of rare childhood diseases. This, coupled with the greater understanding of the importance of early, accurate diagnosis for parents and for their children amongst medical professionals, has created a climate within which rare diseases are more likely to be visible – and more likely to be on the doctor's 'radar' as something to be looked out for than was the case in the past.

With the advent of diagnosis comes the possibility for patients to come together into self-help groups, and (eventually) to develop pressure to promote and conduct research. Even prior to the development of new medicines, accurate diagnosis, coupled with developments in IT make it possible for patients and their doctors to access up to date information on the 'state of the art' in their disease, for registers to be created and expert centres established able to see a 'critical mass' of patients sufficient to generate knowledge and understanding that can become available to the wider patient and professional community.

The fast technical development and availability of transport technology is additional factor that facilitates treatment of even rare diseases in specialized centers and also facilitates face-to-face meetings of affected parents. Other fast evolving areas that facilitate interaction are, e.g., telemedicine that allows the exchange of X-ray pictures, photographs, operation videos, diagnoses and documents within seconds, while years ago such an exchange of information could take weeks.

There needs to be a systematic effort to raise awareness of parents and the public at large about the importance of paediatric research on how clinical trials in children are carried out. If the first contact a parent has with a clinical trial is the patient information sheet, then a valuable opportunity to raise awareness has been lost, and unfortunate pre-conceptions about what is involved may have become fixed and difficult to shift.

Patient organisations represent trusted sources of information for the public. They are keen to disseminate relevant information to their members (and wider afield too if resourced to do so). Given the opportunity they provide a balanced view of the impact of paediatric research, helping to generate understanding amongst the public and facilitating the recruitment and retention of children to clinical trials and other types of research project.

Sustained engagement rests upon ongoing trust:
– that the doctor will apply current scientific understanding wisely,
– that the pharmaceutical industry will give paediatric R&D a sufficiently high priority,
– that there will be incentives to produce novel therapies for rare conditions where market forces alone will not provide sufficient prospects for a return on investment,
– that governments at the European Institutions will develop a proportionate and appropriate regulatory regime and implement it sensitively and in ways that encourage the production of safe effective therapies for children quickly.


**Keeping Up to Date**

It used to be said that you could tell when a doctors qualified by the medicines he or she prescribed. While this may have been a cruel caricature, it did reflect a serious difficulty in keeping up to date, especially with regard to rare conditions where expertise might be located in disparate centres across the globe, prior to the development of modern, efficient means of communication.

Medical textbooks often would carry very little information about individual rare conditions, and that which they did was frequently out of date and of little use when planning care and support for patients and their families. Redundant, obsolete or ineffective therapies would continue to be prescribed long after new knowledge had revealed them to be at best inappropriate, and at worst positively harmful.

Thanks to the internet, and due to a growing partnership between patient groups and expert specialist doctors, it is becoming increasingly feasible for clinicians and families to have access to good quality information about the care and management of a growing number of rare diseases.

There has been another interesting development too. Patient groups have used the internet to set up registers and to bring together resources located in far flung places to facilitate research and to create a more robust infrastructure for researchers to access, and to make developments sustainable over time rather than dependent on a series of short-term projects (as has often been the case in the past)!


**Tradition and Mindsets Coming Together**

Unlike the USA, where access to health care tends to be based on individual entitlements, there by creating a mindset that encourages rights based advocacy, the European solidarity based systems have created a climate within which patients and families have tended to trust that, 'if something can be done it will be'. Whilst American patient advocacy groups will have lobbying and recourse to law to secure what they perceive as their rights at the forefront of their list of options, until recently at least, European groups and organisations have tended to see their role as complimentary to that of the states.

While there was nothing much that could be done for children with serious diseases this reliance on the state health care system was probably alright, doctors did provide a degree of emotional support and organised palliation of symptoms. However, there are now possibilities for intervention (for some at least) and there is a growing realisation that, because of resource constraints, just because something can be done it does not mean that it will be. Parents of sick children in Europe are learning from their American cousins and actively lobbying and campaigning at national and at European level for more research into treatments for childhood diseases, and for the rapid introduction of these novel therapies into clinical practice and their reimbursement by the state's health care system [4].

Europe has a large variety of patient organisations, organised at both disease-specific and umbrella levels; national, European and international (see www.patient-view.com/directories.htm). Patient alliances such as EGAN (the European Genetic Alliances' Network, www.egan.eu), EURORDIS (European Organisation for Rare Disorders, www.eurordis.org) and EACH (European Association for Children in Hospital, www.each-for-sick-children.org) have been actively lobbying the European Commission and Parliament for the introduction of Regulations governing the development of paediatric medicines and paediatric focus of adult medicines. This lobbying has been in association with (but independent from) parallel initiatives by academic associations and industry bodies, all of whom want a clear framework within which they can work, and an appropriate range of incentives to encourage them to enter this field.

## Social Solidarity

Whilst the solidarity-based health care systems of most European states have been one of their great strengths, in that all citizens have had access to a minimum standard of health care, rising demand is putting the consensus on which this provision is based and legitimated under increasing strain. Clearly health care systems cannot afford to respond to patients' wants uncritically, but there is at present a poorly developed system for determining needs and the cost and clinical effectiveness of possible responses to these needs.

High profile innovations, which tend to be expensive and which may only be useful for a small number of patients tend to attract the attention of service planners and those responsible for determining reimbursement policies. Long-established therapies, often used by hundreds of thousands or millions of people do not attract attention and continue to be used, often at substantial cost to the health service, notwithstanding the fact that they may not work, deliver only a marginal benefit or have been superseded by newer, better medicines. Focussing attention on the innovative, whilst turning a blind eye to the rest is inequitable and will disproportionately impact on the likelihood of children getting access to the therapies that they need when these become available. As well as scrutinising new developments, evaluation should be extended across the health care spectrum and a disinvestment strategy introduced to stop paying for things that are of little use. This, if it were to be effectively introduced and policed, might help create the headroom for investment in novel medicines that deliver real health gain but which are beyond the reach of all but the wealthiest without the support of a solidarity based health care system.

## Difficult Choices

We are all aware that medicines may have adverse effects. Therefore, although we are here to talk about medicines for children, we should also look at the health and treatment of children from a broader perspective. This is the reason why the patients' organisation EGAN stresses the importance of early information, early diagnosis, prevention, informed reproductive choices and adequate pre-conceptional and prenatal care. More and more it becomes clear that the perinatal period, including the preconceptional phase, may have significant effects on the child's future health. Environmental and lifestyle factors such as smoking, alcohol, use of medicines, diet, etc. Genetic factors may also be important and without accurate, powerful diagnosis it can still happen that a second or third child with the same severe genetic disease is born in one family, either because the diagnosis in the first child was not made timely, or the diagnosis was made, but the treating physician did not inform the parents of the subsequent reproductive risks. EGAN's objective is healthy children, through the appropriate combination of preventative and therapeutic interventions in ways that reflect the needs of families and which are based on sound science – including safe, effective clinical trials that will produce innovative medicines for currently unmet medical needs.

Whilst animal based research is a topic of increasing contention in many countries in Europe, with non-human priorities being a source of particular concern to many, there can be little doubt about the importance of properly regulated research on animals in the search for therapies for the intractable disease of childhood.

Although such research makes us uncomfortable at times, and the search for replacements to animal-based work must go on, until effective models can be developed that mimic the human situation more closely than their animal counterparts the demand of parents for safe effective paediatric medicines must be respected. Nor should it be forgotten that animal-based research is not an end in itself (unless it is specifically targeted at the creation of veterinary medicines). Rather, it is a step in the direction of being able ethically to begin research in children, one that scientists and clinicians are anxious to achieve as quickly as possible, but not at the cost of further jeopardising the health of already vulnerable people. If you look at the propaganda put out by some of the opponents of animal based work you could be led to believe that it is all cruel and heartless. Most is either not invasive or only minimally so, and although some do cause distress and suffering, this is kept to a minimum in responsible, regulated countries, and the animals are euthanised afterwards.

Given a choice between my child and a mouse – or even a lot of mice – then most parents would opt for a chance for the child, and let the mice be used in research.

**From Hierarchy to Partnership**

The traditional hierarchical model whereby 'doctor knows best' has crumbled, to be replaced by a partnership where parents are stakeholders alongside doctors, nurses, academics, drug companies, etc. in working out the best course of action to improve the outcomes for children with serious diseases. Indeed as children grow and mature, so they too are assuming a greater role in determining the best – or perhaps more often the least worst – way of managing their condition to produce the best possible quality of life.

Patient representatives are taking seats at the tables where decisions are made – not just as observers but as full partners with equal power to the others round the table. At the European Medicines Agency (EMA) for example, patient representatives sit on the Management Board, the Orphan Medicinal Products Committee (COMP), the Committee for Advanced Therapies (CAT) and last but not least the Paediatric Committee (PDCO).

The main responsibility of the Paediatric Committee (PDCO) is to assess the content of paediatric investigation plans and adopt opinions on them in accordance with Regulation (EC) 1901/2006 as amended. This includes the assessment of applications for a full or partial waiver and assessment of applications for deferrals.

The PDCO is composed of five CHMP members appointed by the CHMP itself; one member appointed by each member state; three members representing healthcare professionals and three members representing patients' associations.

Although similar developments of patient participation are taking place at national levels in several EU member states, in many countries and many clinical fields, the value of patient involvement in research and research policy is scarcely recognized. To further explore and stimulate the role of patient organisations in clinical research, especially paediatric clinical research, the PatientPartner project was recently set up within the context of the seventh EU Framework Program (www.patientpartner-europe.eu). Recommendations are expected in 2011.

Patient participation is not confined to membership of committees, important though this is. Patients are also active in lobbying and campaigning for changes in law at national and European level to promote opportunities for research into unmet medical needs, particularly when these affect children or young people who would otherwise be denied the opportunity to grow into adults and take their place in society alongside everyone else. Public awareness is also needed, so that the importance of such paediatric research and development is understood by those not generally affected, and researchers are not put off by ill informed comments that imply that they are simply using children as 'guinea pigs'.

It is useful to contrast the approach of patient and family support organisations for children with serious life-limiting disorders to that taken by some consumer groups. Whilst the approach of the former is to try and stand alongside the research community, acting as a critical friend and being part of the process, the latter can sometimes seem to be taking a confrontational stance – stressing the risks, the danger and the problems and sometimes almost seeming to forget (or at least discount) the fact that everything in the garden is not rosy for those children if no

research is carried out. Without progress, unmet medical needs will remain just that, and children who might otherwise have been treated will remain untreatable, with all the implications that come with it for them and their families.

Of course, paediatric medicine is not an issue that is only relevant to patient organizations. All parents want the best possible treatment for their children when they are sick. We should all be concerned about possible side effects of the current unlicensed and off-label use of medicines in children. Families are no longer willing to accept unquestioningly the fact that a substantial proportion of all medicines that are used in children have not been investigated properly. Instead of the current lack of standards, we need the highest scientific and ethical standards for paediatric research and treatment. Also according to the WHO, children need priority [5, 6]. Much greater investment in the health of children is needed. Properly together some of these may even produce savings later by the avoidance of some of the diseases that now occur during middle or old age.

## Patient Organisations as a Resource

It is sadly still the case that many of the rare disorders that affect children are poorly understood by the academic and clinical community. Little research has been done, and often that which has been carried out has been disjointed, transient and of poor quality. Of course there has been much which is world class, but this tends to be focussed on certain high profile diseases like cystic fibrosis or muscular dystrophy rather than some of the lesser known ones.

For those where little is known, families are often an invaluable repository of first-hand information about the impact of the disease on them and their affected children. The intimate business of providing daily care to the sick child necessarily creates a store of knowledge and understanding that is invaluable if it can only be tapped into effectively. Not only do they have this store of information, but given the opportunity families are eager to share it with anyone who is willing to listen.

This experience can be invaluable in developing training for healthcare professionals, taking hindsight and turning it into a pro-active tool that will enable doctors and others to provide information and support based on what parents and children need and want to know, not what professionals think they ought to know. It can help deliver this in ways that are appropriate and user friendly too, making it more likely that it will be heard, understood and acted on.

It can also guide researchers, contributing positively to the design of experiments and clinical trials, to the selection of appropriate end points and the choice of relevant biomarkers and about the importance of quality of life markers as well as those which reflect physiological or structural changes in the child.

Finally, parents can help to promote awareness of the importance and of the value of novel therapies, once these are licensed, to those responsible for authorising the prescription and/or reimbursement of these drugs by national health care systems, making it more likely that the journey from 'scientific bright idea' to pills in patients will be rewarded by speedy transfer into clinical practice and equitable availability to all the children who need to benefit from the fruits of this research and development.

Parent and patient organizations have a vital role in medical research and development. Patient registries and bio banks, based on uniform diagnostic criteria, will speed up future clinical research and hopefully will stimulate awareness of research possibilities for neglected or rare diseases in academia and industry. Many patient organisations have appointed scientific officers to streamline fragmented research initiatives and to highlight the research needs of their members. Patients should be regarded as a partner in the process towards innovative medicines. Patient's

involvement will help to identify the real therapeutic needs; help to balance urgency, risks and benefits; shorten the recruitment period and increase retention in clinical trials and function as the intermediate between medical science and industry, and the child, his family and society. Consultation with patient organizations at the start of research with children will have added value. This can include participation in trial committees as well as support of development of study protocols, case record forms and patient information sheets, defining quality of life endpoints, adverse event reporting, data confidentiality issues and dissemination of study results.

## Importance of Personalized Medicine and Long-Term Follow-Up

We should not be satisfied that a certain drug at a certain dosage is effective only in 2/3 of the children who take it, but ineffective in the remaining 1/3, Variables that may increase effectiveness, for example age, gender, ethnicity and genetic differences should be taken into account. In order to enhance the effectiveness of targeted interventions including novel medicines, the well-being of children must be our first priority and come before commercial and scientific interests.

We do not know the long-term effects of many medicines in children. Long-term studies should assess possible effects in developing children. Public private partnerships should be set up to secure continuity for those follow-up studies.

The new regulations on paediatric medicine is an opportunity for pharmaceutical industry to prove that commercial research can be combined with the highest ethical standards and improve the health of children currently living with serious diseases. Paediatric research requires the paediatrician, industry and parents working together for the well being of the child. Patient organisations have an important role in bringing all these together in the interests of children today and in the future.

## Conclusions

There is an urgent need for novel therapies to be developed to help treat the unmet health needs of millions of sick children across the world today. Whilst research and development is on going, it is still nowhere near enough, and parents rightly demand that more attention is given to this issue.

Patient organisations and family support groups have a key role to play in helping to produce safe, effective and affordable paediatric medicines available to all who need them on a sustainable basis. They are partners in a multi-stakeholder, trans-national programme that must turn its focus on helping more parents of newborn babies to get the answer they hope for when they ask that first question 'Is my baby alright?'

## References


1   The Voice of 12,000 Patients: Experiences and expectations on diagnosis and care in Europe. Eurordis, 2009. www.eurordis.org.
2   Online Mendelian Inheritance in Man (OMIN). www.ncbi.nlm.nih.gov.
3   Kent A, Oosterwijk C: A patient and family perspective on gene therapy for rare diseases. J Gene Med 2007;9:922–923.
4   It's My Life: A New Revolution. Patient Power. Simon Rozendaal, ASPEKt, 2007.
5   WHO: Priority Medicines for the Citizens of Europe and the World. Geneva, World Health Organisation, 2004.
6   WHO: Make Medicines Child Size. Geneva, World Health Organisation, 2007. www.who.int/childmedicines/en/



Alastair Kent
Director Genetic Interest Group
4D Leroy House, 436 Essex Road
London N1 3QP (UK)
Tel. +44 20 7704 3141, Fax +44 20 7359 1447, E-Mail alastair@gig.org.uk

Rose K, van den Anker JN (eds): Guide to Paediatric Drug Development and Clinical Research.
Basel, Karger, 2010, pp 40–45

# Providing Global Access to Essential Medicines for Children – The WHO Better Medicines for Children Programme

Kalle Hoppu[a] · Suzanne Hill[b]

[a]Poison Information Centre, Helsinki University Central Hospital, and Hospital for Children and Adolescents and Department of Clinical Pharmacology, University of Helsinki, Helsinki, Finland; [b]Medicines, Access and Rational Use, Essential Medicines and Pharmaceutical Policies, World Health Organisation, Geneva, Switzerland

It is estimated that nearly 10 million children under the age of 5 die every year, many of them from treatable conditions. Slightly more than a third of the deaths are in neonates. Undernutrition is present in 35% of under-5 deaths. The main causes of death are pneumonia (19%), diarrhoeal diseases (17%), neonatal severe infections (10%), malaria (8%), measles (3%) and HIV/AIDS (3%). Effective interventions in the form of medicines exist for many of these conditions, but a significant proportion of the children do not have access to these medicines, and even the medicines available for children in the richest countries of the world may not be appropriate for their needs.

While lack of medicines is not the single most important health problem of children, it is clear that the child health goals set cannot be reached without providing children access to appropriate medicines. The work to provide children with better access to appropriate medicines is essential for achievement of the Millennium Development Goals, especially MDG Four: Reduce child mortality and MDG Six: Combat HIV/AIDS, malaria, and other major diseases.

With the paediatric medicines initiatives launched in the US and the EU, in essence public health interventions to improve the health of children, interest in all aspects of paediatric medicines increased and the first positive results have been observed. In order to make the results of these regional initiatives available to benefit all children in the world, the Finnish government proposed in November 2006 that the WHO, as an undisputed expert within the field of global health, should take action in this process. Wide international acceptance of the importance of the issue and the need for WHO actions manifested in the adoption of Resolution WHA60.20 Better Medicines for Children by the World health Assembly in May 2007 [1]. Key points of the resolution are summarized in table 1.

## Children's Access to Medicines – A Global Problem

The lack of availability of medicines for children is a global problem. It concerns all children of the world, even in the richest of all countries, but even

**Table 1.** Key points of the World Health Assembly resolution WHA60.20 on Better Medicines for Children [1]

| |
|---|
| *Urges member states* |
| To take steps to identify appropriate dosage forms and strengths of medicines for children, and to encourage their manufacture and licensing |
| To encourage research and development of appropriate medicines for diseases that affect children, and to ensure that high-quality clinical trials for these medicines are conducted in an ethical manner |
| To facilitate timely licensing of appropriate, high-quality and affordable medicines for children and innovative methods for monitoring the safety of such medicines |
| To encourage the marketing of adequate paediatric formulations together with newly developed medicines |
| To promote access to essential medicines for children |
| To collaborate in order to facilitate innovative research and development on, formulation of, regulatory approval of, provision of adequate prompt information on, and rational use of, paediatric medicines and medicines authorized for adults but not approved for use in children |
| *Requests the WHO Director-General* |
| To promote the development, harmonization and use of standards for clinical trials of medicines for children |
| To revise and regularly update the Model List of Essential Medicines in order to include missing essential medicines for children |
| To ensure that all relevant WHO programmes, including but not limited to that on essential medicines, contribute to making safe and effective medicines as widely available for children as for adults |
| To promote the development of international norms and standards for quality and safety of formulations for children, and of the regulatory capacity to apply them |
| To make available evidence-based treatment guidelines and independent information on dosage and safety aspects of medicines for children, and to work with Member States in order to implement such guidelines |

more those in the developing world. The selection of medicines available to treat children is not comparable anywhere to the choice of medicines available for adults, either in qualitative or quantitative terms [2]. This gap was also true for the WHO Model List of Essential Medicines during the first 30 years of its existence. Some of the main problems of children's access to medicines in the middle- and low-income countries are listed in table 2. Many of the problems are related to general lack of resources locally, but even in these cases, the difference between what is available for adults compared to what medicines are available for children is at least similar or even larger than in high-income countries. In addition to the

specific problems, there is a huge general need for advocacy and education involving all stakeholders in the area of paediatric medicines. The WHO contribution to the advocacy work is spearheaded by the 'make medicines child size' campaign launched in December 2007 [3].

## The WHO Model List of Essential Medicines for Children

Many countries use the WHO Model List of Essential Medicines (EML) to guide drug procurement and supply. It has also been an important

**Table 2.** Examples of the main problems of children's access to medicines in middle- and low-income countries

*Non-availability of many medicines essential for children in a country*

– Medicines essential for children were not in the EML

– Inadequate national procurement of children's medicines even if on EML, and adult medicines procured – children's medicines not available in public and private health care

– National competent authorities do not respond to Marketing Authorisation Applications for paediatric medicines, as they lack experience and expertise to asses them

*Lack of appropriate paediatric formulations*

– Age-appropriate paediatric formulations not produced for many medicines anywhere in the world

– Problems of storing and transporting medicines in areas with high temperatures and humidity

– Liquid formulations expensive and impractical to transport due to bulk and need for cold-chain

– Clean water needed to constitute paediatric formulations not available

– FDCs needed to treat priority diseases like malaria, TB and HIV/AIDS rarely available for children and if available, do not allow age appropriate dosing of all components

*Information and research gaps*

– Appropriate doses needed to account for developmental differences in drug disposition not known for many medicines used to treat priority diseases, especially for newborns, infants and small children

– Nationally adapted paediatric formularies and treatment guidelines needed for rational use of the essential paediatric medicines becoming available

policy and advocacy tool for improving access to important medicines such as the anti-retrovirals. Although the EML has always included some paediatric medicines, children's medicines were not systematically considered each time the list was amended [4]. After a consultation of experts on paediatric essential medicines, the WHO Executive Board established a special Subcommittee of the Expert Committee on the Selection and Use of Essential Medicines to set up a WHO Model List of Essential medicines for Children (EMLc). As a result, the 1st EMLc [5] was adopted in October 2007 and the updated 2nd EML was approved in April 2009. The 2nd Model List includes for the first time a special section on specific medicines for neonatal care. Although a separate paediatric subcommittee no longer exists, measures have been put in place that allows appropriate development of the EMLc also in the future. It is possible to influence the EMLc by sending an application for inclusion, change or deletion of a medicine to the secretary of the committee.

## The WHO Better Medicines for Children Program

The WHO Model List of Essential medicines for Children and a commitment to develop it are a milestone in the WHO paediatric medicines activities [6], but only a starting point for all the other actions needed by all stakeholders to make appropriate medicines available for children at country level. In collaboration with UNICEF, the WHO has developed a program to improve access for essential medicines for children through addressing issues of availability, safety, efficacy and price. It is not possible to describe all the planned actions in detail, but selected areas will be highlighted.

## Paediatric Formulations

Many documents describing the current status of developing appropriate paediatric formulations have been produced recently. Such documents describe the common and tried pharmaceutical formulations that are currently available and considered most suitable for children. The majority of these formulations are in some liquid form, provided as syrups or solutions, or powders that have to be dissolved in water. However, the practical experience from the children, their caregivers, nurses, pharmacists, and prescribing physicians from all over the world is that the existing paediatric formulations are not optimal when it comes to dosing, dispensing, and administering the medicines to children. This problem of lack of age-appropriate paediatric formulations has been widely recognized, including the US and EU paediatric initiatives, and those initiatives include measures designed to try to alleviate the problem.

The problems of paediatric formulations are even more difficult in resource-poor settings, and especially in areas of the world where high temperature and humidity combined with problems of transport make logistics and storage a real challenge. Great global benefit could be achieved if, in the development of new and better paediatric formulations, an aim would be appropriateness for global use. To this end the WHO convened an expert meeting in December 2008 which identified the dosage forms of medicines most suitable for children with particular attention to conditions prevailing in the developing countries, and flagged future areas of research required in this area [7]. The most important proposal of the group was a shift from the traditional paradigm of liquid paediatric formulations to flexible solid dosage forms, which has subsequently been endorsed by the Paediatric Committee of the European Medicines Agency and others. Important research needs were also identified, including: what particle sizes can be comfortably and safely ingested at different ages and developmental stages in children; what standards should be set for granularity and texture or mouth feel, taste and smell, at different ages and developmental stages to optimize the acceptability of dosage forms; what evidence exists to define optimal frequency of dosing (and pill burden) in terms of impact on adherence and clinical outcomes.

## Modelling Existing Data for the Development of Paediatric Medicines for Priority Diseases

In adults, the approach to first-line treatment of malaria, TB and HIV/AIDS is use of fixed-dose combination products. For children, however, very few fixed-dose combination products are currently available that are of good quality and formulated for treating children. In addition, evidence-based information on proper dosing to account for the developmental differences in handling of the individual active substances of drug combinations is needed, but seldom available.

To ensure optimal treatment of TB in children, the dosage recommendations for the first-line drugs required reassessment. In particular, pharmacokinetic studies of first-line drugs needed to be collated to determine whether current WHO dosage recommendations are likely to result in plasma concentrations that are sufficient for a therapeutic effect in children of all ages. The existing pharmacokinetic evidence on pyrazinamide, isoniazide and rifampicin in both adults and children was therefore compiled in a literature review and considered at an expert meeting in July 2008 [8]. The experts concluded that it is likely that the recommendations for doses of rifampicin, isoniazide and pyrazinamide will need to be changed to recommend higher doses per kilogram per day in children up to 12 years of age. Additional work is needed to ensure that the higher doses are safe and that the FDC products reflecting new recommendations become available. The approach used to come up with the new dose recommendations, and definition of optimal age-appropriate FDC strengths to cover all relevant age groups could be useful for development of new medicinal products of old medicines for children, and help to avoid unnecessary trials. Existing published pharmacokinetic data, from old studies with many weaknesses, were combined with pharmacokinetic modelling based on modern understanding of the principles of developmental pharmacology to simulate relevant concentration-time relationships in several age groups using different weight adjusted doses. Once the dose-range proposed as providing concentrations acceptable for efficacy and safety was determined for each medicine, further modelling was used to arrive at optimal FDCs to cover all relevant ages with a minimum of products of different strengths. Clinical trials will still be needed to confirm the true efficacy and safety of the FDCs proposed. A similar approach could be used, as relevant, for other priority diseases, and could be used in many other conditions to avoid unnecessary duplication of clinical trials already performed.

## Development, Harmonization and Use of Standards for Clinical Trials of Medicines for Children

Clinical trials in children are necessary to provide the data needed for safe and effective use, and labelling of medicines in all relevant paediatric age ranges. In children data are needed to cover all ages, from newborns to adolescents. Getting the necessary clinical trials performed is required for success of the US, EU and WHO paediatric medicines initiatives. Studies in children, a most vulnerable population, have to fulfil the highest ethical criteria, including appropriateness of the scientific methods used. Due to several factors, including cost and the increasing complexity of regulations, paediatric clinical trials are now being performed in low and middle income settings, where such trials are economically feasible. This redistribution of paediatric clinical pharmacological research from developed to developing countries can be positive, if it is relevant to the setting where it is performed. However, it may also lead to dissociation of risks and benefits into different paediatric populations if the medicinal products studied will not be available to the population where the trials were performed.

To safeguard children all over the world from harm in inappropriate clinical trials, a comprehensive global consideration of the potential consequences of these developments is needed. Performance of high-quality paediatric trials requires an appropriate framework of legislation and guidance on the ethics; regulators to oversee the research and investigators interested in and trained to perform the trials. Harmonisation of the requirements for clinical trials to demonstrate the safety and efficacy of medicines in children to the extent possible would help in reducing unnecessary trials and facilitate children's access to appropriately labelled medicines worldwide. The WHO is currently also working in this area to develop standards for clinical research in children.

The next 5 years offers an opportunity to address many of the gaps in access to medicines for children. However, success will depend on changing attitudes and interests of many different groups including manufacturers and researchers. Perhaps the most important change that is needed is increased expectations from consumers and carers. If they begin to demand better medicines for children, then the supply is likely to improve. Without that change it is likely that children will remain 'therapeutic orphans' and we will continue to offer second-best treatment to a third of the world's population.

# References


1 World Health Assembly: Resolution WHA60.20 Better Medicines for Children, 2007. Available from: http://www.who.int/entity/childmedicines/publications/WHA6020.pdf.

2 Hoppu K: Paediatric clinical pharmacology: at the beginning of a new era. Eur J Clin Pharmacol 2008;64:201–205.

3 WHO Global Campaign: Make Medicines Child Size, 2007 [cited 2008 11.9.2008]. Available from: http://www.who.int/childmedicines/en/index.html.

4 Hill S, Gray A, Weber M: Setting standards for essential children's medicines. Bull WHO 2007;85:650.

5 WHO: 1st Model List of Essential Medicines for Children 2007. Available from: http://www.who.int/childmedicines/publications/EMLc%20(2).pdf.

6 Zucker H, Rago L: Access to essential medicines for children: the world health organization's global response. Clin Pharmacol Ther 2007;82:503–505.

7 WHO Report of the Informal Expert Meeting on Dosage Forms of Medicines for Children, 2008. Available form: http://www.who.int/selection_medicines/committees/expert/17/application/paediatric/Dosage_form_report-DEC2008.pdf

8 Hill S, Regondi I, Grzemska M, Matiru R: Children and tuberculosis medicines: bridging the research gap. Bull WHO 2008;86:658.



Kalle Hoppu, MD, PhD
Poison Information Centre, Helsinki University Central Hospital
PO Box 790 (Tukholmankatu 17)
FI–00029 HUS Helsinki (Finland)
Tel. +358 9 471 74 788, Fax +358 9 471 74 702, E-Mail kalle.hoppu@hus.fi

Rose K, van den Anker JN (eds): Guide to Paediatric Drug Development and Clinical Research.
Basel, Karger, 2010, pp 46–50

# Paediatric Clinical Pharmacology: From Bench to Bedside

John N. van den Anker

Division of Pediatric Clinical Pharmacology, Children's National Medical Center, Washington, D.C., USA; Department of Pediatrics,
Erasmus MC, Sophia Children's Hospital, Rotterdam, The Netherlands

## Academic and Clinical Pharmacology

The academic discipline of clinical pharmacology has evolved into playing an important role in promoting the rational use of drugs, in supporting the translation of pharmacological concepts from the bench to the patient, in clinical drug development, and in teaching medical and pharmacy students. The American Society for Clinical Pharmacology and Therapeutics decided in 2006 to define clinical pharmacology as the science of drug discovery, development, regulation, and utilization in the context of the effects of medicines on humans [1]. This differs quite substantially, e.g., from the technical report issued by the World Health Organization in 1970 [2] which stated that the function of the clinical pharmacologist was: (1) to improve patient care by promoting safer and more effective use of drugs, (2) to increase knowledge through research, (3) to pass on knowledge through teaching, and (4) to provide services (e.g. analyses, drug information, and advice in the design of experiments). The role of the clinical pharmacologist in the fields of drug discovery, drug development, and regulatory sciences has significantly changed over the last decades. Specifically, the role of paediatric clinical pharmacology is evolving and changing dramatically. This chapter deals predominantly with paediatric clinical pharmacology in private and academic hospitals where few individuals currently possess the broad-based skills necessary to participate effectively in this arena. The role of clinical pharmacology in drug development is addressed by the chapter of Reigner and co-workers in this book [pp. 51–59].

There are continued and serious concerns about the decline of the discipline of clinical pharmacology and therapeutics in many countries across the globe. The same holds true for the actual number of specialized physicians and pharmacists in clinical pharmacology and therapeutics. There is a fierce debate ongoing whether the discipline of clinical pharmacology is exclusively a medical discipline or also a discipline that needs to be open to other health professionals [3], but there is no discussion about the pivotal role of clinical pharmacologists in ensuring rational use of drugs, in translating pharmacological concepts from the bench to the clinic, in clinical drug development, or in teaching the discipline to medical and pharmacy students. It would be desirable for the academic debate to focus on the need of collaboration between physician and non-physician clinical pharmacologists together with clinical drug and therapeutics experts in academic and hospital surroundings as well as in the industrial process of drug development. In both areas only by the formation of integrated teams consisting of individuals from different disciplines and with complementary strengths it will be possible to reach the ultimate goal of the discipline: advancing therapeutics. With increasing complexity, rational and personalized drug therapy the discipline of clinical pharmacology will consist of physicians, pharmacists and PhDs, who implement and validate advanced bioanalytical techniques, population pharmacokinetics and pharmacodynamics (PK/PD) and PK/PD modeling, pharmacogenetics and pharmacogenomics, pharmacoepidemiology and different aspects of translational research.

Medical specialists, pharmacists and other health-care providers who are trained in the discipline of clinical pharmacology are involved with different aspects of patient care, educational activities and research. They combine basic knowledge in the area of pharmacology and pharmacotherapy with specific knowledge related to the pathophysiology of certain diseases and characteristics of the individuals suffering from these diseases. This aims at evidence-based pharmacotherapy to provide the right dose of the right drug to the right patient. The evolvement of this discipline over the last decades took its point of departure from the investigation of absorption, distribution, metabolisation and excretion (ADME) of available drugs, i.e. drugs on the market, both in adults and children. Specifically in the area of paediatric clinical pharmacology, the knowledge and understanding of ADME in the developing body has exploded and has culminated in many important papers in this arena. The explosion of increased understanding of ADME in children has significantly contributed to the pressure that led to paediatric legislation in the USA in 1997 [4], since then re-authorized and expanded in 2003 and 2007, as well as to the EU paediatric

legislation in force since 2007 [5]. Finally, in 2006 the top representatives of the paediatric clinicians, IPA (International Paediatric Association) [6] and of the International Union of Basic and Clinical Pharmacology, IUPHAR [7] established the International Alliance (IA) [8] for better medicines for children, which was essential in kicking off the WHO paediatric campaign described in this book by the chapter of Hill and Hoppu.

## Multidisciplinary Role of Academic and Clinical Pharmacologists

Knowledge in the areas of pharmacodynamics, pharmacokinetics and pharmacogenetics/genomics of prescribed drugs is more and more integrated with guidelines and other evidence of the effectiveness of these medications. However, the increasing knowledge concerning pharmacotherapy in relation to translational science (use of microarrays, DNA chips, and biomarkers) results in a situation where the integration of this new knowledge into daily pharmacotherapy is getting more and more complicated.

Clinical pharmacologists are trained to deduct from a plethora of information the relevant parts for the individual patient with his or her disease resulting in the optimal choice of pharmacotherapy. Based on patient-specific information there is a continuous search for an optimal balance between the safety and efficacy of the pharmacological treatment.

In addition, clinical pharmacologists have a seat in committees dedicated to the optimal use of medications in many health care institutions because of their specific expertise. Many times they chair these pivotal committees being the expert in pharmacotherapy. In addition, they often are also chairing formulary committees determining which drugs should be on the formulary and which ones not.

The discipline of clinical pharmacology has many connections with other disciplines including medicine and hospital pharmacy and there is increasing interest and interaction with paediatrics, cardiology, oncology, etc. in addition, because of the rapidly expanding field of translational science, there will be a significant increase in visibility of clinical pharmacology in both patient care and education.

In the area of patient care, the discipline of clinical pharmacology is crucial to improve medication safety and patient security. There is clearly a need to initiate clinics in clinical pharmacology where patients treated with several medications (polypharmacy), patients with (severe) adverse medication events, and patients who will need pharmacogenetic consultation can be seen and supported.

There are several major areas of research that ultimately will improve the patient care and the educational activities in the field of clinical pharmacology and several of these are outlined below:

## Pharmacogenetics

Pharmacogenetics is the science dedicated to decipher the impact of genes on the observed variability between individuals in their capacity to handle medications that are administered to them. These variations can be already present at birth or can be acquired later in life. There is increasing evidence that the differences in efficacy and safety of several drugs can be explained and perhaps even predicted by differences in genetic capacity to metabolize drugs or differences in receptor sensitivity to certain medications. More than 10 years ago the prediction was that the new knowledge related to pharmacogenetics would result in a revolution in pharmacotherapy. However, that predicted revolution did not happen and currently only for a handful of medications the usefulness of pharmacogenetics has become clear. However, there are indications that for many more drugs there might be a place for pharmacogenetically guided therapy that will optimize the safe and effective use of medicines in patients with different diseases and with different ages.

There are two major areas of interest. The first one is the more population-oriented approach that tries to link epidemiology with clinical pharmacology in order to investigate genetic determinants of drug response in populations. The second one is much more close to the daily activities of the clinical pharmacologist and is becoming a more and more important part of the discipline of clinical pharmacology: the prediction of the right dose of the right drug for the right person. For that goal it is mandatory to collect prospectively demographic and clinical data from patients combined with PK and PD information. It is clear that to be successful in that endeavor it will be mandatory to build and maintain a close collaboration, in addition to mutual respect and trust, between investigators of the different disciplines. During the early stages of study design, it will be beneficial to sit together with all involved and to delineate how to optimize the way data might be generated that not only will answer the primary question but that will allow for more in depth investigations in individuals who show an aberrant effect or a decreased or increased side effect profile.

Finally, a major challenge for physicians/pharmacists, pharmaceutical companies and regulatory agencies, will be to better understand the relative contribution of genetic variation to the observed variability in drug disposition and response across the paediatric age spectrum from preterm and term neonates, to infants, children and adolescents. To accomplish this goal, studies must be appropriately designed and conducted to generate optimal information.

## Population Pharmacokinetics

Well-known differences exist in the disposition of, and response to, drugs between children and adults and between children of different ages. Yet, because well-designed clinical studies in children are scarce, dosing schemes in children are usually derived in an empirical matter from clinical trials in healthy volunteers and/or restricted adult patient groups, and often based on a linear extrapolation on the basis of bodyweight. However, paediatric dosing schedules should be based on an understanding of the PK/PD relationship of the medicine in children as compared to the empiric-dosing regimen based on body weight alone. To be able to reach this goal, to define effective and safe dosing regimens for children of different ages, detailed information is needed on the PK and PD. Both the PK and PD may change over the continuum of a child's life. Age-related differences in PK may be caused by changes in absorption, distribution, metabolism and/or excretion, whereas age-related differences in PD may be caused by changes in receptor expression, and result in altered target tissue sensitivity or changes in the mechanism governing the drug response.

A useful tool to gather better information is the use of population PK/PD modeling. This involves the application of concepts of 'non-linear mixed effects modeling' (NONMEM) where PK and/or PD parameters are simultaneously estimated in all studied individuals. The final results are population PK and/or PD parameters and estimates for the interindividual variability as well as intraindividual variability. Following this characterization of the variability in PK and PD, the next step is the so-called covariate analysis, in which demographic and pathophysiologic (e.g. weight, age, genetics) predictors are identified. These predictors may serve as the basis for the design of individualized dosing regimens. The most important advantage of this approach is that it allows for the utilization of infrequently obtained samples and observations from patients at time points compatible with clinical care.

A close collaboration between clinicians conducting clinical trials, pharmacists supporting clinical trials and clinical pharmacologists who are trained in the use of population pharmacokinetics will therefore not only decrease the invasiveness of clinical trials, but will increase the value of these investigations by combining a priori determination of the optimal dose to be studied, optimal sampling techniques to minimize the invasive procedures, and sophisticated techniques such as NONMEM analysis and Monte Carlo simulations. These techniques will allow the simultaneous determination of the impact of age, development, disease, genetics and concomitant therapies on the pharmacokinetics of investigational drugs. Finally, the use of these new techniques will allow sophisticated PK/PD modeling that will not only make clinical investigations more aimed at real situations but also will decrease the number of patients needed to get the necessary information to allow labeling of the drug.

**Therapeutic Drug Monitoring**

For drugs with a relatively small therapeutic window (the difference between a drug concentration that is effective and with side effects versus a drug concentration that is effective but associated with side effects) the technique of therapeutic drug monitoring (TDM) has been implemented in daily clinical practice for decades. However, recently there has been a dramatic change in the use of TDM in clinical practice. In the past TDM consisted of the sampling of blood to determine peak and/or trough concentrations of the drug of interest. Based on that information dose adjustments were advised by primarily pharmacists and sometimes these adjustments were implemented by the physicians responsible for the direct care of the patients. Nowadays, based on several new developments, TDM has become much more sophisticated and profits intensively from a team approach (clinicians, pharmacists, clinical pharmacologists, PK-PD specialists). Some of these developments are:

1   The development and implementation of new and very sensitive assays using HPLC and HPLC-tandem MS technology to assure

not only very precise but also very reliable quantitation of the drug of interest.

2 The increase in knowledge about the metabolism of drugs and most importantly, the understanding that several metabolites might not only be clinically relevant and active but even more that the determination of the metabolites allowed us to better understand the developmental changes in metabolizing pathways but also the impact of disease on the metabolizing capacity of the liver and the intestine.

3 Sampling at predetermined times is not necessary anymore because of the availability of population PK techniques that will allow more or less random sampling and still will secure outstanding information derived by these sampling techniques.

4 Single blood sampling might not be the best way to go. In several circumstances it has been shown to be much more adequate to calculate an area under the curve (AUC) value for a certain time period (i.e. first 2 or 2–4 h after the gift) to be in a better shape to predict the change in exposure to the drug after adjustment based on TDM.

5 Urine and saliva might be useful alternatives for blood in circumstances where blood sampling is limited due to environmental reasons or limited access.

6 TDM warrants a multidisciplinary team to assure the optimal use of this technique where pharmacists, clinicians, PK/PD experts and clinical pharmacologists can make a difference: improved efficacy and safety!

Training programs in paediatric clinical pharmacology need to contain modules covering items such as rational pharmacotherapy, pharmacokinetics and pharmacodynamics, therapeutic drug monitoring, pharmacogenomics and genotyping, individualized drug therapy, drug toxicology, teaching, clinical pharmacology research, and good clinical practice. Training programs for physicians/pharmacists/nurse practitioners/physician assistants that allow exchange of experiences and specific knowledge exist already, but they are still far too scarce in comparison with the highly unmet medical and clinical needs.


## References

1 ASCPT strategic plan 2006: www.ascpt.org

2 World Health Organization: Technical Report Series No. 446. Clinical Pharmacology: Scope, Organization, Training. Geneva, World Health Organization, 1970.

3 Reed MD: Team-centered clinical pharmacology practice: is it a remedy for or the basis of our discipline? Clin Pharmacol Ther 2008;83:218–219.

4 www.fda.gov/oc/fdama/default.htm

5 The European Paediatric Initiative: History of the Paediatric Regulation. Available at http://www.ema.europa.eu/pdfs/human/paediatrics/1796704en.pdf

6 www.ipa-world.org

7 www.iuphar.org

8 http://www.ipa-world.org/News/Documents/news02.pdf



Prof. John N. van den Anker, MD, PhD
Division of Pediatric Clinical Pharmacology, Children's National Medical Center
111 Michigan Avenue, NW
Washington, DC 20010 (USA)
E-Mail jvandena@cnmc.org

Rose K, van den Anker JN (eds): Guide to Paediatric Drug Development and Clinical Research.
Basel, Karger, 2010, pp 51–59

# Role of Clinical Pharmacology in the Development of Paediatric Clinical Development Plans

Bruno Reigner · Bénédicte M. Ricci · Xavier Liogier d'Ardhuy

Clinical Research and Exploratory Development and Clinical Pharmacology, F. Hoffmann-La Roche Ltd., Basel, Switzerland

The new regulations in the field of paediatrics, especially in the European Union, have led to a significant increase in interest and resources dedicated to paediatric drug development. Designing a paediatric plan is a challenging and interdisciplinary task which requires input and close collaboration of clinicians with expertise in the disease and in paediatrics, clinical pharmacologists, pharmacometricians, statisticians with expertise in innovative study designs, regulatory affairs specialists, and toxicologists with specific knowledge in the conduct of studies in juvenile animals. A paediatric clinical development plan should not be a new plan modelled after the investigational plan in adults with sequential phase 1, phase 2, and phase 3 studies, but rather should effectively take advantage of all the prior knowledge acquired from adult studies and translate this knowledge into a plan of necessary and informative paediatric studies. One particular challenge is the dose selection in the different age groups. The understanding of the pharmacokinetic/pharmacodynamic (PK/PD) relationship in adults can be of great help here to define the dose or dose range to be studied in paediatric patients. The concept for bridging from adults to paediatrics, or paediatric bridging, is to leverage prior drug knowledge in adults (PK, efficacy, safety,

exposure response relationships) and experience in developing compounds in the same indication to inform the design of the necessary paediatric studies and get approval for a paediatric use in the drug label. When used appropriately, paediatric bridging can streamline paediatric investigations, with fewer children in trials exposed to sub-therapeutic or toxic doses and yield earlier availability of medicines with high medical need in children.

The clinical pharmacologist as a member of the project team in a pharmaceutical company is a key contributor to the paediatric plan discussions, because of his/her in depth knowledge of the PK and PK/PD relationships of the drug in adults and his/her familiarity with bridging techniques, commonly used in other clinical pharmacology fields such as ethnicity assessment or new routes of drug administration.

The objective of this chapter is to describe the general principles in paediatric bridging, provide the reader with important references and resources for implementation of paediatric bridging, and finally illustrate these concepts with several examples. Of note, the present chapter does not cover the rare situation where drug development starts immediately with paediatric trials.

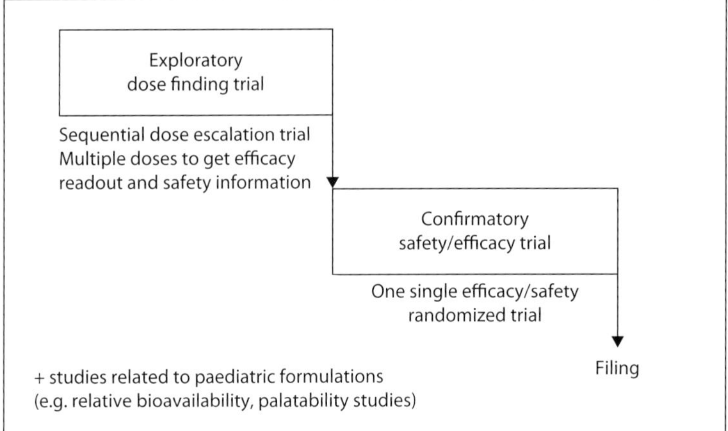


**Fig. 1.** As a starting point for discussion, the schematic representation of a two-step model to design the paediatric development plan.

## A Two-Step Model for the Paediatric Clinical Development Plan

When initiating discussions on the paediatric development plan, we recommend consideration of a 2-step approach composed of an exploratory dose-finding trial with primary efficacy and safety objectives and PK assessments, followed by a confirmatory efficacy/safety trial (fig. 1). One positive confirmatory trial in paediatrics is usually sufficient to get the paediatric indication in the label, as opposed to the general rule of 2 positive pivotal trials to get approval in adults. One exception to the generally accepted rule of one single trial for approval in paediatrics is in the treatment of depression, where the Food and Drug Administration (FDA) indicated in the sample paediatric written request for depression that a paediatric claim would need to be supported by two independent, adequate and well controlled clinical trials in paediatric depression (FDA, Sample Written Request for Antidepressants). In general, the confirmatory trial is the pivotal efficacy and safety study. As such, it is usually a randomized, double-blind trial, comparing the new chemical entity (NCE) to placebo or standard of care. In-depth discussions are needed during protocol development to precisely define the target disease and corresponding patient population (including the age range of patients) and also the clinical efficacy endpoints, which may not be the same as in adults. Another critical point for consideration is the choice of dosing (starting dose, dosing interval, dose adjustment rules when appropriate, maximal dose). The dosing regimen studied in the confirmatory trial, (or the dosing providing the best risk/benefit assessment when more than one dose levels are studied in the confirmatory trial) is usually the dosing recommended in the drug label. This highlights the importance of dosing selection in the paediatric confirmatory trial. When an exploratory dose finding study is carried out, the decision of dosing in the confirmatory trial is not solely informed by extrapolation from adult data, but also from observed data in children. This 2-step approach increases significantly the probability of obtaining a confirmatory trial with a positive outcome, i.e. the trial results are adequate to get regulatory approval. Of note, this 2-step approach could be implemented with 2 distinct clinical trials, or with one larger trial combining the exploratory and confirmatory phases.

The dose finding study is exploratory in nature, and is usually a sequential dose escalation trial, with treatment lasting long enough (e.g. for several weeks) to get an efficacy read out and also safety information in paediatrics. The study starts with a low dose level and once this first dose level is considered well tolerated and safe, a second cohort with a higher dose level is started. If needed, following the same principle to ensure safety of the paediatric patients, a third or fourth dose level may be studied. A randomized dose finding trial, assigning randomly in parallel the patients to 2–4 dose levels would be better to prevent any bias in patient selection and data assessment. However, exposing patients to the highest dose level without prior information in paediatrics at a lower dose level may not be considered acceptable because of the safety risk. Individual up-titration is to be considered in indications where tolerance to side effects is expected to develop; all cohorts could be started with the same low dose, but up-titrated to different target doses. Independently of study design, the endpoints of the exploratory dose finding study should include efficacy (or an adequate biomarker) for optimal use of the bridging strategy. However, should efficacy endpoints not considered an option (e.g. not achievable within a relatively short treatment duration and small sample size), an exploratory dose finding trial would still be very useful for bridging with exposure-safety relationship information. In this scenario, the number and range of dose(s) in the confirmatory trial would be narrowed down based on prior safety information in children.

A dedicated pharmacokinetic trial is not a pre-requisite to start the exploratory dose finding study. Using state of the art techniques like physiologically based pharmacokinetic (PBPK) modelling to predict the pharmacokinetics in paediatrics based on adult pharmacokinetics and knowledge of developmental changes in physiological and biochemical processes, systemic exposure information can be used to select the lowest dose level in the exploratory dose finding trial [1–5]. More information about the approaches and methods that are used to determine the starting dose when the drug is given for the first time in paediatrics is beyond the scope of the present chapter.

Using a single-dose pharmacokinetic trial, in place of an exploratory dose-finding trial, to select the dose in the confirmatory trial has been utilized in several paediatric programs (e.g. adefovir, glimepiride, glyburide) [6], but is not recommended. This sub-optimal approach usually selects a paediatric dose that provides the area under the curve (AUC) observed in adults at the approved therapeutic dose, and assumes that the concentration-response in paediatrics is the same as in adults. We prefer to recommend an approach that does not require this assumption and provides observed data about exposure-response relationship (ERR) in paediatrics after multiple doses before starting the confirmatory paediatric trial. Our recommended approach is more robust as it is appropriate for drugs with or without a similar concentration-response relationship in adults and in paediatrics.

We recommend studying the pharmacokinetics of the drug in the exploratory dose-finding study, using extensive pharmacokinetic profiling, at least in a subset of patients, and sparse blood sampling in all patients to generate the necessary ERR results. A multiple ascending dose study, as typically performed in adults during phase 1 of clinical development, is not necessary in paediatrics and would raise ethical issues when it comes to defining a maximum tolerated dose (MTD) in paediatrics, particularly in view of the vast knowledge already available in adults.

In addition to these paediatric trials, paediatric development plans frequently include studies to support the development and availability of specific paediatric formulations (e.g. tablets of smaller dosage strengths or liquid formulations like syrups or suspensions). Clinical studies to assess the bioavailability of the new paediatric formulation relative to the registered adult formulation are usually conducted in adult healthy volunteers

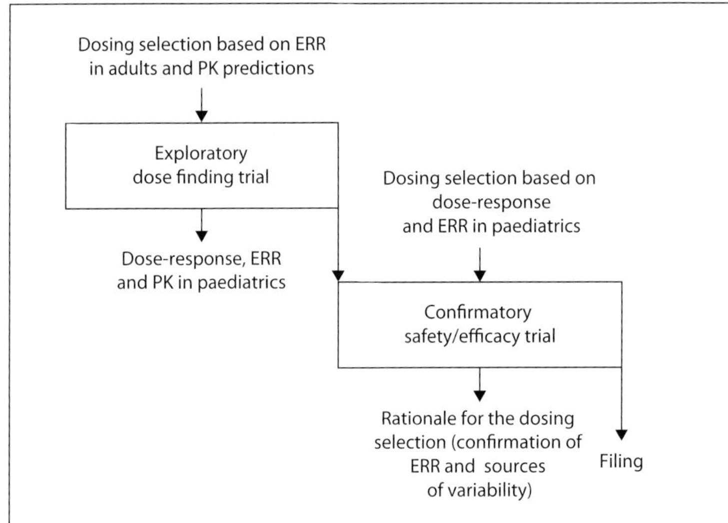



**Fig. 2.** Addition of the paediatric bridging element to the two-step model, and making sure that prior knowledge from adult and paediatric trials is fully utilize to design the confirmatory trial.

[7]. Clinical palatability studies may also be needed when the drug substance has an unpleasant taste that could significantly affect compliance to the prescribed treatment [8, 9]. These studies are most often conducted in an adult population, however one should keep in mind that taste preference are different in adults and in children, and even in children, depending on their culture or age. The paediatric formulation related studies should be conducted before the confirmatory trial to ensure that this pivotal trial is conducted with the final to-be-marketed formulation(s). Different formulations and/or routes of administration may be necessary when the paediatric indication plan covers a large age range [9].

**Adding the Paediatric Bridging Element to the Two-Step Model**

The design of the exploratory dose finding study should be informed with all prior knowledge from adult studies (fig. 2). With regard to the selection of dose levels, the knowledge of ERR in adults together with the prediction of the PK in paediatric patients (on the basis of PK results in adults and developmental pharmacology) is used to select the lowest dose level that is safe and informative from an efficacy point of view, but also to select a second dose level, that ideally should be the dose level, or close to the dose level in the confirmatory paediatric trial (fig. 2). When appropriate or needed, additional dose level(s) can be investigated in the exploratory dose finding study, again using all prior knowledge in adults.

It is also very important to investigate and obtain ERR information in paediatric patients from the exploratory dose finding trial to optimize the design of the confirmatory trial (fig. 2). If ERR is well understood and similar in adults and paediatrics, it will facilitate the dose selection in the confirmatory trial. Conversely, if ERR is different in paediatrics and in adults, then a more careful approach is needed, including the possibility of an extension of the exploratory dose finding trial to fully characterize the dose-response and ERR in paediatrics.

In order to describe the pharmacokinetics and establish ERR in paediatrics at the end of the exploratory dose finding study, it is necessary to implement serial pharmacokinetic blood sampling and assessments of efficacy or disease-related biomarker to describe the time course of the selected endpoint. When appropriate, safety assessments may be implemented to describe the PK-safety relationship in paediatrics. The data collected in the exploratory dose finding study should be sufficient to select with confidence the dosing in the confirmatory study (fig. 2). However, for the purpose of confirmation of the ERR in paediatrics in a larger number of patients, the confirmatory study should also include sparse pharmacokinetic blood sampling in addition to efficacy and safety assessments. The larger number of patients in the confirmatory study should offer the possibility to explore the sources of variability in both PK and ERR. The methodology, commonly called covariate analysis, offers the possibility to study the effect of age and various variables related to body size, which is obviously very important in paediatric drug development. All together, these data provide the scientific rationale for the dosing in paediatrics (fig. 2).

## Paediatric Bridging and Regulatory Guidance/Guideline

The paediatric bridging approach as described in the previous section is not novel and is already well described in regulatory documents from both FDA and European Medicines Agency (EMA).

The bridging approach is described in the FDA Guidance for Industry Document entitled 'Exposure-Response Relationships – Study Design, Data Analysis, and Regulatory Applications' and is summarized as the 'Pediatric Study Decision Tree' [10]. The section addressing paediatrics is part of the sub-section 'new target population':

'A PK-PD relationship or data from an exposure-response study can be used to support use of a previously approved drug in a new target patient population, such as a pediatric population, where the clinical response is expected to be similar to the adult population, based on a good understanding of the pathophysiology of the disease, but there is uncertainty as to the appropriate dose and plasma concentration'.

As of August 2009, the authors are informed that FDA is working on a new guidance about paediatric clinical pharmacology and this would include sections related to the paediatric study decision tree, study design considerations and labelling examples.

This bridging approach in paediatrics is also supported by EMA, as indicated in their Guideline 'The Role of Pharmacokinetics in the Development of Medicinal Products in the Paediatric Population' [11]. It specifically states that:

'Provided that data from adults are considered relevant, pharmacokinetic information can be used to extrapolate efficacy to the paediatric population.
- If similar exposure in adult and paediatric patients can be assumed to produce similar efficacy, pharmacokinetic data alone can be used to extrapolate efficacy.
- If a similar relationship between concentration and clinical efficacy cannot be assumed, paediatric PK/PD (biomarker) data can be used to extrapolate efficacy. In this case, the predictability of the biomarker should have been documented. If this has been performed in adults only, its value for the paediatric population should be adequately justified. Evaluation of the PK/PD relationship in dose-ranging studies or multiple dose level studies is encouraged, as such information may be very valuable for dose selection'.

Both the FDA 'Pediatric Study Decision Tree' and the EMA Guideline describe the possibility to use the PK-efficacy relationship or the PK-biomarker relationship for the paediatric bridging. The example of oxcarbazepine monotherapy for the treatment of partial seizures illustrates the concept of paediatric bridging using the PK efficacy relationship, or more specifically the AUC-seizure frequency relationship. For the monotherapy indication, the dosing recommendations were based on a pharmacometric analysis that compared AUC-seizure frequency relationship in adults, and in children in adjunct therapy. The dosing in paediatrics to match the exposure in adults for monotherapy was derived using the ERR model in adjunct therapy, without the need for specific monotherapy controlled clinical trials [12]. In the same indication, levetiracetam was found to exhibit a consistent AUC-seizure frequency relationship across paediatric and adult patients. As for oxcarbazepine, ERR analysis formed the basis for the dosing instructions in the label [13].

Similarly, sotalol in the treatment of ventricular and supra ventricular tachycardia is a well known example for the use of the PK biomarker relationship in paediatric bridging. As part of the written request, FDA agreed with the sponsor to use heart rate and QTc as biomarkers to derive dosing guidelines in paediatrics such that the effects are consistent with those in adults. The most important paediatric trial studied the drug at several dose levels and included sparse PK sampling and QTc and RR intervals, as biomarkers of the $\beta$-blocking activity. The sponsor was able to demonstrate that the relationship between drug concentration and QTc interval was similar in adults and in paediatric patients with a body surface area greater or equal to 0.33 $m^2$ [12, 14].

**Challenges and Future Directions in Paediatric Drug Development**

Successful trials and approval of a drug in adults in a given indication does not imply that the confirmatory trial in paediatrics will be positive. FDA recently reported about their broad experience in paediatrics, highlighting a large number of negative confirmatory paediatric trials, and concluding that the quality of future paediatric programs needs to improve [15]. It was emphasized that pharmaceutical companies focused solely on the confirmatory trial and did not learn enough from prior trials. In general, the reasons leading to a negative outcome were reported to be (1) poor selection of dose range, (2) poor selection of endpoints, (3) high placebo response rate, and (4) mixing responders and non-/poor responders in the same trial [15]. More specifically in the field of hypertension, a retrospective analysis of paediatric hypertensive trials revealed that poor selection of dose and endpoints, lack of acknowledgement of differences between the adult and paediatric population, and lack of paediatric formulations were associated with failures [16]. Higher placebo response rate in paediatrics than in adults is well illustrated by zolmitriptan results in the treatment of migraine [17]. Roziglitazone in type 2 diabetes can be used as an example of a negative confirmatory trial (verbatim from the US label 'Paediatric: data are insufficient to recommend pediatric use') that can be largely attributed to reason number 4. The study was conducted with a mix of drug naïve patients (n = 85) and previously treated patients (n = 75) who were randomly assigned to roziglitazone or metformin. The results showed a better response in change from baseline in HbA1c (clinical endpoint) for naïve versus previously treated patients but overall, there was an insufficient number of patients to establish statistically whether the observed mean treatment effects were similar or different from metformin [18].

Overall, the unexpected high rate of failure in paediatric confirmatory trials is calling for new and better ways to design paediatric confirmatory trials. The emphasis should be on leveraging prior knowledge from adults and paediatric studies and more specifically, the results of ERR (fig. 3). All attempts should be made to describe these relationships with a pharmaco-statistical model because this methodology provides the possibility to perform paediatric clinical trial simulations (CTS) [19, 20], and, thereby, explore different competing

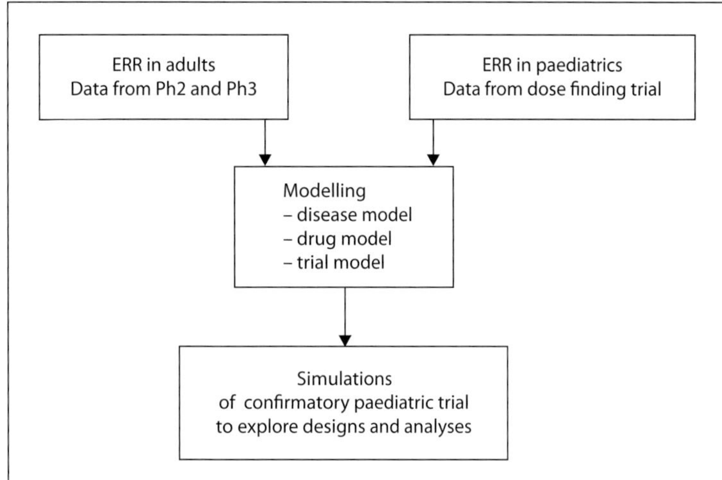

**Fig. 3.** Schematic representation of the use of ERR in adults and in paediatrics to perform modelling and trial simulation of the confirmatory paediatric trial.



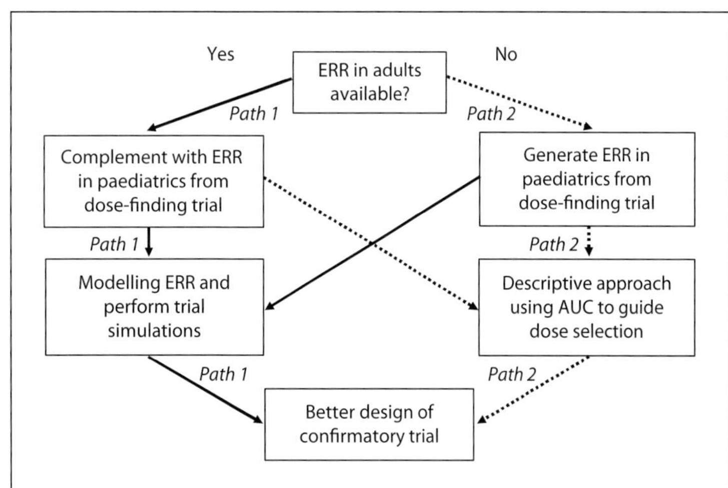

**Fig. 4.** Different ways to implement a bridging approach in a paediatric program. Path 2 (dashed lines) is the most common approach, whereas path 1 (solid lines) is the recommended approach.



designs and data analysis plans before the confirmatory paediatric trial has even started (fig. 3). However, up to now, most of the paediatric confirmatory studies have been designed without trial simulations, and in the best case, using ERR with a descriptive approach (i.e. no modelling), with integrated measures of systemic exposure, like AUC, to guide the dose selection in paediatrics (fig. 4, path 2). The use of trial simulations in paediatric drug development is probably going to increase in the coming years, especially in the pharmaceutical companies that have the necessary and skilful resources in the field of modelling and simulation (fig. 4, path 1). Of interest, one of the strategic goals for 2020 of the Pharmacometric Group at FDA is that 100% of paediatric studies should be designed using simulations, with leverage of prior knowledge to design 'Pediatric Written Request' trials [15]. As an illustration of their focus on paediatrics, the same group recently published a case study of an antihypertensive agent for which the sponsor and FDA conducted CTS, with key data from adult ERR, trial design, placebo-response model, and drop out model, to design a paediatric study with plausible sample size, and support the choice of dose range [21]. In a way, the use of trial simulations to design paediatric trials is an extension of the paediatric bridging, making use of modern tools and methodologies in the field of modelling and simulation in paediatric drug development. The first key input to CTS is the ERR in adults (fig. 4). In adults, the consolidated ERR results are available at the end of Phase 3, with solid findings usually at the end of phase 2B (or dose finding trial). The availability of key data to design the paediatric plan at the end of phase 2B suggests that this is the earliest time point at which a meaningful and reasonably detailed paediatric plan can be developed and discussed with health authorities. Phase 3 results in adults provide consolidated results of ERR in adults and this information should be used to finalize the paediatric study protocols. Again, here the emphasis is on making the best use of prior knowledge, mainly from trials in adults with the same NCE, but also from trials with other drugs of the same pharmacological class or in the same indication. Stressing the importance of studying ERR in both adults and paediatrics implies the collection of blood samples at informative time points in each patient to describe the ERR. Fortunately, sparse blood sampling is sufficient when modelling is used to analyze the data so implementation in the trials is not so difficult. Acceptance of additional blood sampling is sometimes an issue during trial protocol development, but when scientists involved in the clinical trials understand the value of ERR and its potential impact, namely, increasing the probability of obtaining a positive confirmatory trial, then, the required additional blood sampling is accepted.

## Conclusions

Paediatric drug development is a growing and rapidly evolving field. However, a high rate of failure in confirmatory paediatric trials has been reported and now, all efforts must be made to improve the quality of future paediatric programs. Clinical pharmacology can efficiently contribute to this effort, in ensuring optimal use of prior knowledge, especially in the field of ERR in both adults and paediatrics. Further, modelling of ERR and conducting trial simulations to explore competing designs and data analysis plans should be the goal in every paediatric program to optimize the design of the confirmatory paediatric trial and thereby, increasing the probability of a positive outcome, yield rationale dosing recommendations, and useful labelling information in paediatrics.


## References

1 Nestorov I: Whole-body physiologically based pharmacokinetic models. Expert Opin Drug Metab Toxicol 2007;3:235–249.

2 Björkman S: Prediction of drug disposition in infants and children by means of physiologically based pharmacokinetic (PBPK) modelling: theophylline and midazolam as model drugs. Br J Clin Pharmacol 2005;59:691–704.

3 Bartelink IH, Rademaker CM, Schobben AF, Van den Anker JN: Guidelines on paediatric dosing on the basis of developmental physiology and pharmacokinetic considerations. Clin Pharmacokinet 2006;45:1077–1097.

4 Kearns GL, Abdel-Rahman SM, Alander SW, Blowey DL, Leeder JS, Kauffman RE: Developmental pharmacology – drug disposition, action, and therapy in infants and children. N Engl J Med 2003; 349:1157–1167.

5 Haddad S, Restieri C, Krishnan K: Characterization of age-related changes in body weight and organ weights from birth to adolescence in humans. J Toxicol Environ Health [A] 2001;64:453–464.

6   FDA, US Food and Drug Administration: Drugs Development and Approval Process. Medical, Statistical, and Clinical Pharmacology Reviews of Pediatric Studies Conducted under Section 505A and 505B of the Federal Food, Drug, and Cosmetic Act (the Act), as amended by the FDA Amendments Act of 2007 (FDAAA) (http://www.fda.gov/Drugs/DevelopmentApprovalProcess/DevelopmentResources/UCM049872)

7   EMA, European Medicines Agency: CHMP Efficacy Working Party Therapeutic subgroup on pharmacokinetics (EWP-PK). Questions and Answers: Positions on specific questions addressed to the EWP therapeutic subgroup on Pharmacokinetics. Doc.Ref. EMA/618604/2008, London, 2009.

8   Cram A, Breitkreutz J, Desset-Brèthes S, Nunn T, Tuleu C: Challenges of developing palatable oral paediatric formulations. Int J Pharmaceut 2009;365:1–3.

9   EMA, European Medicines Agency: CHMP. Reflection paper: formulations of choice for the paediatric formulation. Doc. Ref EMA/CHMP/PEG/194810/2005, London, 26 July 2006.

10  FDA, US Food and Drug Administration: Guidance for Industry: Exposure-Response Relationships – Study Design, Data Analysis, and Regulatory Applications. Rockville, US Department of Health and Human Services, 2003. (http://www.fda.gov/downloads/Drugs/GuidanceComplianceRegulatoryInformation/Guidances/ucm072109.pdf)

11  EMA, European Medicines Agency: Committee for Medicinal Products for Human use (CHMP): Guideline on the Role of Pharmacokinetics in the development of Medicinal Products in the Paediatric Population. Doc.Ref.EMA/CHMP/EWP/147013/2004, London, 2006. (http://www.ema.europa.eu/pdfs/human/ewp/14701304en.pdf)

12  Bhattaram VA, Booth BP, Ramchandani RP, Beasley BN, Wang Y, Tandon V, Duan JZ, Baweja RK, Marroun PJ, Uppoor RS, Rahman NA, Sahajwalla CG, Powell JR, Mehta MU and Gobburu JVS: Impact of pharmacometrics on drug approval and labeling decisions: a survey of 42 new drug applications. AAPS J 2005;7:E503–E512.

13  Rodriguez W, Selen A, Avant D, Chaurasia C, Crescenzi T, Gieser G, Di Giacinto J, Huang SM, Lee P, Mathis L, Murphy D, Murphy S, Roberts R, Sachs HC, Suarez S, Tandon V, Uppoor RS: Improving pediatric dosing through pediatric initiatives: what we have learned. Pediatrics 2008;121:530–539.

14  Läer S, Elshoff J-P, Meibohm B, Weil J, Mir TS, Zhang W, Hulpke-Wette M: Development of a safe and effective pediatric dosing regimen for Sotalol based on population pharmacokinetics and pharmacodynamics in children with supraventricular tachycardia. J Am Coll Cardiol 2005;46:1322–1330.

15  Goburru JVS: Pediatric drug development: defining quality. ASCPT Meeting in Washington, 2009, oral presentation.

16  Benjamin DK Jr, Smith PB, Jadhav P, Gobburu JV, Murphy MD, Hasselblad V, Baker-Smith C, Califf RM, Li JS: Pediatric antihypertensive trial failures, analysis of end points and dose range. Hypertension 2008;51:834–840.

17  Rothner AD, Wasiewski W, Winner P, Lewis D, Stankowski J: Zolmitriptan oral tablet in migraine treatment: high placebo responses in adolescents. Headache 2006;46:101–109.

18  Avandia US label, PDR 2005.

19  Läer S, Barrett JS, Meibohm B: The in silico child: using simulation to guide pediatric drug development and manage pediatric pharmacotherapy. J Clin Pharmacol 2009;49:889–904.

20  Manolis E, Pons G: Proposals for model-based paediatric medicinal development within the current European Union regulatory framework. Br J Clin Pharmacol 2009;68:4:493–501.

21  Jadhav PR, Zhang J, Gobburu JVS: Leveraging prior quantitative knowledge in guiding pediatric drug development: a case study. Pharmaceut Statist 2009;8:216–224.

Bruno Reigner
F. Hoffmann-La Roche Ltd.
Clinical Research and Exploratory Development & Clinical Pharmacology
CH–4070 Basel (Switzerland)
Tel. +41 61 688 4507, Fax +41 61 688 0415, E-Mail bruno.reigner@roche.com

Rose K, van den Anker JN (eds): Guide to Paediatric Drug Development and Clinical Research.
Basel, Karger, 2010, pp 60–63

# Guide through the EMA Paediatric Website

Klaus Rose[a] · Ulrich Granzer[b] · Oscar Della Pasqua[c]

[a]F. Hoffmann-La Roche Ltd., Pharmaceuticals Division, Basel, Switzerland; [b]Granzer Regulatory Consulting & Services, Munich, Germany; [c]Clinical Pharmacology & Discovery Medicine, GlaxoSmithKline, Stockley Park, UK

The EMA paediatric website (www.ema.europa.eu) is a valuable tool to access relevant information and clarify queries regarding the EU Paediatric Regulation.

The 'Medicines for Children' page can be accessed by clicking on the icon shown on the menu bar on the right-hand side. As most regulatory websites, it is continuously maintained and updated, including many documents that were developed in the years preceding the EU paediatric regulation. Therefore, attention is required when searching for the most recent version of a document. All abbreviations used in this chapter are given in table 1.

The contents of the left menu bar on the main page are given in table 2. Bullet points and subsection numbering have been added to ease the reading in a printed document.

*Introduction*: A short introduction is given about the scope of the EU paediatric regulation. The introduction page also contains a leaflet providing an overview of the EMA's role in the European regulatory environment for paediatric medicines.

*The EU Paediatric Regulation*: An overview of the development and objectives of the paediatric regulation is provided with links to official documents and relevant queries.

*Paediatric Committee*: A short explanation is available about the responsibilities of the paediatric committee (PDCO). Furthermore, it gives the PDCO meeting dates 2008 to 2013 (as of March 2010).

The PDCO section has four main headings, which highlight:
- PDCO's role and responsibility. [Note that the PDCO is not responsible for marketing authorisation of drugs for children, which remains fully within the remit of the EMA CHMP (Committee for Medicinal Products for Human Use). However, the CHMP or any other competent authority may request the PDCO's opinion].
- PDCO composition.
- Rules of procedure.
- Other related documents: The two links available as of March 2010 were: 'Policy on representation of the EMA scientific committees by their members' and 'EMA Policy on appropriate coordination between the scientific committees of the Agency (EMA/124704/2005)'.

*Guidance for applicants*: This item is divided into 7 sections:
1 Scientific advice: Short overview of paediatric scientific advice with a link to the general EMA scientific advice and protocol assistance website.

**Table 1.** Abbreviations

| | |
|---|---|
| Article 7 PIP | PIP for new products not yet registered in the EU |
| Article 8 PIP | PIP for products already registered in the EU |
| CHMP | Committee for Medicinal Products on Human Use: decides about MAAs |
| EuDraCT | European Union Drug Regulating Authorities Clinical Trials, a registry for all clinical trials in the EU |
| MAA | Marketing Authorisation Application |
| PDCO | Paediatric Committee |
| PEG | Paediatric Expert Group, the EMA Paediatric Working Party that preceded the PDCO |
| PIP | Paediatric Investigation Plan |
| PUMA | Paediatric Use Marketing Organisation: special incentives for paediatric research into off-patent drugs |

2   Paediatric Investigation Plans (PIPs), waivers and modifications: A short explanation what a PIP is, a link to list of calls waivers, a link to the EU Commission PIP guideline from 2008, plus a lot of important links, documents and templates:
  – Guidance
  – Templates and forms
  – Deadlines and PDCO meeting dates
3   Standard PIPs on H1N1 pandemic influenza vaccines and a draft standard PIP on allergen extract products for immunotherapy of allergic rhinitis and rhinoconjunctivitis.
4   Paediatric-use marketing authorisations (PUMAs): a short explanation of PUMA PIPs.
5   Annual reports on deferrals including a template.
6   Compliance: Once the PIP  is reported as completed by the respective company, EMA or National authorities will check that all studies and measures have been performed. A successful compliance check will be the condition for an application for marketing authorisation to be considered valid followed by links to key documents in this procedure.
7   Submission of paediatric studies (articles 45–46).

*Opinions and Decisions on PIPs*:
1   Background on the regulation with a guidance on re-examination procedures; a template letter for applicant to waive the right for a re-examination request; the PDCO decision making process on class waivers and the decision-making process of the PDCO for PIPs and product-specific decisions.
2   Class waivers: This list is updated on a regular basis. As of March 2010, two class waivers have been revoked: melanoma as well as menopausal and other peri-menopausal disorders.
3   Product-specific decisions: The subsection on product-specific decisions is probably the fastest growing section in the website. It lists all PDCO decisions since December 2007. The publication list is sorted by decision date, with the newest decisions on the top. This section contains a true wealth of information and gives a flavour of the depth of the demands of EMA and PDCO for the paediatric programme.

*Paediatric-related information*:
1   Paediatric needs: This section describes how the off-label use of drugs in children

is associated with higher incidence of adverse reactions and provides links to key publications on this topic. It is then followed by an inventory of paediatric needs, which includes off-patent medications as well as patent-protected medications and lists currently recognised paediatric needs. The list covers the following therapeutic indications: anaesthesiology, anti-infectious therapy, cardiology, chemotherapy (cytotoxic substances), chemotherapy (supportive therapy), diabetes type 1 and 2, epilepsy, gastroenterology, immunology, migraine, nephrology, obstructive lung disease, pain, psychiatry, and rheumatology. The lists were produced by the EMA Paediatric Working Party (original name: Paediatric Expert Group [PEG]), whose responsibilities have now been shifted to the PDCO. A wide range of paediatric needs have been including issues such as paediatric formulations, dose, efficacy and safety data in specific indications and/ or appropriate age groups, pharmacokinetic data in children and more. The inventory also highlights a list of medications for which no paediatric needs are perceived by the EMA's former PEG, now PDCO.

2. Paediatric clinical trials: All clinical trials performed in the EU are registered in the EudraCT database, which will now include all paediatric trials defined in a PIP, irrespective of the location where it is performed. The paediatric section of EudraCT will be made public. Also details of the results of paediatric clinical trials, including those terminated prematurely, are being made public by the EMA.

3. Priority list of off-patent medicines: a link to the list of recommended studies into off-patent drugs used in children, as well as to the EU 7th Framework Programme for off-patent medicines developed for children.

4. Scientific guidance: This heading refers to the EMA CHMP's scientific guidelines, located in a central repository. They are categorised into quality guidelines, non-clinical guidelines, clinical efficacy and safety guidelines, and multidisciplinary ones.

5. Paediatric formulations: this heading highlights the need for age-appropriate formulations and the issues regarding safety associated with pharmaceutical excipients.

6. Presentations: Presentations made by EMA staff at various public meetings can be found on this page. As of March 2010, one 27-slide power point presentation on the EU paediatric regulation is available.

7. EU paediatric network: As of March 2010, a list of 60 paediatric research networks is available in Europe; two working groups; the Implementing Strategy of the Network of Paediatric Networks at the EMA; a link to EMA workshops.

*Global cooperation*:

1. Member States:
 – List of measures adopted by EU Member States to support research, development and availability of medicinal products for paediatric use.
 – Access to the EU Heads of Medicines Agencies (HMA) website and to a document 'Guidance on the Content and Format of Data to be collected on All Existing Uses of Medicinal Products in the Paediatric Population'.

2. International: Gives a short history of the US paediatric legislations and links to the FDA paediatric website as well as to a press release on intensified collaboration between EMA and FDA on medicines for children.

3. Workshops: As of March 2010, agenda and presentations EMA workshops on:
 – Paediatric development and Juvenile Animal Studies Assessors meeting, July 2009.
 – EU Paediatric Networks, February 2009.
 – Modelling in Paediatric Medicines, April 2008.
 – FP7 and off-patent medicines developed for children, June 2007.
 – Neonates, October 2006.
 – Paediatric pain, October 2004.

4. Related links: As of March 2010, this section contains 3 links:
 – FDA Office of Paediatric Therapeutics.
 – EU Commission website 'Medicines for Children' that gives access to a multitude of additional documents, including a press release on intensified cooperation between FDA and EMA in paediatric drug development and the extended impact assessment that preceded the EU paediatric regulation.
 – EU Commission Directorate-General for Research 7th Framework Programme website.


Klaus Rose, MD, MS
Principal Consultant
Granzer Regulatory Consulting & Services, Zielstattstrasse 44
DE–81379 Munich (Germany)
Tel. +49 89 780 68 98 29, Fax +49 89 780 68 98 15, E-Mail rose@granzer.biz

Rose K, van den Anker JN (eds): Guide to Paediatric Drug Development and Clinical Research.
Basel, Karger, 2010, pp 64–70

# Paediatric Homework: Paediatric Investigation Plan Key Elements

Klaus Rose[a]  ·  Oscar Della Pasqua[b]

[a]F. Hoffmann-La Roche Ltd., Pharmaceuticals Division, Basel, Switzerland; [b]Clinical Pharmacology & Discovery Medicine,
GlaxoSmithKline, Stockley Park, UK

Various aspects ought to be considered during the preparation, submission, negotiation or modification of a paediatric investigation plan (PIP). Whilst regulatory discussions are common in the development of drugs for adult indications, the nature and timing of the interactions for medicines for children are new and still represent a challenge both for sponsors and regulators. In contrast to the market authorisation application (MAA) in adults, the incentive mechanisms associated with this regulatory requirement have triggered a new modus operandi for drug development in the EU. Once the PIP is agreed upon, the execution phase represents a regulatory commitment and should follow strict timelines. In addition, approval of market exclusivity for 6 months by the EMA/PDCO will depend on compliance to the PIP. Please find an overview over abbreviations used in this chapter in table 1.

## Paediatric Homework

The development of new chemical or biological entities and subsequent commercialization of the resulting medicinal product assumes that the new entity will be equal or superior to the available therapeutic options and sufficient evidence is gathered to justify medical utility, regulatory approval and reimbursement.

Historically, portfolio review and life cycle management have not always been aligned with unmet medical needs when considering subgroups within a target patient population or special populations when considering age-specific diseases. The regulatory requirements to address such needs have for a long time been limited to claims and/or restrictions associated with the so-called special populations section of the label (prescriber information in the USA summary of product characteristics in the EU). The legal obligation to include children as target population in this process addresses therefore a long-standing public health issue.

As a consequence, clinical development teams involved with portfolio review and life cycle management must now acquaint themselves with an area that is probably not their key competence. Since January 2007, no drug applications can be submitted in the EU without a paediatric investigation plan (PIP) agreed upon by the EMA and PDCO. Specifically, this new regulatory landscape entails that the sponsor must submit paediatric data together with the adult MAA or have negotiated a deferral of the studies and other development measures, or have applied for and been

**Table 1.** Abbreviations

| | |
|---|---|
| Article 7 PIP | PIP for new products not yet registered in the EU |
| Article 8 PIP | PIP for products already registered in the EU |
| CHMP | Committee for Medicinal Products on Human Use: decides about MAAs |
| EMA | European Medicines Agency, coordinating the EU National Regulatory Authorities |
| FDA | Food and Drug Agency (USA) |
| ICHE11 | Clinical Investigation of Medicinal Products in the Paediatric Population; agreed upon by regulatory authorities and pharmaceutical industry in the USA, EU and Japan |
| KOL | Key Opinion Leader |
| MAA | Marketing Authorisation Application |
| PDCO | Paediatric Committee |
| PIP | Paediatric Investigation Plan |
| PK/PD | Pharmacokinetics/pharmacodynamics |
| R&D | Research and Development |

granted a waiver, i.e. written confirmation by the EMA that there is no need to develop a compound for the specific paediatric indication at all.

Table 2 shows a schematic overview of the key steps involved in the decision making process, which ought to be taken into consideration by the clinical team responsible for negotiating the clinical development plan with the regulatory agency. Although these recommendations are primarily for the preparation of a PIP, general concepts are included which support the development of a global development plan, ensuring duplication of efforts are avoided and unmet medical needs prioritized beyond regulatory boundaries.

These four steps may or may not be sequential. They will also be iterative, i.e. during the PIP preparation the team will have to go through several cycles of these steps.

If the targeted indication is on the list of class waivers, the sponsor can assume that no paediatric development is required. Nevertheless, this must be communicated in writing to the EMA (template letter on the EMA website). Only with written confirmation from the regulatory agency can the company ensure at a later stage that the MAA will not be withheld due to the lack of a PIP.

In contrast to the requirements for new chemical and biological entities, for marketed products (article 8 PIPs), the EMA/PDCO can only enforce paediatric assessment on the same disease for which the compound is registered in adults. Article 7 PIPs refer to later use of a new compound in a paediatric indication. Even if the targeted disease does not exist in children, but a similar or comparable condition exists, the sponsor may be asked by the EMA/PDCO to consider development in that area, e.g. development of a contrast medium for ultrasound investigation of cardiac atherosclerosis does not mean that the compound will not be used for the ultrasound examination of other conditions, e.g. congenital heart abnormalities.

**Table 2.** The four key elements in the preparation of a PIP

- Step 1: Initial reflections/brainstorm

    - Therapeutic agent: Is the compound a new medicinal or biological product for human use? Is the compound already approved for use in adults (article 8 PIP)

    - Therapeutic indication: Is the targeted indication listed in the list of class waivers?

    - Current therapeutic options: Do other products exist for this indication in children?

    - Potential therapeutic use: Do condition(s) targeted by a new compound (article 7 PIP) exist in children?

    - Alternative indications and secondary pharmacology: Is there any other foreseeable use in children for a new article 7 PIP compound?

    - Business opportunities: Is the compound intended for a rare disease? Should an orphan drug application be considered instead?

    - Competitive intelligence: how do published PDCO decisions relate to the new compound?

    - Expert opinion: Consider paediatric scientific advice regarding, e.g. unmet medical needs, diagnosis, epidemiology (prevalence, incidence, morbidity, mortality), endpoints, safety and efficacy measures.

- Step 2: Consider implementation options per age group

    - Non-clinical package: in vitro/in animals/in juvenile animals.

    - Pharmaceutical development: paediatric formulations and devices.

    - Disease prevalence: Are ICH E11 age ranges easily applicable?

    - Clinical Pharmacology: dose rationale, PKPD relationship, modelling and simulation, bridging studies.

    - Requirements for 'confirmatory' trials: choice and validation of efficacy and safety endpoints, duration of the trial, long term safety requirements.

    - Other potential limiting factors: feasibility , recruitment, patient retention, expertise availability, professional training.

- Step 3: Timing of measures, waivers, deferrals by age group

    - Single vs. multiple indications: pros and cons of submitting separate PIPs.

    - Clinical development plan: investigational protocols, deferrals, waivers.

    - Regulatory requirements and incentives: what is the impact of development timelines relative to patent expiration and availability of generics. Commercial factors can affect patient recruitment and availability.

- Step 4: Global clinical development; thinking ahead

    - Timing differences: Is the FDA willing to consider paediatric development at an early stage?

    - Country specific requirements/preferences: Can an FDA opinion be obtained on, e.g., preferred species in juvenile animal studies.

    - Cultural/country differences in clinical practice: Reality check of preliminary assumptions with key opinion leaders/advisory board.

    - Acceptance of foreign data: What are the limitations for including foreign patients in the development programme?

Age-specific requirements are one of the main challenges and risk factors in the development programme for a paediatric indication. A balance must be found between unmet medical needs and feasibility issues, such as age boundaries for disease prevalence and availability of age-friendly dosage forms. These considerations may become the cause of debate or even disagreement between sponsor and regulators, in particular with respect to implementation timelines and the application for deferrals. From a company's standpoint investment issues need to be accounted for which may not be reflected at all in a regulatory discussion, e.g. it does not make much sense to develop a liquid formulation for newborns before evidence for efficacy and safety is available from a proof of concept. The EMA/PDCO may be of a different opinion.

Given the considerably new implementation of the legislation, understanding is still lacking within companies and EMA about the implications of the paediatric regulation for life cycle management. At a given time point in the development of a compound, a company might plan to submit an application for indication A now and consider indication B only 3 or 5 years later.

Whilst the regulation encourages an all-encompassing investigational plan, including all potential indications for a compound, in practice this may lead to unmanageable complexities. For instance, if both indications are included in the same PIP, the sponsor will be stuck with it even if for business reasons the pursuit for indication B is discontinued. Instead, if paediatric development plans for these indications are proposed in two separate PIPs, they can be executed in parallel without confusion and interference. Often handling different indications in separate PIPs also enables more focussed interactions with advisory groups, external experts and the EMA/PDCO. Of course, it is important to be clear about a company choices regarding portfolio management. The EMA will request a company to consider further indications other than the one for which the PIP has been submitted. Hence, in presenting separate PIPs full consideration must have been made about secondary indications. The main advantage of this approach is that an indication can be dropped or adapted to suit both medical and business needs at a later time point. Companies and sponsors should insist on their right to develop and implement investigational plans separately.

For implementation purposes, sponsors are advised to devote special attention to the nature of the clinical programme, i.e. which questions need to be addressed and handled independently from pharmaceutical and nonclinical aspects. One of the opportunities offered by existing guidelines is to use a bridging approach to extrapolate exposure, and eventually efficacy/safety data from adults. Furthermore, observational data, PK/PD relationships and modelling and simulation techniques are valuable tools for addressing clinically relevant questions and coping with practical and ethical limitations imposed by paediatric trials. These tools are also particularly effective in supporting queries about age-specific requirements, such as dose selection and role of covariates.

Under the current legislation, the PDCO is meant to represent existing European regulatory and academic knowledge about drug development and paediatric diseases. Whereas this objective is highly desirable, members of the PDCO may not always have previous experience in the pharmaceutical industry or in drug development. At present, only a minority of the members seem to have such expertise. Nevertheless, it is the PDCO which make decisions about the requirements for a PIP, based on the expertise of its own members or, if applicable, through feedback they may have received from academic key opinion leaders (KOLs). Part of the preparation of the PIP must therefore include an overview of the most influential academic representatives for a specific disease area. It is likely that earlier or later these KOLs may participate in formal discussions with the EMA/PDCO.

**Paediatric Scientific Advice and Pre-Submission Meetings**

The paediatric scientific advice is planned to become an integrated part of the work of EMA and PDCO. However, in the first year of the EU paediatric regulation, key processes had to be established and both EMA and PDCO members were overwhelmed with the amount of work submitted by applicants. Until now, most requests for paediatric scientific advice occurred after the initial PIP submission. In the future, sponsors are advised to consider scientific advice well before putting together a formal PIP.

Even though the EMA has no capacity for pre-submission meetings on specific compounds, it may allow a portfolio meeting if several PIPs are to be discussed. In the future, the EMA plans to have enough capacity for pre-submission meetings on individual compounds.

**PIP Submission**

Before a PIP is formally submitted, applicants are requested to inform the EMA about the intention to submit it. The deadline for this letter of intent is 40 days before the planned date of submission. This is to allow resource planning by the EMA. The template for the letter of intent can be obtained on the EMA paediatric website.

**PIP Negotiation**

Once the PIP is submitted, a pre-defined set of processes and procedures is triggered:
- The EMA paediatric coordinator will write a summary report that will form the basis for the PDCO rapporteur. Applicants have just two days to answer validation questions arising during the preparation of the summary report.
- After 30 days, the PDCO rapporteur will present the PIP proposal to the PDCO and a summary report will be sent to the applicant.
- An oral explanation of the report may be considered by the applicant up to a maximum of 30 days after receipt of the summary report.
- At day 60, a clock stop of up to a maximum of 30 days starts. This period is meant to allow time for answering queries from the PDCO or to react to requests for modification.
- After restart of the clock stop, the PIP will be discussed again by the PDCO at day 90. If the submission meets the revised requirements and an agreement can be reached, the PDCO formally issues a positive recommendation for the implementation of the plan.
- If after restarting the clock stop the requests for modification are unresolved, an oral explanation may be scheduled.
- On day 120 the PIP is discussed for the third time in the PDCO.
- If the applicant disagrees with the PDCO recommendations, he can ask for a re-examination. The deadline is no later than 30 days after receipt of the report.
- The overall procedure may take approximately 1 year, but longer timelines are not excluded.
- After an initial period of grace, negative recommendations have become increasingly more often. The potential consequences for the applicant is delay in the submission of the marketing authorisation application for the adult indication, which cannot progress without an agreed PIP.
- Should the applicant want to avoid a formal negative recommendation, the PIP can be retracted even during the day of the oral explanation. This brings the ongoing submission process to a close. A new PIP has to be submitted to ensure validation by the EMA.

**PIP Modification**

There are specific procedures for a PIP modification. It is shorter to modify a PIP than to write and submit it completely from scratch again.

Currently, it is unclear how the agency will manage feasibility issues, in particular those relative to patient recruitment and technical limitations such as formulations and devices. The legislation is clearly aimed at shortening the timelines between the approval of the adult indication and the availability of the medicinal product for the paediatric population. In this sense, opposition may be expected to proposals which lead to further delays in agreed timelines for deferrals.

Another important consideration regards the growing number of in-licencing and out-licencing activities in pharmaceutical R&D. The terms of agreement between the agency and the applicant are formally binding. However, the regulation has not anticipated the implications of R&D activities such as in-licensing or out-licensing. Depending on portfolio considerations (e.g. development for another indication) and other business related decisions (e.g. different delivery device or route of administration), the buyer may request a revision of the previously agreed PIP if necessary.

When contemplating the need for modification of an agreed PIP, it is also critical to bear in mind the implications for the MAA submission. Also important are the implications for the timing of the studies for the incentives for market exclusivity.

**PIP Execution**

So far, only a few PIPs have formally reached full completion. Despite that, the first compliance checks have been performed by the agency. Depending on the therapeutic indication and terms of agreement, the execution of a PIP can take many years. Sponsors should bear in mind that much of the EMA's positions are based on FDA experiences in the USA. E.g. patient recruitment

can be poor for different reasons. For instance, if the inappropriate study centres have been selected, the EMA will expect the sponsor to take corrective action. On the other hand, if the study protocol has been rejected by all ethics committees, EMA will have to agree with the request for modification of the PIP.

Whatever changes occur to a PIP during its execution phase, they need to be carefully documented in order to show the sponsor's commitment and compliance to the agreed plan. If compliance cannot be warranted or deviations occur, this must be communicated to the EMA as soon as possible. Under no circumstances should sponsors assume that the EMA will accept an explanation years later and agree with the modified programme.

**Compliance Check**

Not all details of the process and procedures for compliance checks have been outlined, which may be required to claim potential regulatory incentives once the PIP has been completed. However, it is important to note that the applicant will need a statement of compliance for the national patent offices in every single EU member state. It is the patent office that issues the SPC extensions.

**EMA and FDA**

Discussion of paediatric development with the FDA before submission is voluntary, and so far the FDA divisions were not keen to discuss paediatric development plans as early as beginning of phase 2. With the increasing paediatric cooperation between EMA and FDA this should change over time. At present, both FDA and EMA emphasise their strong cooperation and collaboration, aiming at a common global development plan. These statements contrast with recent industry experience showing that not only the minimum regulatory requirements are different, but also the interpretation of the findings can vary between the EU and USA (e.g. one vs. two species for the evaluation of juvenile animal toxicity).

## Additional Channels of Communication

In addition to formal procedures, there are several channels of communication between regulators and sponsors: official meetings, unofficial meetings, e.g. during a conference, phone calls for clarification, etc. The more these channels are used, the easier it will be to explain an applicant's position. Public communication channels are particularly important to clarify strategic, clinical and scientific choices in a given disease or therapeutic area. These mechanisms should be used to generate debate and ensure best practices are shared and understood by all parties, including patients and/or their representatives.

## Conclusions

The preparation, submission, negotiation, execution and examination for compliance of a paediatric investigation plan involves a series of rather complex interactions between applicant and regulators. In addition to the scientific and technical difficulties associated with the development of a paediatric indication, not all procedures pertinent to the regulatory review are fully implemented. From an operational perspective, these activities are usually coordinated by the regulatory affairs department within every single company. Without sufficient background knowledge and without a clear communication strategy, the development of medicines for children may become unnecessarily complex. It may cause severe delays to the MAA submission and ultimately cause delayed access to novel therapeutic options.


Klaus Rose, MD, MS
Principal Consultant
Granzer Regulatory Consulting & Services, Zielstattstrasse 44
DE–81379 Munich (Germany)
Tel. +49 89 780 68 98 29, Fax +49 89 780 68 98 15, E-Mail rose@granzer.biz

Rose K, van den Anker JN (eds): Guide to Paediatric Drug Development and Clinical Research.
Basel, Karger, 2010, pp 71–74

# Ethics in Paediatric Research: Three Years after the Introduction of the European Regulation

Dirk Matthys[a] · Klaus Rose[b]

[a]Department of Pediatrics, Ghent University, Ghent, Belgium and [b]F. Hoffmann-La Roche Ltd., Pharmaceuticals Division, Basel, Switzerland

Ethics seeks to give guidance on protection of adults and children as it relates to participation in clinical research. For more reading on this topic, we would like to refer to several recent publications [1–7]. Overprotection of children in the past has resulted many times in exclusion of children from participation in clinical investigations resulting in less access of children to new treatment modalities or medications. In that sense, children's overprotection in the past might currently be perceived as in appropriate and even unethical. The high number of publications on ethics in clinical research in paediatrics reflect this shift of paradigm.

Three years after the introduction of the EU paediatric legislation, we would like to discuss a few practical issues:

1 Did Regulation 1901/2006 provoke 'the launch' [5] of paediatric research in Europe?
2 Is the existing ethical framework in Europe sufficient?
3 Which new challenges do we observe today and will we observe in the future?

*(Ad 1):*
We begin with an example. The figures in table 1 demonstrate for a University Hospital that there was indeed an increase in clinical studies in infants and children after the publication of the EU regulation. The decline in the first semester of 2009, may be related to the worldwide financial crisis. Although these figures may not be completely representative, communication with other academic colleagues have confirmed this trend.

Looking at the EMA website, it is obvious that a high number of PIPs has been submitted, many have been approved and the first ones have been finalized. For detailed statistics, see numerous presentations published on the internet, e.g. http://www.dgra.de/fortbildung/pdf/kongresse/2008/kongr2008-brasseur.pdf

*(Ad 2): Is the existing ethical framework in Europe sufficient?*
We refer for background reading to recent key publications [1–7]. Two additional key documents are the EU Clinical Trials Directive 2001/20/EC contains article 4 on clinical trials in minors, and, following Directive 2001/20/EC, the 'Ethical Considerations For Clinical Trials On Medicinal Products Conducted With The Paediatric Population', submitted for comments from the public in 2006 and finalized in 2008 [8].

On the one hand, we observe that the existing ethical framework has not restrained clinical research in children so far. On the other hand, the

**Table 1.** Clinical trials approved by the Ethics Committee of the University Hospital of Ghent, Belgium, per year/ per first semester

| Years | |
| --- | --- |
| 2006 | 55 |
| 2007 | 91 |
| 2008 | 128 |
| First semesters | |
| 2006 | 26 |
| 2007 | 39 |
| 2008 | 76 |
| 2009 | 56 |

first author as member of his hospital's ethics committee sees many present and future challenges.

## Informed Consent/Assent

Although article 4 of the EU Clinical Trials Directive does not use 'assent', it is clear that 'the minor's presumed will' can be considered as 'assent'. Initially, at the University Hospital of Ghent many researchers had problems with different informed consent and assents sheets for different age categories. In the mean time, it has become standard to submit separate sheets for parents/ legal representatives (informed consent) and assent for minors aged 12–18 years, and for minors younger than 12 years.

## Benefit/Risks

To minimise risks some progress has been made in reducing the volumes of blood sampling (see dedicated chapter), but less in the use of alternatives for blood sampling (saliva, urine, breath tests). Researchers in the field should be made aware of the development of new technology in clinical chemistry.

*Special Populations*

In addition there is still a lot of work to be done in the field of specific paediatric populations such as neonates. Also particularly vulnerable patients such as mentally retarded children should only be included into clinical trials if they can benefit from them.

## Role of Ethics Committees

In Europe philosophical/religious/ethical standards are extremely different from Oslo to Palermo and from Dublin to Warsaw. The increasing number of member states contributes to this diversity. This is in particular the case in end of life decisions. However, in clinical trials, coordination and mutual consultation are possible. In testing the Influenza A H1N1 vaccine no preliminary European consultation of ethics committees has been done. However, later on, due to a non-formal cooperation a similar standpoint was taken by two countries. The example stated here makes obvious that a pan-European assessment of protocols for children would be desirable.

Ethical testing of protocols goes mainly through three axes: the equipoise (weighing the possible harm of the child versus the knowledge to get obtained), the rules of informed consent and assent of the patient and legal representative and the financial agreements.

The equipoise if tested in a pan-European panel would be very easily performed by a small group of external experts. If the preliminary examinations could be done by the EMA, a per member state testing of the informed consent and the financial agreement would make procedures a lot easier. In contrast to the equipoise principle, the rules of informed consent/assent and the financial agreement can be different from one member state to another.

Again, we conclude that the existing ethical norms have not been a major obstacle for the feasibility of clinical trials in minors. However, many challenges remain and new ones will evolve.

**What Do We Need?**

In some research hospitals, the financial crisis is one of the reasons of skipping a considerable part of clinical academic research in children. Furthermore, young paediatricians should be encouraged to get involved in clinical research trials. The diversity of routine clinical work is more attractive than designing clinical trials. Clinical paediatric pharmacology is a discipline with very limited attraction to young people. However, we need experts in designing paediatric clinical trials [6]. This is mandatory not only to create new medicines for children but also to test 'off-patent' drugs.

**Clinical Trials Networking**

The EMA organised a conference in early 2009 to bring different national research network organisations into contact. It is clear that there is a need for transnational networking.

*(Ad 3): Which new challenges do we observe today and will we observe in the future?*
Never has child research been so exposed to the private pharmaceutical development sector. This is enforced by the EU paediatric regulation and offers many good research opportunities. Here are some reflections on the potential challenges.

- Where several companies compete for a small patient population, the potential for unethical means to promote study inclusion might evolve. No such observations are available, but ethics committees should have that potential in the back of their minds.

- With the increased public interest in paediatric research, it is extremely important that clinical paediatric pharmacologists should be trained in a common academic-industrial setting.
- The PDCO may in a specific rare disease advise large randomized, double-blind, placebo-controlled clinical trials, while the local ethics committee might object to this approach based on daily clinical practice and other ethical concerns. At present, the ethics committee can ask for a protocol modification, which is challenging in a multicenter clinical trial, or reject it, which might exclude children from a promising new therapeutic approach. A stronger networking between the EU ethics committees and specifically between those involved in paediatric trials would be desirable.

**Conclusion**

The European regulation 1901/2006 resulted in an increase in clinical trials in minors. Researchers have become more a familiar with the ethical guidelines. The increased exposure of children to modern biopharmaceutical research has a high potential to allow them earlier access to innovative medicines. There are multiple ethical challenges in this process, for which the existing ethical framework in Europe is partially sufficient. New challenges will require new approaches and an open-minded discussion. Europe is not yet one uniform research landscape but still a region with many different approaches, laws and customs. Eventually, Europe will move towards more uniform conditions within Europe and also compared with other global regions. The debate on ethics in paediatric research will hopefully contribute considerable to this transformation process.

# References


1 Gill D, et al: Guidelines for informed consent. Eur J Pediatr 2003;162:455–458.
2 Royal College for the Ethical Conduct of Medical Research Involving Children. Arch Dis Child 2000;82:177–182.
3 Gill D, et al: Ethical principles and operational guidelines for good clinical practice Eur J Pediatr 2004;163:53–57.
4 Sauer PJ: A report of the Ethics Working Group of the CESP. Eur J Pediatr 2002;161:1–5.
5 Ramet J: What the paediatricians need – the launch of paediatric research in Europe. Eur J Pediatr 2005;164:263–265.
6 Sammons H: Ethical issues of clinical trials in children: a European perspective. Arch Dis Child 2009;94:474–477.
7 Tan J, Koelch M: The ethics of psychopharmacological research in legal minors. Child Adolesc Psychiatry Ment Hlth 2008;2:39.
8 Ethical Considerations For Clinical Trials On Medicinal Products Conducted With The Paediatric Population. http://ec.europa.eu/enterprise/pharmaceuticals/eudralex/vol-10/ethical_considerations.pdf



Klaus Rose, MD, MS
Principal Consultant
Granzer Regulatory Consulting & Services, Zielstattstrasse 44
DE–81379 Munich (Germany)
Tel. +49 89 780 68 98 29, Fax +49 89 780 68 98 15, E-Mail rose@granzer.biz

Rose K, van den Anker JN (eds): Guide to Paediatric Drug Development and Clinical Research.
Basel, Karger, 2010, pp 75–82

# Consent and Assent in Paediatric Clinical Trials

M.R. Simar[a] · P.A. Fowler[b]

[a]INC Research, Austin, Tex., USA; [b]Danemount Consulting, Hertford, UK

The need for informing research participants about research risk was recognized as early as 1900 when Spanish and English consent forms were used during studies of yellow fever in Cuba [1]. Nearly half a century later, standards for voluntary agreement were initiated under the Nuremberg Code in 1946. Further guidelines addressed the fundamental rights of vulnerable populations, such as children, to decide about research participation [2, 3]. This chapter will describe the consent process for research involving children and review practical considerations for study sponsors.

## Framework of Paediatric Consent

Clinical trial participation is predicated upon a process whereby potential volunteers receive information on risks and benefits and then decide on whether or not to volunteer. The progression from disclosure by an investigator to decision-making by the participant is the core feature of the informed consent process. The process begins with the initial invitation to participate and extends for the duration of the study.

The process assumes that an individual has the intellectual capacity to make informed decisions based on personal goals and values and that the decision is free of excessive influences [4].

Consent can only be given for oneself, and cannot be given on behalf of another person. Within this framework, a parent or legal guardian could not consent for their child. Children are limited in their capacity for decision-making and are precluded from consent for themselves. Because agreement to participate is a condition for human research, applied principles of informed consent have been modified to allow inclusion of children. Ethical guidelines and international requirements [5–7] have evolved over the past 15 years and given rise to a framework whereby children are included with parents in the decision to participate. The requirement (with few exceptions) to include children constitutes a dyad of consent for paediatric studies, whereby consent is given by the parent and assent by the child.

## Parents (or Legal Guardian)

Parents can only consent for themselves so 'informed permission' has been adopted by some paediatric advocates to describe the role of the parent [5, 8]. More often, 'parental consent' is the term applied to the process. A parent reviews trial information with the investigator then decides whether or not to allow their child to participate. The disclosure by the investigator, followed by open dialogue between investigator and parent are essential to the process. Consent requirements in some regions and cultures may extend beyond the role of parents to family elders, tribal leaders or other community representatives in accordance with local customs [9].

Regulations do not specify whether or not the child should be included in the initial process. Most advocates suggest engaging the parents, then the child. Others suggest independent discussions, especially in the case of adolescents with a long history of illness. Separate discussions afford the opportunity to advise the adolescent about confidential issues ordinarily protected by clinical standards that may be altered by research protocols (e.g. study requirements for contraception). The investigator should judge the most appropriate scenario to support informed decisions within the context of the family.

Provisions of the process assume that parents will evaluate risk and benefit, then render a decision that protects the well-being of their children. If an investigator perceives that a parent is not acting in the best interests of the child, the investigator is expected to withdraw the invitation to participate in the study. Investigators should not only disclose information but also encourage questions related to:

- The purpose of the research and why their child has been selected.
- The potential for benefit and likelihood of risk for their child.
- Differences in treatment for their child under standard medical care compared to study participation.
- Study requirements that will impact activities of daily living (e.g. school absences for clinic visits).
- Medical care for unexpected events.
- Rights for participants (e.g. withdrawal without penalty).

Consent from two parents is required under some country-specific regulations unless a parent is not reasonably available or is without legal responsibilities. For example, in the US, research involving greater than minimal risk that does not hold out the prospect of direct benefit to the child requires permission from both parents [8]. The two-parent requirement varies across EU Member States [10]. Even if two parents are not required by regulation, study sponsors and investigators should consider involving both parents for several reasons. Most obvious is that the risk of disputes once the child is under treatment is minimized if one parent has reservations about participation. Additionally, compliance is more likely if both parents have been fully engaged about the study commitment.


## Child Assent

Assent is a willingness (and not just a lack of dissent) by a minor to participate following age-appropriate disclosure. Assent supports the principles of respect established by the Declaration of Helsinki in which a person should be given the right to choose and that groups with limited autonomy be given special protections [11]. The EU Clinical Trials Directive requires that a child's will be 'considered,' but the guidance recommends assent from the child and, in the absence of assent, the process and child's response should be documented [10].

Assent is required in most cases in the US unless the ethics committee determines that the research is expected to directly benefit the child and the treatment can only be obtained in a research setting [8]. In these cases, investigators must weigh the desires of parents and the child and may choose to engage an independent party in the consent conference. All events related to the decision should be well-documented. Despite these exceptions, stakeholders generally agree that knowledgeable agreement should be obtained from children capable of giving assent.

Philosophical distinctions regarding the rights of children impact regional requirements for assent. A recent review of a case study on enrolling children in Kenya is a reminder that traditions and social practices must be considered for assent [12]. Kenyan leaders reasoned that ability to assent would vary widely depending on whether the child lived in an urban or rural area. In some cases, Kenyan children are still an important means of labour within the family unit and are expected to follow adult decisions. Children in such a context may be hesitant to respond negatively about a study. Researchers must be aware of local attitudes that might differ from international standards when conducting studies in multi-cultural settings to ensure that the right to assent is protected.

*Age*

The age at which meaningful assent can be accomplished has been widely debated with some advocates suggesting that even very young children can understand medical procedures [13]. Others recommend that assent should be delayed until age 14 years when abstract concepts related to the purpose of research and reasons to participate are more likely to be understood [14]. Cultural attitudes toward the role of a child in the family and society contribute to the debate on the appropriate age [12].

In practice, ethics committees most often require assent by age 6 or 7 years although local requirements in some regions defer the requirement until adolescence. Local requirements also differ on the age and conditions for allowing an adolescent to consent for themselves [10, 15]. Adolescents are most often eligible to consent for research upon reaching the age of majority or achieving emancipation (e.g. marriage, military service).

Regardless of limits on age, child advocates recognise that many factors apart from chronological stages impact a child's ability to make decisions. Developmental stage, intellectual capacities, psychological state, and life experience contribute to a child's ability to assent. Children's competency to make decisions also varies by the degree of influence of their parents or doctors. Broome described the collective social, psychological and cognitive differences that impact the means for engaging children in the process [13]. For example, younger children are more likely to defer to authority to avoid punishment rather than voicing their opinion. Therefore, investigators should take sufficient time to ensure that the child's motivation reflects their own desires to the best extent possible. Because abstract concepts are more difficult for younger children, pictures and/or demonstration of the study procedures will enhance understanding. On the other hand, many adolescents have the ability to evaluate alternatives with less influence of their parents. They should accordingly be engaged about risks and benefits in terms they can understand.

Competency can be further influenced by the type or severity of the child's condition. The impact of diseases or medications on cognition should be considered, as well. Impaired decision-making and attention are associated with schizophrenia, impulse disorders and ADHD. Neurological diseases such as epilepsy may alter understanding, suggesting the need for simpler forms and information sheets for some children. In most cases, the impairments will be evident to the investigator who takes requisite time to fully assess the child or adolescent.

*Dissent*

Ethicists and authorities generally agree that reluctance or refusal ('dissent') by a child should be respected [2]. Investigators should seek to understand the reason for unwillingness. Reasons could vary considerably depending on age and prior experience with medical procedures. Wendler [14] suggests that research staff should adopt a strategy of 'stop, assess and address'. Where research distress is temporary and the child well prepared for the procedure, usually assent is not a problem – especially as children have been shown to perform research for altruistic reasons [16]. Nonetheless, at the first sign of distress and dissent the procedure should be stopped. A short pause to allow the child to feel in control, to provide further explanation and to assess the situation may be all that is needed to reassure the child. For example, a child's distress over a painless ECG if they fear that electricity will be put into them might be overcome by a simple explanation. Often it is not the procedure they object to, but restraint or fear of separation from the parent during the procedure. Children can be indirectly assessed for agreement by gauging their response for routine clinical care. A child who is needle phobic would not be a good candidate for a trial involving multiple venepunctures.

## Vulnerability of Children and Parents

Vulnerability surrounding a decision to participate in a research trial applies not only to the child but also to the parent. A variety of issues can impair understanding and these should be considered when designing the consent and assent forms, supplemental information and procedures to support the process. Primary factors include timing and prior experience with medical settings.

### Timing of the Process

The ICH E6 Guideline states that sufficient time between disclosure and decision should be allowed but does not define the interval [17]. Inadequate time to ask questions and consider options has often been cited as a barrier to parental comprehension of study procedures and to stimulating parental interest in participation [18]. Ethics committees may require an explanation if less than 24 h is allowed. Ideally, a family should be given time away from the clinic to make a decision. A staged approach has been suggested for chronic conditions where a short delay in treatment does not impose risk [19]. The additional time allows for more careful consideration of risk, benefits and overall time commitment. Sufficient time is particularly important when consent is requested shortly after a new diagnosis.

An obvious dilemma arises when an acute condition requires rapid intervention and a standard treatment would exclude an otherwise qualified participant. Particularly problematic is consent in an emergency setting. Some experts suggest that recruitment in an emergency room should only be done if absolutely necessary [20]. In these cases, investigators should follow disclosure about the study with an assessment of understanding using open-ended questions ('What will happen to your child during the study?'). Indeed, the perceived value of written assessment has led some ethics committees to include questions on consent forms.

### Experience

Prior experience with the medical condition and/or research will influence the consent process. Implicit to a new diagnosis is the inherent stress for the family and the child as they seek to understand the illness and implications of research participation [21]. For this reason, sufficient time for informed decision-making is essential to an ethical process of permission and assent. Even in the case of acute treatment mentioned above, the process should be conducted in a supportive manner that engenders reflection without coercion to quickly decide. Katz and Fox [20] remind us that the approach 'demands a level of engagement beyond mere information transfer'.

Perceptions about research will differ considerably among families naïve to research compared to those whose children who have participated, possibly multiple times, in a clinical study. However, familiarity does not imply willingness, so investigators should initiate the discussion with all families as an invitation, not an expectation that they will agree. Full disclosure even for those with research experience is important. Some parents who previously granted permission may determine that the added burden of research procedures is no longer appropriate for their child. Parents and children may differ in opinion on perceived burden and willingness to participate. In such cases, an individual apart from the research team may be more suited than the investigator to resolve differences.

**The Forms**

Regulations on informed consent focus on the consent/assent form and signature requirements. The form describes the purpose, procedures, risks, alternative treatments and other details mandated by national and local regulations. The basic elements contained in the forms have gained international acceptance, as well as the requirement that language should be at an educational level appropriate for the parent and child. These general agreements leave considerable latitude in the content, format, and means of presentation of the forms.

The form is the conduit for summarizing the study and documenting disclosure about the study. It should be perceived as an adjunct to the primary means for informing participants – meaningful discussion. However, forms have increasingly evolved into a detailed description of every event, often in language beyond the recommended levels of ethics committees. One reason that experts and advocates have called for improvements is that understandable language fulfills the basic tenet for *informing* parents. Another reason, on a practical level, is that simple explanations overcome a barrier to participation sometimes cited by parents. Lengthy and overly technical forms may deter rather than motivate parents to consider enrolling their child [18].

Ability to focus on the content of the form can be impaired not only by stressful events surrounding their child's initial diagnosis or progressive illness, but by distraction of increasing paperwork associated with medical visits. Difficulties in grasping the differences in treatment under standard care versus a clinical trial are inevitable, especially for families facing a life-altering condition. For this reason, parental consent forms should attend to the distinctions between standard care and research to avoid misconceptions about the purpose and benefits of the study. Secondly, the right for withdrawal without penalty should be highlighted, so that parents fully understand that participation is an ongoing choice throughout the duration of the study.

Content for the assent form should be appropriate for each age group or level of understanding. As such, one study may need more than one version of the assent form The EC recommends that terms be 'honest, but not frightening' [10]. A very simple explanation that the doctor wants to learn about their condition and that the study doctor and parents will explain what will happen may be sufficient for 6- to 8-year-olds. Older children and adolescents need information on the purpose of the study and why they are being asked to participate. Some ethics committees allow that the parental permission form be used for adolescents. A better practice is to design a form that addresses the adolescent directly, since the parental form often cites 'your child'. Matters of confidentiality that differ from clinical practice should be transparent. If the outcome of pregnancy testing will be shared with parents, then the form should explicitly state how the information will be conveyed.

The lay-out of the consent and assent form can also impact understanding and interest. Most experts suggest arranging information so that it appears less like a contract and more like educational material. Wide margins, larger text, flow-chart or other graphics, distinct headings and two-column formats can improve communication. Pictures are recommended for young children.

The means of presentation of the forms is a critical element of the process. A verbal overview of the trial should be the first step before handing over the form. A staff member should then review the form, explaining its purpose and highlighting key points from the overview. Lastly, families should be given time to review alone but with staff available to answer questions. As mentioned above, a period for decision-making at home is ideal whenever possible.

The complexities of many study designs suggest that another step may be important to an informed decision. Given the tendency of sponsors and ethics committees to require more, not less, information in the consent forms, supportive materials may be a solution for enhancing comprehension. The materials may take the form of patient information leaflets, video presentations, or brochures. Scripts to direct site staff through key points can also be useful for engaging parents and children about their initial concerns prior to reviewing the form. The materials can be individualised for educational levels, languages and dialects, and other specifics relevant to the targeted study population. All materials must be reviewed by the ethics committee.

## Documentation of the Process

Ethics committees are charged with deciding how the process should be documented. A signature of one parent is required on the consent form and, as noted above, two parents may be required for some studies with significant risk and by some authorities. Documentation for an oral consent process involving interpreters in paediatric trials is the same as for other studies.

Unique to the paediatric process is the documentation of assent. FDA and EMA regulations defer to ethics committees on the requirement, whereas most sponsors mandate signatures. Some guidelines suggests that signature by a young child may not be appropriate if they are without experience [22]. The child may not perceive the symbolic meaning or could be intimidated by the request [23]. Another guidance suggests that the child should be invited, not required, to sign [6]. Some ethics committees have recently changed their policy on signature requirements for assent by replacing the signature line with statements verifying assent by the individual conducting assent [24]. Regardless of requirements for signature, the process of discussing with the child and their decision regarding participation should be documented by the investigator. Sponsors and investigators should be mindful of older adolescents who reach the age of majority and would require documentation of consent prior to study completion.

## Practical Matters for the Role of Sponsors in Paediatric Consent

Trial sponsors share the obligations for paediatric consent with ethics committees and investigators for ensuring an ethical process in accordance with applicable regulations. Key responsibilities for sponsors are summarized in figure 1. Additional considerations for aligning efforts with stakeholders are presented below.

### *Ethics Committees*

Compliance with consent and assent regulations can be challenging when study teams encounter variable requirements from ethics committees. Imposing or ignoring requirements are likely to invoke multiple rounds of review. Avoid delays by knowing the regional regulations and anticipating committee concerns about the content or layout of the forms, advertising materials and supporting documents. Investigators are often willing to offer suggestions on the documents to enhance approvals by their local committees.

### *Investigator Training*

The conundrum for industry to manage paediatric consent is that the process itself cannot be directly

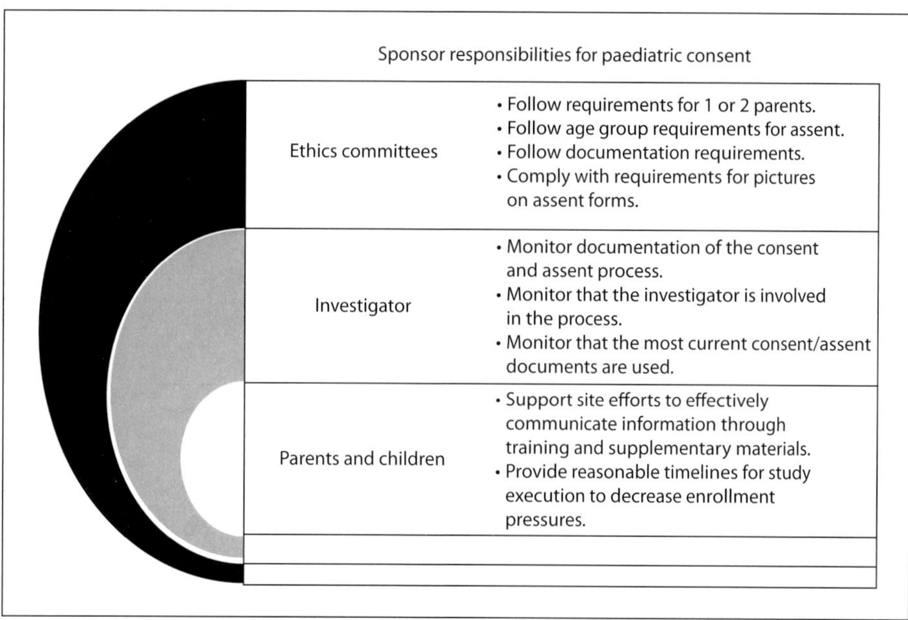



**Fig. 1.** Sponsor responsibilities for paediatric consent.

assessed by the sponsor. The sponsor's purview is limited to monitoring form approval by the ethics committee and investigator documentation of the process. That sponsors are a step removed from the event suggests an obligation for site training on consent and assent for each study. Investigators may be averse to consent training, but the exercise demonstrates the sponsor's commitment to ensuring highest standards of paediatric consent. Rather than limiting instruction to iteration of the requirements, a lively discussion on the unique elements of the study that will impact willingness to participate can be important to subsequent planning for recruitment of parents and children.

*Impact of Timelines on Parents and Children*

Concerns about investigator pressure from sponsors [25] regarding enrolment merit special attention for studies in children. Although the practice of competitive enrollment may generate acceptable competition in some studies, sponsors should reflect on the implications for paediatric studies. Scrutiny is greater for all aspects of research in children and motivations for enrolling children should be of the highest standards. Sponsors risk undermining the special protections afforded children and their parents when competition for subjects becomes a central focus of study activities.

**Conclusions**

Consent and assent is a challenging but essential element in paediatric clinical trial management. Foremost to an ethical and well-documented process is careful planning and a family centred approach. Enrolling children into a clinical trial should begin with an invitation to participate that is commensurate with their development, respectful of their privacy and acknowledges family dynamics. Given the increasing information on factors important to the process, study sponsors have the opportunity to enrich the process through improved consent materials, training and attention to local requirements.

## References


1 University of Virginia Health Sciences System Historical Collections: The United States Army Yellow Fever Commission (1900–1901). Available from: http://etext.virginia.edu/healthsci/reed/commission.html.
2 International Conference on Harmonisation, Clinical Investigation of Medicinal Products in the Pediatric Population: Step 4CH Consensus Guideline, 2000.
3 National Commission for the Protection of Human Subjects of Biomedical and Behavioral Research, Report and Recommendations: Research Involving Children. Washington, Department of Health, Education & Welfare, 1977.
4 Brody BA: Making meaningful consent meaningful. IRB Ethics Hum Res 2001: 23:1–5.
5 American Academy of Pediatrics: Committee on bioethics, informed consent, parental permission, and assent in pediatric practice. Pediatrics 1995;95:314–317.
6 Gill D, et al: Guidelines for informed consent in biomedical research involving paediatric populations as research participants; the Ethics Working Group of the Confederation of European Specialists in Paediatrics (CESP). Eur J Pediatr 2003;162:455–458.
7 Council for International Organizations of Medical Sciences: International Ethical Guidelines for Biomedical Research Involving Human Subjects. Geneva, 2002.
8 Food and Drug Administration, 21 CFR Subpart D: Additional Safeguards for Children in Clinical Investigations of FDA-Regulated Products: Interim Rule. Federal Register, 2001, p 66 FR 20598.
9 Eder M: Testing drugs in developing countries: pediatric research ethics in the international context; in Kodish E (ed): Ethics and Research with Children. New York, Oxford University Press, 2005, pp 241–261.
10 European Commission: Ethical Considerations for Clinical Trials on Medicinal Products Conducted with the Paediatric Population. Final, 2008.
11 World Medical Association: Declaration of Helsinki: Ethical Principles for Medical Research Involving Human Subjects. 52nd WMA General Assembly, Edinburgh, 2000.
12 Vreeman R, Nyandiko W, Meslin E: Pediatric assent for a study o antiretroviral therapy dosing for children in western Kenya: a case study in international research collaboration. J Empir Res Hum Res Ethics 2009;4:3–16.
13 Broome M: Consent (assent) for research with pediatric patients. Semin Oncol Nurs 1999;15:196–213.
14 Wendler D: Assent in paediatric research: theoretical and practical considerations. J Med Ethics 2006;32229–234.
15 Institute of Medicine Committee on Clinical Research Involving Children, Understanding and Agreeing to Children's Participation in Clinical Research; in Field J, Behrman RE (eds): The Ethical Conduct of Clinical Research Involving Children. Washington, National Academy of Sciences, 2004, pp 146–210.
16 Wolthers OD: A questionnaire on factors influencing children's assent and dissent to non-therapeutic research. J Med Ethics 2006;32:292–297.
17 International Conference on Harmonisation, Consolidated Guideline: Good Clinical Practice, 1997.
18 Chappuy H, et al: Parental consent in paediatric clinical research. Arch Dis Childh 2006;91:112–116.
19 Eder ML, et al: Improving informed consent: suggestions from parents of children with leukemia. Pediatrics 2007; 119:e849–e859.
20 Katz A, Fox K: The Process of Informed Consent: What's at Stake? Boston, Children's Hospital, Department of Social Medicine, Harvard Medical School, 2004.
21 Simon C, et al: Groups potentially at risk for making poorly Informed decisions about entry into clinical trials for childhood cancer. J Clin Oncol 2003;21:2173–2178.
22 US Department of Health and Human Services, FDA Guidance for Industry and FDA Staff: Premarket Assessment of Pediatric Medical Devices, 2004.
23 Ungar D, Joffe S, Kodish E: Children are not small adults: documentation of assent for research involving children. J Pediatr 2006;149(1 suppl):S31–S33.
24 Western Institutional Review Board. Pediatric Assent Changes. 2007; available at: http://www.wirb.com/content/foot_wirb_news_latest.aspx
25 Office of Inspector General, O.o.E.a.I., DHHS, Recruiting Human Subjects: Pressures in Industry Sponsored Trials. 2000, OIG, OEI, DHHS.



Renee Simar, PhD
Principal Strategist, Pediatrics, INC Research
3321 Bee Caves Road
Austin, TX 78746 (USA)
Tel./Fax +1 512 858 4928, E-Mail rsimar@incresearch.com

Rose K, van den Anker JN (eds): Guide to Paediatric Drug Development and Clinical Research.
Basel, Karger, 2010, pp 83–96

# Study and Protocol Design for Paediatric Patients of Different Ages

O. Della Pasqua[a] · L.B. Zimmerhackl[b] · K. Rose[c]

[a]Clinical Pharmacology & Discovery Medicine, GlaxoSmithKline, Stockley Park, UK; [b]Department of Pediatrics I, Medical University Innsbruck, Innsbruck, Austria; [c]F. Hoffmann-La Roche Ltd., Pharmaceuticals Division, Basel, Switzerland

## Introduction

*Study Protocol and Protocol Rationale*

A clinical study protocol is the key document and backbone of every single clinical trial. In principle, there are no differences between an adult and a paediatric protocol. It has to describe what is planned, as well as why, when and how to achieve it. It has to include a high-level study rationale and should list operational details. Clinical research is now expanding from the adult population where basic principles are well established to the paediatric population where many key players are relative newcomers. A practicing paediatrician has in-depth knowledge of the physiology and mindset of a child. However, he will often be less knowledgeable in designing multi-centre international trial protocols. Vice versa, an industry scientist well experienced in writing adult study protocols will have to learn a lot about children when he is assigned to write a clinical protocol for a paediatric indication. One of the reasons paediatric clinical research is more work intensive is because the implementation of study protocols requires careful considerations regarding feasibility. Another hurdle are ethical committees, which sometimes have less experience with children and might block or at least slow the approval of paediatric trials. Several specific challenges are covered in other chapters of this book, including blood volume, parental informed consent and child's assent, appropriate paediatric formulations and others.

The study rationale is crucial in making the trial justifiable. It should explain the objectives of the study in a language that can be understood by all members of an ethical committee, including those that are not MDs, PhDs or PharmDs. It should explain the key characteristics of the investigational drug in adults, compare the targeted disease(s) in adults and in children, give a high-level assessment of the therapeutic options available at present, and explain the expected therapeutic benefit as well as the expected scientific learning of the planned trial. As healthy children do not generally participate in clinical trials, the objective of every paediatric clinical study is always twofold. First, the children to be included in the trial have a health problem that might be positively influenced by the study participation. Second, scientific lessons are expected to be learned from the study participation. A balanced assessment of potential risks and benefits needs to be part of the study rationale. Failure to address these key issues will often result in additional questions from the ethical committee and/or in additional conditions

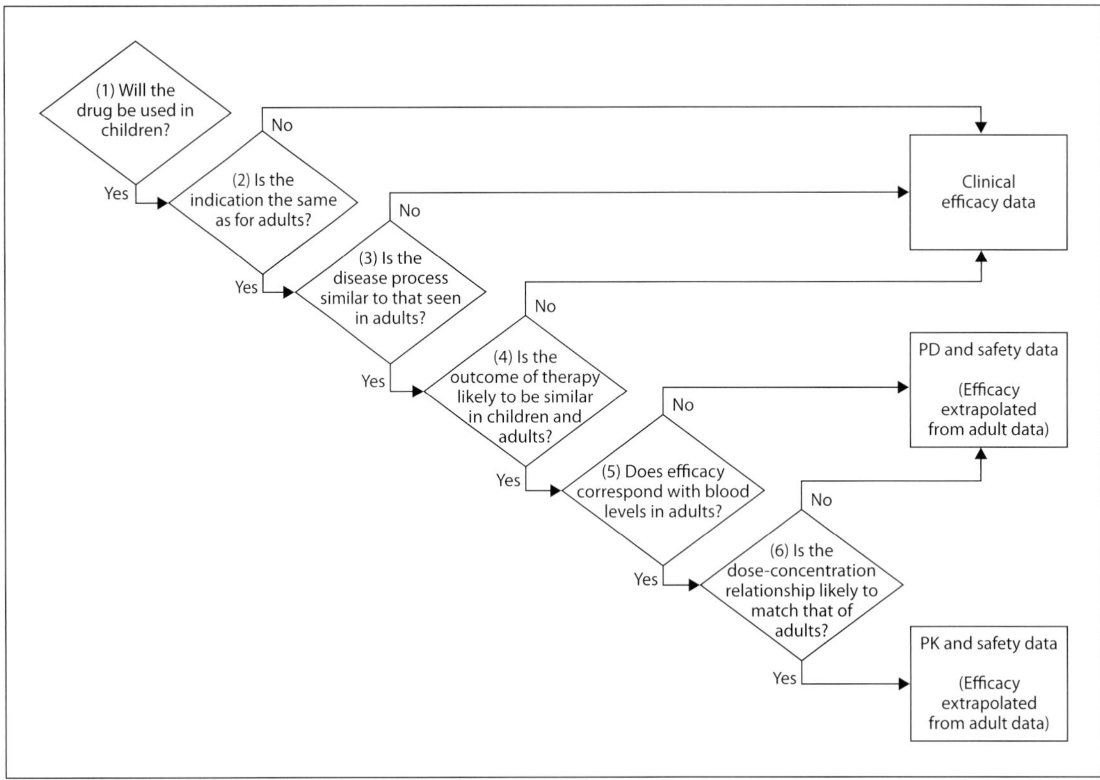


**Fig. 1.** Decision tree for the identification of clinical study requirements in a paediatric drug development program.

that have to be met before the study can start. A good rationale will cost time at the beginning and will save time during study preparation and performance. It is also highly recommended to have paediatric protocol reviewed by a paediatrician or a person otherwise competent in paediatric drug development.

*Study Planning*

Before operational details are planned, the study essentials should be discussed in the framework of the general clinical development plan with an appropriate expert. The following conditions need to be checked (fig. 1).

*Flow Sheet*

In the planning phase and in particular during the study period itself, the development of a flow sheet supports the surveillance and execution of the study activities and procedures.

## Study Population

The ICH guideline ICH E 11 suggests five different age groups (table 1). Since this system defines only age as a descriptor of size and function, it disregards the evidence that multiple physiological processes develop beyond the proposed age boundaries, which determine, for example,

| ICH strata | Range |
| --- | --- |
| Pre-term neonate | <37 weeks' gestation |
| Term neonate | 0–27 days |
| Infants and toddlers | 28 days to 23 months |
| Children | 2–11 years |
| Adolescent | 12–18 years |

homeostatic mechanisms and drug metabolism. Understanding how these factors change over time is essential for dose selection across the different phases of development. Furthermore, in many instances disease incidence and/or severity may be age-dependent, but not in agreement with the current ICH classification.

These developmental differences make the criteria for selecting the study population and dose rationale in a paediatric study more complex than in adult studies. Population stratification must be carefully considered in conjunction with aetiology and epidemiology aspects, instead of solely relying on ICH strata. On the other hand, patient selection will depend upon evidence for safety and tolerability across the different age groups. Whilst the dosage form is constant in an adult study, the availability of a suitable formulation will also play an important role in defining the study population.

*Healthy Subjects versus Patients*

Whilst healthy subjects are enrolled in most studies in early clinical development for adult indications, this option is generally not possible and ethically unacceptable for paediatric indications. A few exceptions exist in vaccine trials and when adolescents (>16–18 years of age) are legally granted adulthood status. However, even in such circumstances careful consideration of medical risk/benefit ratio is needed to decide on the enrolment of healthy subjects.

*Stratification versus Balanced Population*

Often supporting data on safety and epidemiology will impose staggering or stratification of the study population. The challenge is to identify a priori which factor or covariate best describes the developmental changes and hence which treatment arms or dose levels should be investigated. Common practice has been geared to stratification by age and/or weight. However, this approach disregards the role of other relevant physiological variables that may underlie the changes in function in the paediatric population.

In principle, it may be preferable to enrol groups of patients across a wide range of age, weight, or physiological variable (e.g., haematocrit, creatinine clearance).

The need to stagger the clinical development across different age groups will be discussed later in conjunction with other safety aspects. The feasibility of such an approach will depend upon whether the necessary pre-clinical toxicology studies in animals have been performed and whether evidence is available for efficacy and safety in adults. These data will also be used as the basis for justification of the dosing rationale.

*Medical History and Disease Status*

Whilst it is commonly accepted that the development of a paediatric indication may be safer if progression is based on evaluation of older patients before exposing younger children to the investigational drug, this approach overlooks the aetiology of disease. Depending on the age of onset, disease status may be worse or severity of symptoms more pronounced in older age groups.

**Study Design**

*Development Phases*

For many years, clinical research has been based on sequential development, with rather well-defined stages and designs for the transition of a molecule from first-time-in-humans to a full pivotal efficacy trial. New approaches trying to reduce time and number of patients needed to complete a study are rapidly evolving. In addition, paediatric study protocols have to cope with specific requirements in that an even less strict separation between the different study phases may be necessary and desirable. Such a requirement may impose the need for flexible or alternative study designs. The ability to identify these differences is crucial to the success of a clinical study. Also, patient recruitment and overall incidence of disease in the target population ought to be taken into account when selecting study designs. Often the difficulties to recruit patients across a relevant range (based on age, weight or any other relevant physiological variable) are overlooked and have become the cause of frequent protocol amendments.

*Early versus Late Clinical Development Studies*

As stated above, there is a less strict separation of the study phases when it comes to paediatric development, as one would not necessarily progress through clinical development by stand-alone studies aimed at single and multiple ascending dose escalation for pharmacokinetics, safety and tolerability, followed by a proof-of-concept, a phase IIb dose ranging study followed by a pivotal efficacy trial. Paediatric protocols must address relevant clinical development questions efficiently. It is not advisable to perform stand-alone studies.

First, there will be feasibility and ethical hurdles in running a study which has as primary objective the characterisation of pharmacokinetics and safety and tolerability only. One must be aware of the patient's needs and find a compromise between scientific rigour to derive accurate information about pharmacokinetics, pharmacodynamics, safety and tolerability with the potential benefits of treatment in the target population. The selection of any given study design should take into account the location and shape of the concentration-response curve. From a statistical point of view, clinical efficacy study designs can be categorised according to the classification proposed by Palmer [4]. Whilst most clinical study protocols in adults can be based on a randomised, double-blind, placebo-controlled, parallel group design with fixed sample sizes, such a protocol may turn out to be inappropriate or unethical in a paediatric indication.

These limitations may be overcome by the use of so-called data-dependent designs, which have been applied not only in exploratory research but also in confirmatory (regulatory) clinical studies. Data-dependent study designs were introduced progressively in clinical research in the early 1940s, and consist of sequential, group sequential, adaptive interim, response-adaptive and Bayesian adaptive designs.

*Minimal Detectable Difference*

The minimal detectable difference is the smallest difference between the treatments or strength of association that one wishes to be able to detect. In clinical trials this is the smallest difference considered to be clinically important and biologically plausible. In a study of association, it is the smallest change in the dependent (outcome variable, response), per unit change in the independent (input variable, covariate) that is plausible.

*Parallel Design*

A parallel-designed clinical trial compares the results of a treatment on two separate groups of patients. The sample size calculated for a parallel design can be used for any study where two groups are being compared.

### Crossover Study

A crossover study compares the results of a two-treatment regimen in the same group of patients. The sample size calculated for a crossover study can also be used for a study that compares the value of a variable after treatment with its value before treatment. The standard deviation of the outcome variable is expressed as either the within-patient standard deviation or the standard deviation of the difference. The former is the standard deviation of repeated observations in the same individual and the latter is the standard deviation of the difference between two measurements in the same individual.

### Study to Find an Association

A study to find an association determines if one variable, the dependent variable, is affected by another, the independent variable. For instance, a study to determine whether blood pressure is affected by salt intake.

### Success/Failure

The outcome of the study is a variable with two values, usually treatment success or treatment failure.

### 'Smart' Designs

Data-dependent designs offer alternatives to clinical research protocols that may be more efficient, i.e. giving a surer answer about the location and shape of the exposure-response curve, providing important data for subsequent regulatory studies. The objective of these designs is to increase the proportion of subjects allocated to effective treatment levels. In fact, these concepts can be widely applied in adult and paediatric protocols.

These include:
- enrichment approaches;
- titration design;
- the randomised withdrawal study.

### Enrichment Approaches

Prospective use of any patient characteristic – demographic, pathophysiologic, or genetic, and others – as inclusion criteria for selecting patients in a study is usually done to obtain a study population in which the drug effect is supposedly more likely to be detected. This practice, whilst not necessarily explicit, occurs all the time in clinical medicine. Enrichment designs can decrease heterogeneity, identifying a population capable of responding to the treatment and thereby increasing the rate of response, or increasing the number of events that will occur in the study. A higher number of responders to treatment increases statistical power. Enrichment can thus greatly facilitate 'proof-of-concept' studies. Implementation of enrichment design requires an interim evaluation of response, as defined by a biomarker or clinical endpoint. Non-responders are subsequently withdrawn from the trial or randomised to a different dose level or treatment. In paediatric protocols this approach warrants shorter duration of exposure of patients who do not respond to an ineffective treatment arm.

### Concentration-Controlled (Titration) Design

In traditional efficacy studies, patients are randomised to a dose level. However, this procedure ignores the role of individual pharmacokinetic factors, yielding drug exposures that do not cover the thorough concentration-response curve,

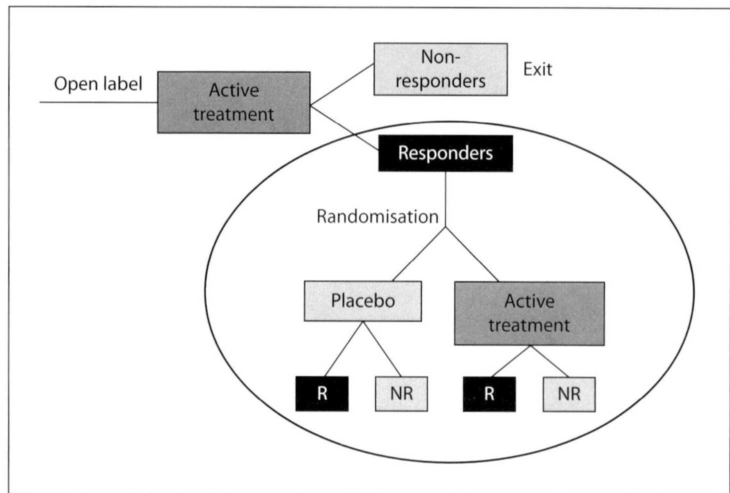



**Fig. 2.** Randomised placebo withdrawal study design. R = Responders; NR = non-responders.

i.e. one of the key objectives of early clinical development. The titration design eliminates this limitation, as it is based on the allocation of a patient to a concentration range, rather than a dose level [5]. Implementation of this design requires a monitoring phase under steady-state conditions to ensure compliance to randomization levels. A placebo or complementary dose level is subsequently used to titrate the patient to the allocated concentration range. Requirements for monitoring of drug concentration and dose adjustment are based on sparse sampling of pharmacokinetics and simulation techniques. Details of the data analysis methodology will be discussed in another section (see 'Data Analysis and Statistical Considerations').

*Randomised Placebo-Withdrawal Design*

In some circumstances, enrichment can be achieved by evaluating the drug effect by withdrawal of treatment in patients who have been identified as responders (fig. 2). This approach can be particularly useful to identify treatment outcome associated with symptomatic improvement [6].

From a practical point of view, randomised placebo-withdrawal studies offer every patient an opportunity to experience the potential benefits of active treatment. This results in better patient accrual in indications for which the use of a placebo arm may not be suitable or ethically acceptable (fig. 2).

A few points must be considered for the implementation of a randomized placebo withdrawal study, which may limit its application in early drug development. First, the use of parallel designs is often not possible due to varying disease features. Second, it cannot be used in testing drugs with a very long half-life (months) or drugs that induce irreversible changes. Third, it has limited value in unstable diseases and is not recommended for studying serious or life-threatening diseases.

*Adapted Three-Stage Design*

In therapeutic indications such as rare diseases, accrual of patients becomes the main risk factor for the success of a clinical study. The concept of placebo withdrawal followed by re-randomisation

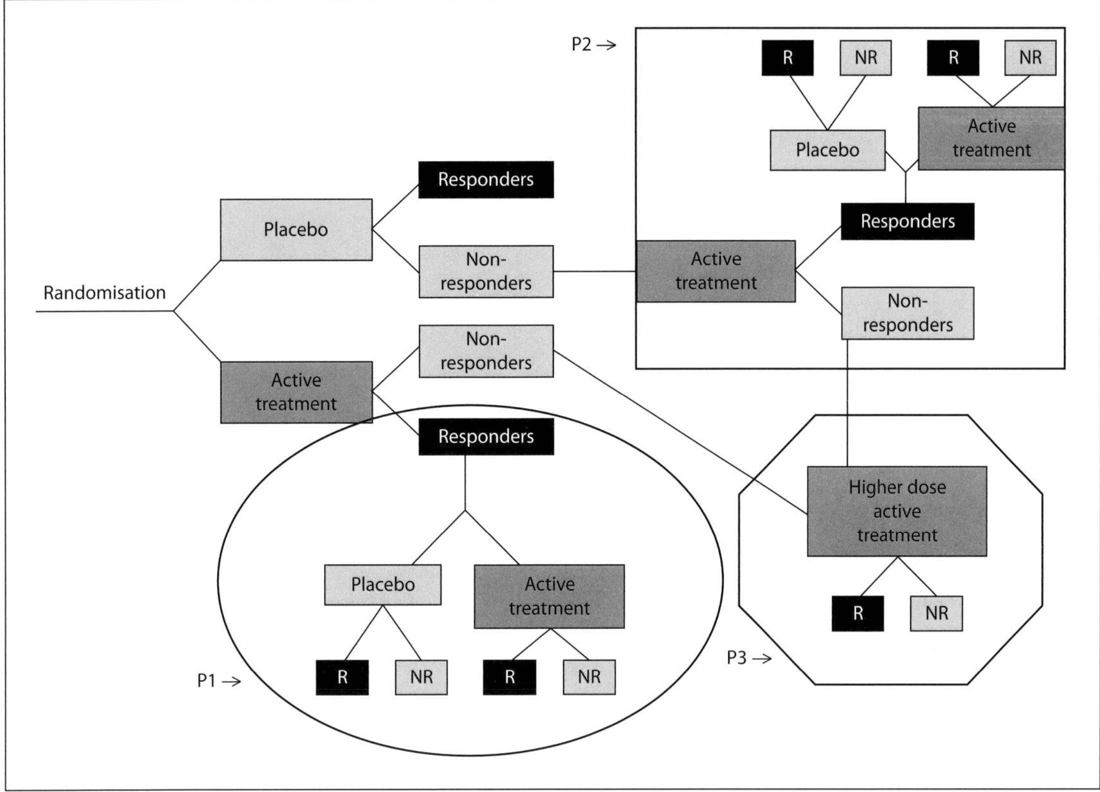

**Fig. 3.** Adapted three-stage design. R = Responder; NR = non-responder. P1, P2 and P3 indicate the points at which the statistical analysis of response is performed.

of non-responders to a subsequent treatment level offers a very attractive alternative to standard designs. In a three-stage trial, all patients receive the active medication at a given stage of the trial, which consists of a sequence of three placebo-withdrawal stages (fig. 3). The main advantage of the approach is that non-responders are not excluded from the study, but are re-randomised to a different treatment level.

The formal statistical assessment of efficacy incorporates three separate stages, increasing the power of the study. In practice, the increase in statistical power results in a reduction in sample size of approximately 20–30%. The study design is, however, only applicable to chronic, stable conditions.

## Randomised Placebo Phase Design

The randomised placebo phase design (RPPD) was proposed initially to assess the effect of monoclonal antibodies which produce permanent response or remission of disease. These treatments cannot be studied by placebo withdrawal or crossover designs. Design limitations are even more important in the context of rare diseases or special population groups. RPPD was developed to investigate disease-modifying therapies using survival endpoints.

Patients entering a RPPD study are not formally randomised to a placebo treatment arm, but to a randomised period during which placebo doses replace the active medication. The dependent

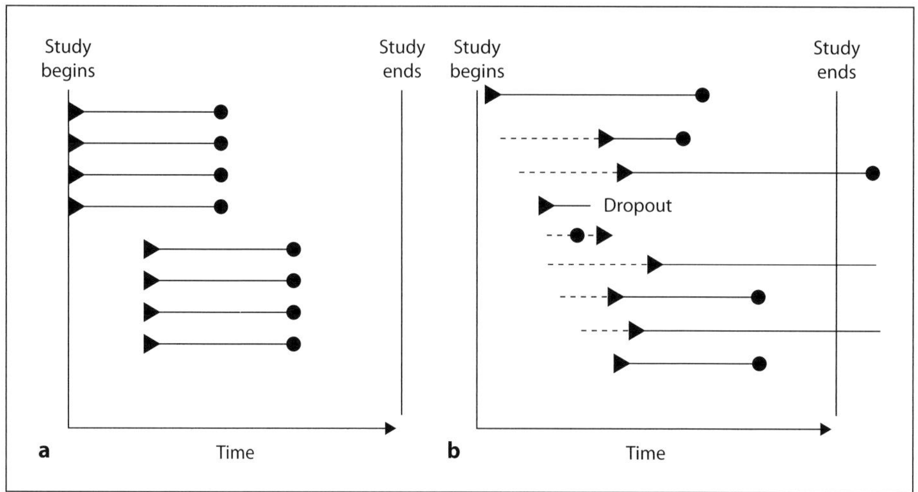


**Fig. 4.** Randomised placebo phase design. **a** In standard clinical trials the duration of treatment with the active compound is fixed. The vertical bars represent the start and finish dates of the clinical trial. Each horizontal line represents one study subject. The triangles indicate the start of active treatment, whilst solid lines represent the treatment duration. Subjects are followed until they respond (closed circle). **b** Features of the randomized placebo-phase design (RPPD) trial. Subjects enter the trial at various times in the accrual phase. Subjects are randomly assigned a period of time on placebo treatment (broken line). At the randomly determined time subjects blindly switch to active treatment (triangles). Subjects who do not respond during the trial (third, sixth and eighth subjects from top), and those who drop out (fourth subject from top) are censored. Some subjects may respond spontaneously while still on placebo (fifth subject from top). Adapted from Feldman et al. [7].

variable is time from entry into the study to the time of a response (time to event). The independent variable is the time from entry into the study to the time of starting active treatment. The length of the placebo phase will predict the overall time to response if treatment is truly efficacious (fig. 4). Some subjects are censored if response occurs after termination of the study and dropouts may occur randomly or be related to treatment effect. The statistical significance of the treatment effect is based on a Cox proportional hazards regression (fig. 4).

*Adaptive Designs*

The use of enrichment approaches, concentration-controlled designs, placebo withdrawal and randomised placebo phase design presumes some knowledge and confidence about the location and shape of the concentration-response curve, as the allocated treatment levels are defined a priori, during the planning phase of the protocol. In many cases, however, there may not be enough understanding or confidence about the exact location and shape of the concentration-response curve.

Therefore, performing studies with predefined, fixed doses or exposure levels may result in a higher development risk with potential failure to identify treatment effect in the target population. The possibility to make adjustments as one learns about the concentration-response curve may be very appealing in paediatric indications. Adaptive designs enable the implementation of adjustments in a formal manner, with statistical rigour and validity.

**Table 2.** Rules for an adaptive design

| | |
|---|---|
| Allocation rule | how subjects will be allocated to available treatment arms |
| Sampling rule | how many subjects will be sampled at the next stage |
| Stopping rule | when to stop the trial (for efficacy, for harm, for futility) |
| Decision rule | interim decisions (to update the model, to change endpoint, to modify initial plan) |

**Table 3.** Opportunities and limitations of adaptive designs: adaptive designs enable adaptations to be real without losing credibility, transparency and rigour

| Opportunities | Limitations |
|---|---|
| Enhance design efficiency by conducting the trial | complex logistics for learning as you go |
| Flexibility with respect to sample size | need for short-term endpoints |
| Options for early stopping and/or required | fast data capture and analysis change the initial design |
| Decrease costs associated with number of patients | more sophisticated statistical methodology |
| More accurate information with less  resources | 'accrual' and time bias; knowledge of design can cause operational bias (later patients have higher probability of optimal treatment) |
| Additional breakpoints for checks of consistency | population drift |

An adaptive design requires the trial to be conducted in several stages with access to the accumulated data. An adaptive design may have one or more rules (table 2).

At any stage, the data may be analysed and subsequent stages redesigned taking into account all available data. During interim adaptation patient recruitment is not interrupted. A summary of the opportunities and limitations is presented in table 3. From a statistical point of view, the main differences between a standard randomised, double-blind, placebo-controlled, parallel-treatment group and an adaptive design include re-randomisation throughout the study and consequently an unbalanced distribution of patients across treatment arms. It also allows for variations in sampling schemes.

Not surprisingly, the ability to formally adapt a study results in similar logistics issues pertaining to traditional group-sequential designs, in particular, drug supplies. Adaptations should be performed by an independent third party with no conflict of interest, i.e. an Independent Data Monitoring Committee (IDMC) (table 3).

*Pharmacokinetic Studies*

As indicated previously, formal 'bridging' studies can be devised to explore dosing regimens associated with efficacious concentration levels. However, it is not recommended to set pharmacokinetics as the only objective in a paediatric clinical trial. Ethically, it is not easy to defend a trial without any potential benefit to the child.

To overcome this limitation, it is advisable to combine pharmacokinetic sampling with an open efficacy and tolerability study. The study is rolled out in two phases, each of which has a specific set of objectives.

Pharmacokinetics can be assessed after single dosing and at steady state in the same patient population. The main difficulty associated with paediatric studies is related to the requirement for frequent, serial blood sampling. This requirement derives from the use of non-compartmental pharmacokinetic analysis to derive information about drug exposure (AUC, area under the concentration-time curve) and other parameters, such as observed peak concentration ($C_{max}$) and the time associated with it ($T_{max}$). In fact, the same type of problem arises when serial sampling is required for efficacy and safety endpoints.

These limitations can be overcome by sparse sampling and limited population size in conjunction with a more sensitive data analysis methodology, which provides predicted population pharmacokinetic estimates instead of individual observed parameters. The population approach is a parametric statistical method, based on non-linear regression techniques that yield population parameter distributions with estimates of a typical value for the population as well as providing a measure of inter-individual variability. Details of the population approach are provided under 'data analysis and statistical considerations'.

**Endpoints**

The primary variable ('target' variable, primary endpoint) should be the variable capable of providing the most clinically relevant and scientifically accepted evidence to support the primary objective of the trial. There should generally be only one primary variable and the one used when estimating the sample size. Pharmacokinetic parameters derived from drug exposure data, such as plasma concentrations, are also primary variables required to demonstrate safety, tolerability and efficacy.

In principle, the choice of the primary variable often relies on experience gained either in earlier studies or in the published literature, which shows whether or not a given variable is reliable and validated. This requirement, however, cannot be met in many paediatric indications due to the lack of experience with randomised clinical trials or clinical understanding of disease. The issue becomes evident in areas for which only subjective clinical scales or health outcome measures are available. Many subjective questions may not be easily extrapolated to the context of a young child or an infant, who may not even be able to understand such questions properly. This situation imposes an open dialogue between investigators, clinical research scientists and regulatory agencies about the validity and acceptance of certain endpoints as proof of safety and efficacy for the purposes of a regulatory submission. Another important problem related to the validation of endpoints is the choice for alternatives where extrapolation is not possible. For instance, whilst FEV 1 is undoubtedly an ideal measure of efficacy for asthma, this endpoint is not reliably measurable in children under the age of 3.

In many cases, assessment of clinical outcome may not be straightforward and should be carefully defined. For example, it is inadequate to specify mortality as a primary endpoint without specifying whether proportions alive at fixed points in time or distributions of survival times over a specified interval will be compared. Similarly, when the endpoint is a recurring event, the measure of treatment effect may be defined in different ways, such as any occurrence during a specified interval, time to first occurrence, and rate of occurrence (events per time units of observation). The assessment of functional status over time in studying treatment for chronic disease presents other challenges in selection of the primary variable. There are many possible approaches, such as comparisons of the assessments done at the beginning and end of the interval of observation, comparisons of slopes calculated from all assessments throughout the interval, comparisons of the proportions of subjects exceeding or declining beyond a specified threshold, or comparisons based on methods for repeated measures data. Whatever the choice is, it is critical to specify in the protocol the precise definition of the primary variable as it will be used in the statistical analysis, including the clinical relevance and associated measurement procedures. These procedures may differ considerably from the adult population and should be highlighted in the protocol.

Secondary endpoints are either supportive measurements related to the primary objective or measurements of effects related to the secondary objectives. The correlation between primary and secondary endpoints in the paediatric population may not resemble findings in adults.

Pre-definition and explanation of the relative importance and roles of secondary endpoints is essential for the interpretation of trial results. They are not important for the sample size calculation, but may influence the study design, the planning of patient visits, sample collection and statistical considerations.

## Dosing Rationale

### Evidence for Safety and Tolerability

It is essential to consider whether the necessary pre-clinical toxicology studies in animals have been performed and whether evidence is available for efficacy and safety in adults. Depending on available evidence, staggering or stratification of the study population may be required (grouping by age, weight or any other relevant physiological variable).

### Concentration-Effect Relationships

Dose selection for the paediatric indication must be based on pharmacokinetic-pharmacodynamic (PK/PD) relationships. Scaling factors for size must be treated as covariates. If the disease mechanisms and the clinical endpoint do not differ from the adult population, there will be many cases in which the concentration-effect relationship will be similar in both populations. In these circumstances, bridging is the appropriate strategy for the clinical development of the paediatric indication. The rationale for dose selection should be such as to explore the exposure ranges that yield evidence of minimum and maximum clinical benefit.

If disease mechanisms are the same as in the adult population, but the endpoint is different or there is evidence for potential differences in PK/PD relationships, then doses should be evaluated that allow for characterisation of the concentration-effect curve.

### Requirements for 'Bridging'

A bridging strategy is applicable for indications for which evidence is available on the aetiology of disease and similarities in the concentration-effect relationship in the adult population. The principle underlying bridging studies is based on identifying a dosing regimen that produces drug levels in children that are equivalent to the exposure associated with efficacy in adults. Bridging approaches and adaptive designs can be implemented by modelling and simulation techniques. Such studies are cost-effective and have high informative value.

## Data Analysis and Statistical Considerations

Most statistical requirements ensure appropriate group size and frequent sampling. As previously described, the operational limitations associated with paediatric drug development impose careful consideration about data analysis prior to the start of the study. A particularly important issue is how to accurately estimate parameters of interest or draw conclusions about the statistical significance of treatment effect based on a sparse sampling or reduced group size.

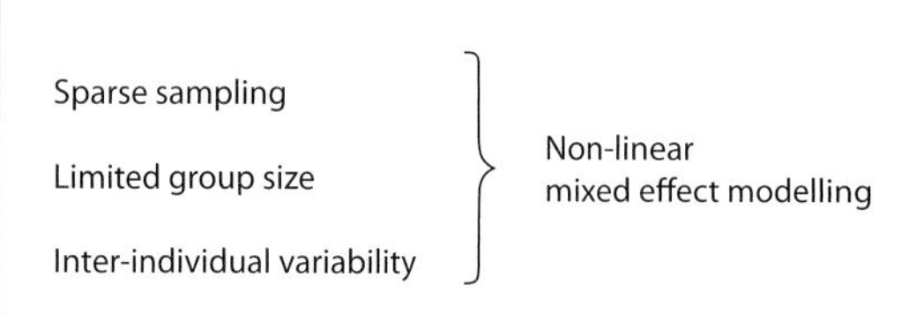


**Fig. 5.** Data analysis limitations due to small group size and sparse sampling can be overcome by the population approach. The method lends itself to the identification of the sources of inter-individual variability in pharmacokinetics and pharmacodynamics.

The methodology of choice for data analysis is the population approach, which is also known as non-linear mixed effects modelling. The population approach allows characterisation of the sources of variability in drug concentrations or treatment response among individuals receiving clinically relevant doses of a drug of interest.

The use of the population approach to evaluate drug pharmacokinetics in the paediatric population is the subject of specific guidelines from the ICH, FDA and CHMP. Despite the focus of guidelines on pharmacokinetic studies, the population approach can be extended to the assessment of pharmacokinetic-pharmacodynamic relationships and efficacy (fig. 5).

Population pharmacokinetics seeks to identify the measurable pathophysiologic factors that cause changes in the dose-concentration relationship and the extent of these changes so that, if such changes are associated with clinically significant shifts in the therapeutic index, dosage can be appropriately modified. Patient demographics, pathophysiology and other therapeutic features, such as body weight, excretory and metabolic functions, and the presence of co-medication, can regularly alter dose-concentration relationships.

Using the population pharmacokinetic approach in drug development offers the possibility of gaining integrated information on pharmacokinetics, not only from relatively sparse data obtained from study subjects, but also from relatively dense data or a combination of sparse and dense data [8–10]. The population approach allows the analysis of data from a variety of unbalanced designs as well as from studies that are normally excluded because they do not lend themselves to the usual forms of pharmacokinetic analysis.

The use of the population approach for pharmacokinetic data analysis requires special consideration to be given to the following aspects in the study design:

- Where feasible, the study population, sample size, and age distribution should be adequate, either in a single study or several studies, to provide information on all the paediatric age groups for which the drug is intended.
- If other factors affecting the pharmacokinetics of the drug are to be studied (e.g. the effect of a concomitant medication or the presence or absence of a disease), sufficient numbers of subjects with and without the factor should be included in the study.
- The sampling scheme should be carefully planned to obtain the maximum information using the minimum number of samples.
- Some knowledge of the pharmacokinetics of the drug to be investigated from previous adult or paediatric experience may be used to develop the sampling scheme.

The following covariates should ordinarily be obtained for each subject: height, weight, body surface area, gestational age and birth weight for neonates, and relevant laboratory tests that reflect the function of organs responsible for drug disposition. Concomitant and recent drug therapy should also be recorded. The relationship between these parameters and the pharmacokinetics of the drug of interest should be examined using suitable statistical techniques and study designs.

In bridging studies, when evaluating relevant pharmacokinetic and pharmacodynamic parameters, one should assess whether the estimated parameters in children originates from a different distribution, as compared to the adult or other reference population.

*Additional Considerations*

*Adolescence*

In addition to puberty itself, several clinically specific elements should be considered. As an example, growth criteria may not be useful in pubertal populations. Furthermore, since endocrinological changes occur during puberty, they might influence clinical and biochemical parameters. In this age group non-adherence is high. Therefore, psychosocial interactions are already important in the planning phase.

*Pregnancy*

In most studies, pregnancy may interfere with study medication. In phase II/III studies usually pregnancy has to be excluded before study entry and has to be controlled during the study. Common gestational problems of the study population have to be evaluated. Therefore, special consultation with paediatric gynaecological expertise is advised.

*Compliance/Adherence*

Non-compliance/adherence is of particular importance in all clinical studies. However, in the paediatric study population this depends not only on the patient but also on their parents (child caregiver). In addition, divorced parents as well as families with a single caregiver are frequent and may represent an additional risk for non-compliance. These specific situations need to be considered when planning paediatric clinical studies.

*Support from and Liaising with Paediatric Research Networks*

Many diseases in children have low incidence and prevalence. In these cases, only a multicentre trial makes recruitment of a sufficient number of patients possible. Paediatric research networks can support the realistic planning of clinical studies and help with their execution. Most subspecialties have a contact address with the Confederation of European Specialists in Paediatrics (CESP) that has changed its name to European Academy of Paediatrics (EAP). CESP/EAP is part of the European Union of Medical Specialties (UEMS) of the member countries of the European Union (EU) and the European Free Trade Association (EFTA). It is governed by the provisions of these statutes, grouping together paediatricians irrespective of background or therapeutic expertise (www.cesp-eap.org). Several national paediatric research networks have been built up In addition, there are several disease-specific networks in Europe. The first steps are undertaken by the EMA to establish a network of these paediatric research networks [11]. A complete list of all European paediatric research networks is posted on the EMA website [12].

These networks are prepared to help with strategic advice on paediatric development plans as well as with the support of executing individual studies. There is general agreement that study networks should be implemented by the European paediatric Societies. The future will show to what degree these networks will be established to perform this role.

## Conclusions

Responsibility for study and protocol design for paediatric patients require not only solid knowledge of the methodology of adult clinical trials, but also in-depth understanding of child physiology, child psychology, the social embedding of children, as well as about the way institutions that take care of children work, and many other factors. It is rare that all this knowledge can be found within a single person or organisation. Usually, it requires a dedicated team with specialists in different specialties and a dedicated leader for the entire project. The execution of the study demands close collaboration between academic researchers, industrial sponsors, and, if applicable, a dedicated clinical research organization.

## References


1 Stephenson T: How children's responses to drugs differ from adults. Br J Clin Pharmacol 2005;59:670–673.
2 Benedetti MS, Baltes EL: Drug metabolism and disposition in children. Fund Clin Pharmacol 2003;17:281–299.
3 Johnson TN, Rostami-Hodjegan A, Tucker GT: Prediction of the clearance of eleven drugs and associated variability in neonates, infants and children. Clin Pharmacokinet 2006;45:931–956.
4 Palmer CR: Ethics, data-dependent designs, and the strategy of clinical trials: time to start learning-as-we-go? Stat Methods Med Res 2002;11:381–402.
5 Holford N, Hashimoto Y, Sheiner LB: Time and theophylline concentration help explain the recovery of peak flow following acute airways obstruction: population analysis of a randomised concentration controlled trial. Clin Pharmacokinet 1993;25:506–515.
6 Giannini EH, Lovell DJ, Silverman ED, Sundel RP, Tague BL, Ruperto N: Intravenous immunoglobulin in the treatment of polyarticular juvenile rheumatoid arthritis: a phase I/II study. Pediatric Rheumatology Collaborative Study Group. J Rheumatol 1996;23:919–924.
7 Feldman B, Wang E, Willan A, Szalai JP: The randomized placebo-phase design for clinical trials. J Clin Epidemiol 2001;54:550–557.
8 Meibohm B, Läer S, Panetta JC 1st, Barrett JS: Population pharmacokinetic studies in pediatrics: issues in design and analysis. AAPS J 2005;7:E475–E487.
9 Knibbe CA, Zuideveld KP, DeJongh J, Kuks PF, Aarts LP, Danhof M: Population pharmacokinetic and pharmacodynamic modeling of propofol for long-term sedation in critically ill patients: a comparison between propofol 6% and propofol 1%. Clin Pharmacol Ther 2002;72:670–684.
10 Coad DS, Rosenberger WF: A comparison of the randomized play-the-winner rule and the triangular test for clinical trials with binary responses. Stat Med 1999;18:761–769.
11 http://www.ema.europa.eu/pdfs/conferenceflyers/Workshop_16022009/10569009en.pdf
12 http://www.ema.europa.eu/pdfs/human/paediatrics/24883409en.pdf



Oscar E. Della Pasqua, MD, PhD
Clinical Pharmacology & Discovery Medicine
GlaxoSmithKline, Stockley Park West
Uxbridge UB11 1BT (UK)
E-Mail odp72514@gsk.com

Rose K, van den Anker JN (eds): Guide to Paediatric Drug Development and Clinical Research.
Basel, Karger, 2010, pp 97–110

# Points to Consider when Planning the Collection of Blood or Tissue Samples in Clinical Trials of Investigational Medicinal Products in Children, Infants and Neonates

Daniel B. Hawcutt[a,b] · Andrew C. Rose[a] · Sabine Fuerst-Recktenwald[d] · Tony Nunn[b] · Mark A. Turner[a, c]

[a]University of Liverpool, [b]Alder Hey Children's Hospital, and [c]Liverpool Women's Hospital, Liverpool, UK; [d]F. Hoffmann-La Roche, Basel, Switzerland

## Background

This chapter describes how blood and tissue samples should be collected in paediatric and neonatal clinical trials. Practice in this area is guided by several documents including the US Food and Drug Administration (Guidance for Industry E11 Clinical investigation of medicinal products in the Pediatric population [1]), the European Union (Ethical Considerations for Clinical Trials on Medicinal Products Conducted with the Paediatric Population [2]), the European medicines agency (EMA) (Guideline on the investigation of medicinal products in the term and preterm neonate [3]) and, in the UK, the Royal College of Paediatrics and Child Health (RCPCH) (Guidelines for the ethical conduct of medical research involving children [4]). Any mention of blood tests in a trial protocol should take account of these documents.

This chapter provides some points to consider based on a representation of what constitutes a reasonable body of opinion and should not be considered as a definitive guide to practice. Practice varies between centres and across age ranges. It is essential that sponsors and their representatives have detailed discussions with paediatricians and other relevant members of the multidisciplinary team (e.g. nurses, nurse practitioners, play specialists and/or phlebotomists, depending on the type and location of patients to be recruited to the study) at every stage of the research from initial concept to ongoing monitoring. Practice can vary considerably between sites and with time. For example, sampling from a scalp vein may be appropriate in some cultural settings, but would not be appropriate in contemporary UK practice. When planning research in children, it is not sufficient to ask a few representative experts about the feasibility of a project. It is essential to make contact with clinicians at a representative number of sites where blood sampling will occur, so that study design can fit in with sampling procedures. Furthermore, it is essential to continue dialogue with all study sites during a study since circumstances and practice can change during a trial. This chapter aims to provide background information for these discussions. Institutional review boards or ethics committees may recommend different or additional recommendations in regard to blood sampling.

Similar approaches to blood sampling may apply when sampling blood from children in order to compile 'normal ranges' that are used to provide a context for clinical trials, or for research studies that are not clinical trials. If a child is having a clinically indicated blood sample, then the considerations outlined here are relevant. Blood sampling for ascertainment of immune response during immunisation studies may be warranted, but will need careful justification and adherence to best practice outlined below.

*Volumes of Blood Sampling*

Recommendations about the volumes of blood to be taken from children and neonates have been produced by a number of different bodies in Europe and the United States. The European Commission has included some guidance in the document 'Ethical Considerations for Clinical Trials on Medicinal Products Conducted with the Paediatric Population' (section 13.2) which is also included in the EMA guidance on studies in neonates (section 9.6). This states:

The following blood volume limits for sampling are recommended (although they are not evidence-based). If an investigator decides to deviate from these, this should be justified (in the protocol and application for ethical review). Per individual, the trial-related blood loss (including any losses in the manoeuvre) should not exceed 3% of the total blood volume during a period of 4 weeks and should not exceed 1% at any single time. In the rare case of simultaneous trials, the recommendation of 3% remains the maximum. The total volume of blood is estimated at 80–90 ml/kg body weight; 3% is 2.4 ml blood per kg body weight.

A US-based guideline produced by the University of Pittsburgh Institutional Review Board [5] suggests slightly different values, with a maximum single blood sample of 2.5% total blood volume and a maximum that can be taken in a 30-day period of 5% of the total blood volume. Due to the small circulating volume seen in a neonate for example, the difference in blood volume collected between the 2 protocols is actually very small. In a 4-kg infant (average weight newborn), this equates to (European) 3.2 ml for a single sample or 9.6 ml over 4 weeks or (US) 8 ml for a single sample and 16 ml over 30 days. For an 8-kg infant (e.g. a small 1-year-old girl), this equates to (European) 6.4 ml per sample or 19.2 ml over 4 weeks or (US) 16 ml for a single sample or 32 ml over 30 days.

The key point is that there is a very limited amount of blood available for testing in small children, and the values presented here are maximums not targets. When writing protocols for studies in children, investigators must consider as many ways as possible of minimising the volume to be taken. Interpretation of the various guidance documents presented here with regard to the clinical condition of the child, and potential for other blood sampling to be occurring at the same time, is a necessity. In our opinion, it would be very hard to justify a study taking the maximum recommended volumes of blood in, for example, unwell neonates who may require daily, clinically necessary, blood tests.

## Paediatric and Neonatal Blood Sampling

Blood tests in children are appropriate if there is a favourable risk-benefit balance, but investigators should always consider whether the blood test is really necessary (could the same result be achieved with salivary samples or urinalysis?). Whenever possible, collection of blood samples for clinical research should be performed at the same time as a clinically needed blood draw to avoid extra sampling procedures. Liaison with the clinical team (including paediatricians and other members of the multi-disciplinary team who may take blood, for example, nurse practitioners or phlebotomists) at the participating centres can identify these opportunities to minimise additional and unnecessary blood sampling episodes.

The risk-benefit balance will depend on factors such as how sick the child is expected to be at the time of sampling, the importance of the medication under study and the scientific need for the level of precision (e.g. how many samples are required for adequate pharmacokinetic data). This risk balance is ultimately the responsibility of the ethics committee/institutional review board, but the sponsor and investigators can profitably consider the issues in advance of ethical review. Risk to the child does not relate solely to the severity or seriousness of the condition, but can also relate to the impact of the sampling procedure on the child. For example, children who are very unwell are likely to have regular blood tests and may have venous and/or arterial access (for example, ventilated and sedated in the intensive care setting). The taking of an additional sample in conjunction with routine phlebotomy in this situation would be less distressing than for a relatively well child who needs a finger prick. For the affected child: the question of 'how' blood is taken is much more important than 'how much'. Another example comes from children or babies on extracorporeal membrane oxygenation (ECMO), where the effective circulating volume is increased considerably as part of the procedure. In this case, the sampling volume may be less critical than in other situations.

The use of population pharmacokinetics and sparse sampling based on optimal sampling theory to minimize the number of samples obtained from each patient is desirable in paediatric studies. In sparse sampling approaches (where each patient contributes as few as 2–4 observations at predetermined times), an overall 'population area-under-the-curve' can be assembled without an individual child having too many samples. Population pharmacokinetic analysis can be carried out using the most useful sampling time points derived from modelling of adult data [6].

For all children in research, it is always necessary to get the informed consent of the parent/guardian of the child. Documented assent should also be obtained for all children participating in clinical trials who are judged by the investigator to be old enough to comprehend the study. This level of understanding will depend on the age, underlying illnesses, medications taken by the child, the current clinical condition of the child participating, as well as the complexity of the study. As a general rule, school-age children who are educationally age appropriate and not taking sedative medication should be assented.

*Ethical Points to Consider with Regard to Blood Sampling*

The RCPCH statement and guidance in Eudralex indicate that blood sampling is a 'low risk' procedure that can be included in a research project if it can be justified. This justification will be required on a study-by-study basis. The criteria will depend on the importance of the medication and the reason for doing the blood test.

While it is possible to argue that a separate procedure to obtain blood is ethical for some research studies, it is preferable to obtain blood during a procedure that would otherwise happen. That is, it is better to take 'extra blood' during a routine sampling episode than have sampling episodes especially for a trial. In order to optimise the design of the trial, it is highly desirable to collaborate with the hospital that will conduct the study, since the frequency and practice of routine sampling episodes can vary from hospital to hospital.

Blood volumes should be justified in protocols. Institutional review boards or ethics committees review and may define the maximum amount of blood (usually on a ml/kg or percentage of total blood volume basis) that may be taken for investigational purposes (especially neonatal studies: see below). Parent and patient information leaflets should explain what is going to happen to the sample once it has been taken (for example being frozen for later analysis) to help delineate the difference between the research being undertaken and the routine clinical care of the child.

Samples should be taken at the same time as samples for clinical purposes whenever possible. The clinical sample takes precedence when blood is difficult to draw. It may be possible to use part or all of a sample retained by Pathology Departments for logistical or quality assurance purposes, so it is important to liaise closely with this department. When sampling is over and above that which occurs in routine clinical practice, the risks of any procedures must be clearly explained to the carers/child as part of the recruitment process.

*Acceptability to Children and Families*

Approval by an ethics committee does not guarantee that all families will consent to a procedure. For example, some families may consent to a trial that includes retaining extra blood during routine sampling episodes, but decline consent for extra sampling episodes.

Methodologies and sample size estimates should account for the possibility that blood samples may not be available from all children at all time points. For example, a child may not want/ allow a test to be performed on a particular occasion despite parental agreement (and if it is a research blood test and not directly affecting the child's health then it may have to be abandoned).

*Practicalities in Children Aged more than One Month*

See tables 1 and 2 for a list of possible sampling strategies in infants (1–24 months) and children

(2–18 years), respectively. In general, blood volumes should be limited and as few samples as possible should be taken (consider sparse data methods) [5]. Typically 250–500 µl of whole blood is suitable for assays involving plasma.

Finger pricks are often more acceptable to children than a venous sample (especially if a single sample is all that is required). However, if haemolysis affects analysis, a venous sample should be obtained. Larger volumes (> approximately 2 ml) are difficult to obtain from a single finger prick. Blood should only be drawn by an experienced person and the number of sampling attempts that will be acceptable should be limited to 2 or 3 in the study protocol to avoid subjecting the child to unnecessary discomfort.

Existing peripheral or central catheters should be used where present, as long as the study drug will be delivered through a separate infusion. It is crucial to not use the same catheters for infusion of the study drug and consequent blood draws for kinetic purposes. Cannulae and 'butterfly' needles can be used to reduce the need for venepuncture, but they may not be suitable for extended sampling periods. Freshly sited 24 g cannulae can be used for venous sampling for approximately 12 h after insertion if this is required for the protocol, has been approved by the ethics committee, the parents give consent and a child gives assent. Younger children may need to have butterfly needles or cannulae bandaged lightly with a small bandage (as the sight of a cannula can be upsetting for some children) and supported with a light splint (as young children may not keep a hand or foot in the correct position despite not being in discomfort). Local policy should be consulted to guide practice relating to the method of covering and managing the cannula and the frequency of observation of the cannula site when in use. All children who have a cannula or butterfly inserted for research purposes need to be attended by clinical staff with experience in the relevant age-group. It should be recognized that some children will not tolerate a cannula/butterfly for



Hawcutt · Rose · Fuerst-Recktenwald · Nunn · Turner

**Table 1.** Potential routes of blood sampling in infants (1–24 months)

| Route of sampling | Availability | Amount that can be obtained | Practical issues | Comments |
|---|---|---|---|---|
| Venous | Entire age range | 0.1–5 ml | Most commonly done using 'butterfly needle'. 23 g ('butterfly') is most appropriate for this age group. Local anaesthetic cream application should be applied 30 min (AMETOP®) or 1 h (EMLA®) prior to use. Needle (23 g) and syringe may be used for single samples, but are more difficult to use in young children as they may move around. Indwelling cannulae may be used instead of a butterfly, only if there is no alternative to multiple samples being taken in a short time frame. | In long-stay patients, the supply of veins can become limited due to repeated sampling and use for cannulae. In patients at risk of having a limited supply of veins, it may be unethical to draw blood from a vein for trial-related sampling that is not coupled with sampling for clinical purposes. When samples are obtained at the same time as clinically-indicated samples, priority must be given to samples required for clinical management. In extreme circumstances, it may not be possible to sample blood at all. In other circumstances, non-clinically required samples may not be allowed by staff or families for a period of time. Design and analytic plan must be able to take account of this possibility. |
| Finger/ heel-prick | Entire age range | 0.1–2.0 ml | Fingers are used in older infants, heels in infants who are not walking. Blood is dropped from finger/heel into bottle. Some units use petroleum jelly to enhance drop formation. This minimises the duration of the procedure and the volume of blood actually lost by the child. On the other hand, the use of petroleum jelly may affect analysis by increasing viscosity of blood or adding chemical moieties. This aspect may need formally addressing in the context of a particular trial. | In long-stay patients, the fingers/heels can become sore due to repeated sampling. In patients at high-risk of repeated sampling, it may be unethical to draw blood for trial-related sampling that is not coupled with sampling for clinical purposes. When samples are obtained at the same time as clinically-indicated samples, priority must be given to samples required for clinical management. In extreme circumstances it may not be possible to sample blood at all. In other circumstances, non-clinically required samples may not be allowed by staff or families for a period of time. Design and analytic plan must be able to take account of this possibility. |
| Paper | Entire age range | 0.1–0.3 ml | Blood is dropped from finger/heel onto paper card. | The suitability of dried blood spot testing for the investigations needed in the trial would need to be established prior to deciding on this technique and the method validated for the drug concerned |
| Peripheral arterial | During periods of critical illness | 0.1–5.0 ml | Arterial lines usually have a maintenance infusion of heparinised saline. This requires adequate flushing which can lead to infusion of significant amounts of fluid. Use of this sampling method would need a stronger justification than for other sampling routes. | Insertion of a peripheral arterial line purely for research purposes has greater risks than other forms of sampling. It is classified as high risk in the RCPCH guidelines. |

| Route of sampling | Availability | Amount that can be obtained | Practical issues | Comments |
|---|---|---|---|---|
| 'Surgical' long lines, e.g. Broviac lines | Only placed when other forms of access are impossible, or certain chronic conditions (e.g. oncology) | 0.1–5.0 ml | Painless access in those children in whom they are placed. Often sole access, so would need to establish if would get accurate drug levels if the medication is also administered by this route. | Each sampling episode introduces the risk of systemic infection. |
| Percuta-neous long lines | During periods of critical illness or times of prolonged drug administration (e.g. 2 weeks of antibiotics) | | | Cannot be used to sample blood. |
| Femoral lines | During periods of critical illness | 0.1–5.0 ml | | Each sampling episode introduces the risk of systemic infection. |

the whole of a planned period. Clinical staff will remove cannulae/butterflies if a child is unhappy with the procedure. The threshold of discomfort for removal of a cannula/butterfly will be lower in a research setting than the threshold used in clinical practice. Protocols should be planned with this in mind and make allowance for missing samples.

The volume of blood withdrawn should be minimized in paediatric studies. Use of sensitive assays for parent drugs and metabolites to decrease the volume of blood required per sample will assist in this, as will use of laboratories experienced in handling small volumes of blood for pharmacokinetic analyses and for laboratory safety studies (blood counts, clinical chemistry). On occasion, dried blood spots (20 µl of blood per spot) can support analytical techniques, with blood collected on a Guthrie card. Typically, 2 blood spots are collected at each sampling time.

Methods of transport, recovery and assay must be validated.

As for adult studies, the type of tube used for storage of blood/plasma can be very important. Some drugs are strongly adsorbed on to certain plastics. In addition, components of the plastic can contaminate samples and subsequently interfere with analytical techniques. It is therefore best to carry out preliminary work. Clearly, it is also important to confirm that different study sites are using the same sample tubes, etc.

Sponsors and investigators should be aware of the potential for non-negligent harm to arise during these procedures. For example bruising and some discomfort may arise during blood sampling even if there is no negligence. Sponsors who are not able to offer indemnity in advance for non-negligent harm (e.g. UK NHS Trusts) should ensure that this is made clear to participants during the recruitment process. Sponsors who are not

**Table 2.** Potential routes of blood sampling in children (2–18 years)

| Route of sampling | Availability | Amount that can be obtained | Practical issues | Comments |
|---|---|---|---|---|
| Venous | Entire age range | 0.1–10 ml*<br><br>*greater volumes for older ages only | Most commonly done using 'butterfly needle'. Local anaesthetic cream or 'cold spay' should be applied 30 min (AMETOP®), 1 h (EMLA®) or immediately (ethyl chloride) prior to use. Needle (23 g) and syringe may be used for single samples, but are more difficult to use in young children as they may move around. Indwelling cannulae may be used instead of a butterfly, only if there is no alternative to multiple samples being taken in a short time frame. | In long-stay patients, the supply of veins can become limited due to repeated sampling and use for cannulae. In patients at risk of having a limited supply of veins, it may be unethical to draw blood from a vein for trial-related sampling that is not coupled with sampling for clinical purposes. When samples are obtained at the same time as clinically-indicated samples, priority must be given to samples required for clinical management. In extreme circumstances it may not be possible to sample blood at all. In other circumstances, non-clinically required samples may not be allowed by staff or families for a period of time. Design and analytic plan must be able to take account of this possibility. |
| Finger-prick | Entire age range | 0.1–2 ml | Fingers are used rather than heels in these children. Blood is dropped from finger/heel into bottle. Some units use petroleum jelly to enhance drop formation. This minimises the duration of the procedure and the volume of blood actually lost by the child. On the other hand, the use of petroleum jelly may affect analysis by increasing viscosity of blood or adding chemical moieties. This aspect may need formally addressing in the context of a particular trial. | In long-stay patients, the fingers/heels can become sore due to repeated sampling. In patients at high risk of repeated sampling, it may be unethical to draw blood for trial-related sampling that is not coupled with sampling for clinical purposes. When samples are obtained at the same time as clinically-indicated samples, priority must be given to samples required for clinical management. In extreme circumstances it may not be possible to sample blood at all. In other circumstances, non-clinically required samples may not be allowed by staff or families for a period of time. Design and analytic plan must be able to take account of this possibility. |
| Paper | Entire age range | 0.1 – 0.3 ml | Blood is dropped from finger onto paper card. | The suitability of dried blood spot testing for the investigations needed in the trial would need to be established prior to deciding on this technique and the method validated for the drug concerned. |

| Route of sampling | Availability | Amount that can be obtained | Practical issues | Comments |
|---|---|---|---|---|
| Peripheral arterial | During periods of critical illness | 0.1–5.0 ml | Arterial lines usually have a maintenance infusion of heparinised saline. This requires adequate flushing which can lead to infusion of significant amounts of fluid. Use of this sampling method would need a stronger justification than for other sampling routes. | Insertion of a peripheral arterial line purely for research purposes has greater risks than other forms of sampling. It is classified as high risk in the RCPCH guidelines. |
| "Surgical" long lines, e.g. Broviac lines | Only placed when other forms of access are impossible, or certain chronic conditions (e.g. oncology) | 0.1–5.0 ml | Painless access in those children in whom they are placed. Often sole access, so would need to establish if would get accurate drug levels if the medication is also administered by this route. | Each sampling episode introduces the risk of systemic infection. |
| Percutaneous long lines | During periods of critical illness or times of prolonged drug administration (e.g. 2 weeks of antibiotics) | | | Cannot be used to sample blood |
| Femoral lines | During periods of critical illness | 0.1–5.0 ml | | Each sampling episode introduces the risk of systemic infection. |

able to offer indemnity for non-negligent harm need to ensure that consent to participation includes accepting that no compensation will be automatically be paid in the event of non-negligent harm.

*Pain Relief*

For venous samples, topical local anaesthetic should be offered to all children. Various preparations are available including EMLA® (1 h to be effective), AMETOP® (30 min to be effective) and 'Cold Spray' (ethyl chloride, effective once evaporated).

Children have preferences about whether finger prick or venous, so should be given the choice, if possible. Older children may not want AMETOP®, so cold spray or nothing should be available options. The more flexible the protocol, the greater the likelihood of success.

If anaesthesia is required, it may be possible to take samples then or to place a cannula for blood sampling at that time.

Children who are hospitalised may have an indwelling cannula that, depending on whether it is being used for drug administration, may be used to get multiple samples for kinetic studies.

Children with chronic conditions (e.g. oncology patients) may have a Broviac® line or similar permanent line inserted, which may be used to obtain multiple samples. For both cannulae and permanent access, caution must be taken if the same line is used to administer the medication under investigation as artefactually high levels may be found.

There are evidence-based approaches to minimizing the pain and distress that children experience during blood sampling procedures. These include distraction and combined cognitive-behavioural interventions [7]. If any of these techniques are mentioned in the protocol, sponsors and investigators must ensure that these techniques are available in centres at which recruitment will take place. Sponsors and investigators cannot assume that all relevant techniques will be available in all centres.

*Site of Sampling*
In order of preference, the normal sites for venous sampling:
1   antecubital vein of the arm,
2   dorsal metacarpal veins of the hand,
3   veins of the foot (some countries prefer scalp veins to foot veins, but this is not acceptable in other countries, e.g. UK).

Children may have very firm ideas about where they want the samples to be taken from, and investigators should adhere to their wishes. The more flexible the protocol, the greater the likelihood of success.

*Applicability across Different Units*
Children admitted to specialist units (e.g. oncology) can receive care in more than one hospital (e.g. chemotherapy will be given in the tertiary centre, but neutropenic sepsis may be seen at the child's local district general hospital). Data collection (including blood samples) required for a trial should be practicable at all the sites that a particular child could be transferred to.

## Additional Considerations for Neonatal Blood Sampling

The information given in the paediatric and neonatal blood sampling section above is applicable to neonatal studies, but there are additional factors to consider in this population.

Blood tests in neonates are appropriate if there is a favourable risk benefit balance and total volume of blood removed is not excessive. The risk-benefit balance will depend on factors such as how sick the child is expected to be at the time of sampling, the impact of the sampling procedure on the mental or physical state of the baby, the importance of the medication under study and the scientific need for the level of precision (e.g. how many samples are required for adequate pharmacokinetic data).

Total volume of blood is discussed in the EMA guidelines (section 9.6) [3]:

'The following blood volume limits for sampling are recommended (not evidence-based). If an investigator decides to deviate from these, this should be justified. Per individual, the trial-related blood loss (including any losses in the manoeuvre) should not exceed 3% of the total blood volume during a period of 4 weeks and should not exceed 1% at any single time. The actual situation of the neonate (sleep/activity, severity of anaemia, and haemodynamic state) must permit such blood sampling. The total volume of blood is estimated at 80–90 ml/kg body weight; 3% corresponds to about 2.4–2.7 ml blood per kg body weight'.

For a 500-gram infant, this corresponds to 0.4 ml per sample and 1.2 ml over 4 weeks.

Timing of blood samples is also discussed in the EMA guidance:

'Monitoring of actual blood loss is routinely required in preterm and term neonates. Expected blood loss is to be detailed in the trial protocol. Sampling should be performed by trained staff. The number of attempts for sampling should be limited. Techniques to minimise blood loss due to sampling should be used, and re-administration of void blood can be considered if acceptable under local healthcare provisions. Timing of sampling and number of sampling attempts should be defined in the protocol. Timing of sampling should be co-ordinated as far as possible to avoid repeat procedures and to avoid repeat sampling during the day in order to minimise pain and distress, and the risk of iatrogenic complications.'

*Practicalities*

See table 3 for a list of possible sampling strategies and when they might be relevant.

Important general points are:

- Practical issues vary between units and so the specifics in the protocol should take account of the circumstances in the units in which the sampling will take place. It is absolutely essential to involve all relevant units in the planning of sample collection.
- Statistical methodologies and sample size estimates should account for the possibility that blood samples may not be available from all infants at all time points (particularly in critically ill preterm infants).

*Pain Relief*

The pain and distress of venepuncture/capillary sampling may be reduced by comfort measures and/or sucrose/glucose. The applicability of these measures varies between situations and units. The discussion of pain relief in the protocol should be developed with the units in which the research will be done. Topical anaesthesia is not routinely used for venous procedures in preterm infants in many units. There are significant differences between best practice in older children and in neonates, particularly preterm neonates. In addition, there are differences depending on the gestational age and the chronological age of a baby. Sucrose/glucose is unlikely to be appropriate for an infant born at 24 weeks of gestation who is 2 weeks old. The same infant would benefit from sucrose when they are 12 weeks old, i.e. at 36 weeks of gestation.

*Applicability Across Different Units*

Babies admitted to neonatal units can receive care in more than one hospital. Data collection (including blood samples) required for a trial should be practicable in all the units that a particular baby could be transferred to. One example is of a trial that recruits extremely preterm infants close to birth. Such a trial may involve an end-point 3 months later when the child may be in a different hospital, or may have been discharged.

*Ethical Points to Consider with Regard to Blood Sampling*

Due to the unique issues in obtaining blood from neonates, particularly critically ill preterm babies, it is difficult to separate ethical issues from practical issues and protocol development should consider both aspects in parallel. Involvement of clinicians who will be responsible for sample collection during early stages of protocol development is essential.

The RCPCH statement and guidance in EudraLex indicates that blood sampling is a 'low risk' procedure that can be included in a research project if it can be justified. This justification will be required on a study-by-study basis. The criteria will depend on the importance of the medication and the reason for doing the blood test.

While it is possible to argue that a separate procedure to obtain blood may be ethical for some research studies (e.g. pharmacokinetics), it is preferable to obtain blood during a procedure that would otherwise happen. That is, it is better to take 'extra blood' during a routine sampling episode than have sampling episodes especially for a trial. Population pharmacokinetic approaches may obviate the need to sample blood at fixed intervals after a dose is given. These approaches will be preferred if they mean that a study-specific blood sampling episode can be avoided. In order to design the trial, it is necessary to collaborate with the units in which it will take place since the

**Table 3.** Potential routes of blood sampling in neonates (preterm to 28 days)

| Route of sampling | Availability | Amount that can be obtained | Practical issues | Comments |
|---|---|---|---|---|
| Venous | From birth onwards | 0.1–2 ml | Most commonly done using 'modified broken needle technique' (see http://www.vygon.com/document/NeoSafe.pdf relating to one supplier). Some units use an unmodified needle and allow the blood to collect in the hub of the needle where it can be collected using a separate need and syringe. 'Butterfly and syringe' is not usually used because suction pressure may cause veins to collapse and thus prevent reliable sampling [8]. Indwelling cannulae are not recommended as sources of blood because of problems obtaining adequate flushes and because suction pressure may cause veins to collapse and thus prevent reliable sampling[1]. | In long-stay patients, the supply of veins can become limited due to repeated sampling and use for cannulae. In patients at risk of having a limited supply of veins, it may be unethical to draw blood from a vein for trial-related sampling that is not coupled with sampling for clinical purposes. When samples are obtained at the same time as clinically-indicated samples, priority must be given to samples required for clinical management. In extreme circumstances it may not be possible to sample blood at all. In other circumstances, non-clinically required samples may not be allowed by staff or families for a period of time. Design and analytic plan must be able to take account of this possibility. |
| Heel-prick / "capillary" | From birth onwards | 0.1–2 ml | Blood is dropped from heel into bottle. Some units use petroleum jelly to enhance drop formation. This minimises the duration of the procedure and the volume of blood actually lost by the child. On the other hand, the use of petroleum jelly may affect analysis by increasing viscosity of blood or adding chemical moieties. This aspect may need to be formally addressed in the context of a particular trial. | In long-stay patients, the fingers/heels can become sore due to repeated sampling. In patients at high-risk of repeated sampling, it may be unethical to draw blood for trial-related sampling that is not coupled with sampling for clinical purposes. When samples are obtained at the same time as clinically indicated samples, priority must be given to samples required for clinical management. In extreme circumstances it may not be possible to sample blood at all. In other circumstances, non-clinically required samples may not be allowed by staff or families for a period of time. Design and analytic plan must be able to take account of this possibility. |
| Paper | From birth onwards | 0.1–0.3 ml | Blood is dropped from heel onto paper card. | This is done routinely as part of neonatal screening (7–10 days after birth for term babies; at various time points including 36 weeks corrected gestational age in babies born at extreme prematurity). The method must be validated for the drug concerned. |

| Route of sampling | Availability | Amount that can be obtained | Practical issues | Comments |
|---|---|---|---|---|
| Peripheral arterial | During periods of critical illness | 0.1–2.0 ml | Arterial lines usually have a maintenance infusion of heparinised saline. This requires adequate flushing which can lead to infusion of significant amounts of fluid (compared to circulating volume). This means that extra sampling episodes would need a stronger justification than for other sampling routes. | Insertion of a peripheral arterial line purely for research purposes has greater risks than other forms of sampling. It is classified as high risk in the RCPCH guidelines, and so would be not permissible in the newborn. |
| Umbilical arterial | For 2–3 days following birth if the child is critically ill | 0.1–2.0 ml | Arterial lines usually have a maintenance infusion of heparinised saline. This requires adequate flushing which can lead to infusion of significant amounts of fluid (compared to circulating volume). This means that extra sampling episodes would need a stronger justification than for other sampling routes. | Insertion of an umbilical arterial line purely for research purposes has greater risks than other forms of sampling. It is classified as high risk in the RCPCH guidelines, and so would be not permissible in the newborn. |
| Umbilical venous | For 2–3 days following birth if the child is critically ill | 0.1–2.0 ml | Umbilical venous lines are often used to administer medication. This requires adequate flushing which can lead to infusion of significant amounts of fluid (compared to circulating volume). This means that extra sampling episodes would need a stronger justification than for other sampling routes. | |
| "Surgical" long lines, e.g. Broviac lines | Only placed when other forms of access are impossible | 0.1–2.0 ml | | Each sampling episode introduces the risk of systemic infection. |
| Percutaneous long lines | | | | Cannot be used to sample blood. |
| Femoral lines | | 0.1–3.0 ml | | Similar to umbilical lines. |

[1] This is a problem specific to preterm infants and illustrates how age-specific application of guidance is required – cf. section 2.6.5 of ICH E11.

frequency of routine sampling episodes can vary from unit to unit. The clinical sample takes precedence when blood is difficult to draw. It may be possible to use part or all of a sample retained by pathology departments for logistical or quality assurance purposes, so it is important to liaise closely with this department in each participating unit.

*Acceptability to Children and Families*

Approval by an ethics committee does not guarantee that all families will consent to a procedure. For example, some families may consent to a trial that includes retaining extra blood during routine sampling episodes, but decline consent for extra sampling episodes.

Methodologies and sample size estimates should account for the possibility that blood samples may not be available from all infants at all time points.

## Tissue Sampling

Tissues sampling might occasionally be applicable in paediatric clinical trials, e.g. with liver or kidney biopsies, bone marrow aspiration, collection of fluids such as cerebral spinal fluid (CSF) or bronchial fluids, or sampling within endoscopic examinations. All these are invasive procedures that should only be used when clinically necessary and not outside standard medical care. Any sampling procedure must be done by a clinician with appropriate technical expertise and the ability to obtain a good cosmetic result. In many cases this means that a paediatric surgeon is required for tissue sampling. Samples obtained during a specific procedure must be obtained with the least trauma compatible with a reliable sample (e.g. consider whether fine needle biopsy is preferable to open biopsy).

For most of theses procedures not only analgesia (see previous chapter), but also sedation will be required (especially in young children), and safe sedation of children undergoing diagnostic and therapeutic procedures has to be ensured. If tissue sampling is not urgent, consideration should be given to combining it with any other general anaesthetic requiring procedure(s) planned. Routine clinical practice in each recruiting centre has to be evaluated as there may be significant differences between centres.

As in adult studies, it is important to liaise with relevant laboratories well in advance to ensure correct tissue handling and storage. As with all clinical research, time should be given to the participants and parents to understand the implications of participating and give fully informed consent/assent.

Non-invasive sampling procedures, such as urine and saliva collection, may suffice if the correlation with blood and/or plasma levels has been validated [8–10]. Examples include theophylline therapy in asthmatic children where both saliva and urine can be used with high reliability in pharmacokinetic research. Saliva has also been used as a non-invasive method of measuring drug concentrations, e.g. gentamicin and for collecting DNA samples in pharmacogenetic studies.

## References


1 Guidance for Industry E11 Clinical investigation of medicinal products in the pediatric population FDA ICH. http://www.fda.gov/cber/gdlns/ich-clinped.pdf
2 http://ec.europa.eu/enterprise/pharmaceuticals/eudralex/vol-10/ethical_considerations.pdf
3 http://www.ema.europa.eu/pdfs/human/paediatrics/53681008enfin.pdf
4 Guidelines for the ethical conduct of medical research involving children. Arch Dis Child 2000;82:177–182. http://adc.bmj.com/cgi/content/extract/82/2/177.
5 University of Pittsburgh Institutional Review Board, Adapted by Rhona Jack, PhD, August 2001;Children's Hospital and Regional Medical Center Laboratory, Seattle, Wash., USA. http://www.childrensmercy.org/Content/uploaded-Files/Medical_Research/Office_for_Research_Integrity/Guidelines%20for%20Blood%20Sampling.doc
6 http://www.ema.europa.eu/pdfs/human/ewp/8356105en.pdf
7 Uman LS, et al: A systematic review of randomized controlled trials examining psychological interventions for needle-related procedural pain and distress in children and adolescents: an abbreviated Cochrane Review. J Pediatr Psychol 2008;33:842–854.

8   Brown RD, Campoli-Richards D: Anti-
    microbial therapy in neonates, infants
    and children. Clin Pharmacokinet 1989;
    17(suppl 1):105–115.

9   Butler D, Kuhn R, Chandler M: Pharma-
    cokinetics of anti-infective agents in
    paediatric patients. Clin Pharmacokinet
    1994;26:374–395.

10  FDA, CDER, CBER, Draft Guidance for
    Industry, November 1998: General con-
    siderations for pediatric pharmacoki-
    netic studies for drugs and biological
    products. http://www.fda.gov/down-
    loads/Drugs/GuidanceComplianceRegu-
    latoryInformation/Guidances/
    UCM072114.pdf

Dr. Daniel B. Hawcutt
Clinical Lecturer in Paediatric Pharmacology
University of Liverpool
Alder Hey Hospital, Eaton Road
Liverpool L12 2AP (UK)
Tel. +44 151 282 4730, Fax +44 151 282 4719, E-Mail d.hawcutt@liverpool.ac.uk

   Hawcutt · Rose · Fuerst-Recktenwald · Nunn · Turner

Rose K, van den Anker JN (eds): Guide to Paediatric Drug Development and Clinical Research.
Basel, Karger, 2010, pp 111–116

# What Constitutes Adequate Strength of Evidence?

Simon Day

Roche Products Ltd., Welwyn Garden City, UK

In evaluating therapies, few would argue that the randomised, double-blind controlled clinical trial is probably the gold standard method. Of course, a trial can be performed badly or problems such as highly variable adherence to treatment schedules or extreme amounts of missing data may mean that a trial's result might not be reliable – but so too is the fate of any form of research. At least the randomised controlled clinical trial has the *potential* to provide gold standard evidence.

The purpose should not be to strive towards 'minimum' standards or cutting corners, but rather to focus on what are 'necessary' standards in different settings, in different diseases, with different therapies, different measures of success, and so on. We need to keep an open mind to appropriate methods of obtaining reliable evidence in the light of opinions such as '…the brilliant success of the randomised controlled trial has now become a form of intellectual tyranny' [1] and '… the view that randomised clinical trials are the only scientifically valid means of resolving controversies about therapies is mistaken…' [2].

## Different Types of Problems

In many forums where diseases of children and very rare diseases are being discussed, there is much overlap or confusion of thinking. Separating the thinking about problems that are separate from each other, whilst recognising problems that are associated with each other, should help set the background and so help in making progress in addressing particular problems. Figure 1 illustrates this overlap in the form of a Venn diagram. Each of the circles represents a different problem – one for diseases that are rare, one for diseases that are serious, and one for diseases that show dramatic response to treatment.

Doing clinical trials in children need not always be particularly difficult or challenging. Clearly, not all diseases in children are rare, nor are they all particularly serious. Mild-to-moderate eczema is not uncommon, nor are trials in that condition. The disease is certainly distressing (for child and carer) but in mild forms cannot be said to be serious. As with all trials in children, those in mild-to-moderate eczema should conform to the very highest ethical standards but it is usually not difficult to recruit sufficient numbers of patients, or to allocate them in a blinded fashion to alternative therapies by some suitable randomisation process. Even use of 'placebo' can be considered – particularly when placebo is, in fact, an emollient being used as the vehicle for carrying a new experimental agent. In short term trials, with appropriate allowance and availability for 'rescue medication', such a study could be acceptable. Equally, not all rare conditions are serious or life threatening.

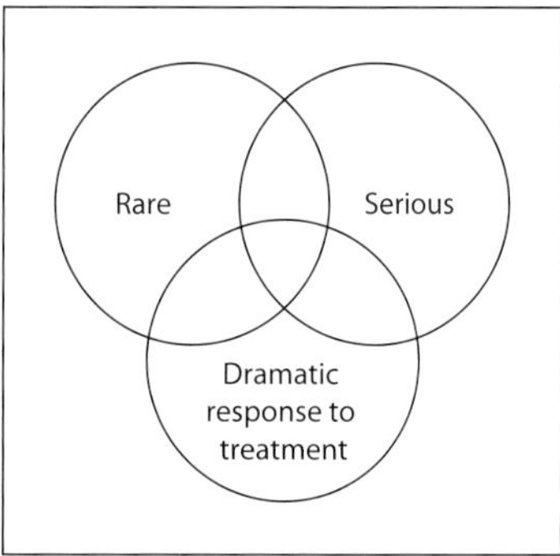



**Fig. 1.** The box represents the set of all possible diseases in children. A subset of all diseases are those that are rare, another subset represents the serious diseases, and the third are those in which dramatic treatment effects may sometimes be seen. 'Rare', 'serious' and 'dramatic effect' are, of course, all relative terms.

Of course, and unfortunately, not all serious and life-threatening diseases are rare. But from here we can learn valuable lessons, not least the fact that trials even in common conditions do not necessarily need to be large in order to be convincing. The size of a trial (if it is to be adequately 'powered') is dependent on the magnitude of the treatment effect to be detected. Treatments that have very large ('dramatic') effects typically do not need many patients to demonstrate those effects. Even in rare conditions, appropriately designed and sufficiently large (even if not always very large) trials can still be possible. The study by Eng et al. [3] of α-galactosidase A replacement therapy in Fabry's disease is an excellent example. They randomised 58 patients to either active or placebo arms. Twenty of the 29 patients in the active arm met the primary endpoint of no microvascular endothelial deposits after 20 weeks compared to none in the placebo group. Cuervo and Clarke [4] have surmised that, 'Randomised controlled trials are the best way to evaluate small to moderate effects in healthcare interventions...'. This is probably true but such trials may not be necessary – nor even necessarily the best approach – in

rare diseases where, sometimes, very substantial effects of treatment can be seen. Arguably, the study by Eng et al. [3] may have been convincing even without a placebo control group. Braiteh and Kurzrock [5] rationalise why large and dramatic treatment effects in rare diseases may not necessarily be surprising. The overlap area in figure 1 of the rare and serious diseases (as in Fabry's disease) is, of course, the most important but need not necessarily always be the most challenging.

## Arguments to Randomise

Whether in children or in adults, when no adequate treatment exists for a condition that has an inevitably fatal outcome, the argument for trying any potential treatment as a 'last resort' with 'nothing to lose' seems compelling. Here we need to contrast individual ethics and collective ethics. Collective ethics is perhaps easiest to argue first.

Patients consent to take part in trials for a variety of reasons. For many, the reasons are substantially altruistic – helping to develop medicines for patients in the future. Even when existing therapies exist, some patients are still willing to put themselves forward in this way. Altruistic attitudes of adults towards helping to develop therapies for children can be even stronger. But adults can give their own *informed* consent; children can not; and healthy children's voluntary participation in research *only* (or even *substantively only*) for altruistic reasons is not allowed at present.

If we follow the line of behaviour intended to do the greatest good for the greatest number of patients, why should we not carry out randomised controlled trials? Rarity of the condition being investigated and the ensuing inevitability of 'under-powered' studies is not an argument that can withstand much criticism. Studies of extracorporeal membrane oxygenation (ECMO) typically show mortality benefits of the order of 30 to 60% [6]. Perhaps in some special unique population, we might wish to see if we can reduce mortality rates from 80 to 60%; this would need about 100 patients in each group to have reasonable power for a significance test at the 5% significance level. Such a study size would be extremely challenging – so what are the alternatives? As the sample size in each group reduces to (say), 75, or 50, or 25, the power to detect the same size treatment benefit reduces to approximately 75, 60 and 35%, respectively. For some, such low power is their justification for using no control group. But a study with no control group has *zero* power to detect the treatment benefits we are searching for – whether the study is of 1,000 patients or 10 patients, it still has *zero* power. Worse than this, a study with no control group has zero power to detect treatment benefits of *any* size, however big. How can a study with low power be worse than one with zero power? It is easy to argue (as many have, see for example [7]) that underpowered studies are unethical. Despite this ease of argument – and the fact that counter-arguments need more careful consideration – counter-arguments can be made [8, 9].

Concern for the individual patient seemingly needs little justification – that is what a doctor should be thinking when treating every patient. Even when acting as an investigator in a randomised trial, the health of each patient must be paramount. So in an acutely serious condition with an inevitably bleak prognosis, when there is no existing therapy, what should be our approach towards a new experimental therapy? For adults, the fact that they may have 'nothing to lose' seems, superficially, to be persuasive. In the United States in November 2005, Senators Brownback and Inhofe tried to introduce the Access Act – a three-tiered system of approvals to make experimental therapies (drugs, biologics and devices) available without the need for confirmatory evidence [10], although it never became law. But there are dangers both in terms of individual and collective interests to such an access approach.

Chalmers has argued with increasing vigour [11–13] to 'randomise the first patient'. In summary his justification is that, if we do not randomise

right from the outset, then we may never get good evidence for safety and efficacy of new therapies. Instead they will come to be considered the best standard of care. It then becomes extremely difficult ever to do proper trials to test their effects and, furthermore, they can hinder the ability to carry out future trials of future experimental therapies; patients and their doctors being unwilling to risk not getting the assumed (although unproven, and in fact untested) beneficial therapy which has become the agreed best standard of care.

Whilst ever hopeful that new therapies can be discovered, at early stages of drug development the pharmaceutical and bio-tech industries' track records in developing them are rather poor. Kola and Landis [14], for example, quote attrition rates of new products between phase I studies and registration as being 89%, ranging from 80%, (the best they quote) in cardiology to a depressing 95% in oncology. In the year 2000, although 20% of products were discontinued for commercial reasons, a further 20 and 12% were discontinued for toxicology or clinical safety reasons, and 27% for lack of efficacy. Similarly, DiMasi [15] reports primary reasons for attrition being efficacy (37.6%) and safety (19.6%). In short, more than half the products initially tested in man turn out to have a *negative* benefit-risk profile. This is not saying 'no better than placebo' but rather '*worse* than placebo'. Spodick's comment [16] on Chalmers' urge to randomise the first patient is:

'[it is always possible to do a randomized trial]… in the search for a real answer, and ensures an ethical approach that gives every patient a 50–50 chance to get best treatment, that is, not to get the new medicine at a time when its precise effects and risk–benefit ratio are not understood.'

To emphasise his point, he is arguing patients deserve a 50–50 chance *not* to get the new experimental treatment. Patients deserve this chance, particularly when they are offering themselves for altruistic reasons; hard evidence tells us that more than half of all these 'hopeful' products are worse than placebo. Pushing always for early (premature) introduction of new and inadequately tested therapies can be harmful.

## Levels of Evidence and Cases where We Might Not Randomise

'Evidence-based medicine' does not always mean randomised, blinded, controlled clinical trials. As Sackett and Wennberg [17] state: 'It's time to stop squabbling over the "best" methods'. It is over 10 years since they wrote this but the insistence of randomised controlled trials seems to be growing ever stronger. It is always easy to identify problems that can (and frequently do) result from studies that have not used concurrent, randomised controls but if other types of controls are used selectively and appropriately, then reliable conclusions may still sometimes be drawn. As long ago as 1965, Bradford Hill wrote lucidly about strength of association and what indicators might help associations be identified. Although this was in the context of observational data, that – of course – is what an uncontrolled study is. These 'indicators' (my term) have been greatly misinterpreted as 'criteria' (as in 'the Bradford Hill criteria') but he never saw them as strongly as this; rather he referred to them as 'viewpoints' – which needed a good deal of careful and critical thinking to go with them:

'None of my nine viewpoints can bring indisputable evidence for or against the cause-and-effect hypothesis and none can be required as a sine qua non. What they can do, with greater or less strength, is to help to make up our minds on the fundamental question – is there any other way of explaining the set of facts before us, is there any other answer which is more likely than cause and effect?' [18].

Emphasising the need for careful, critical thinking, he wrote:

'What I do not believe – and this has been suggested – is that we can usefully lay down some hard-and-fast rules of evidence that *must* be obeyed before we accept cause and effect' [18].

The dangers of not randomising are rife, but not necessarily universal. When the natural course of disease is well characterised – and almost uniform across all patients – then this helps us to know the answer to the question 'What would have happened if... [we had not treated, or we had used placebo, or we had used current best standard of care, etc.]?' Even this characterisation may not always be sufficient. We need to know the current prognosis of patients that we might treat, not just that of their historical or otherwise contemporary counterparts. Improvement in diagnosis, for example, seems to demonstrate that patients live longer today with their disease than they used to. But, in fact, it may simply be that they live longer *post-diagnosis* then they used to. Indeed, in a long term study, we really need to know the *future* prognosis of these patients since other factors (environmental or therapeutic) may subsequently impact the course of disease (positively or negatively). Whilst including a concurrent randomised control group does nothing to ensure uniformity of prognosis, we can still make valid comparative inferences despite this. Oncology is an area that historically had very poor prognosis and in which treatments were of very limited success. But even in this area, Pocock [19] used data from a series of trials to show just how unreliably predictive historical survival data from 'the last trial' can be of survival in 'the next trial'.

Of all Bradford Hill's viewpoints, some may be more useful in developing therapies than others and, although every situation should be considered individually, table 1 presented here offers some suggestions on their relative degrees of convincingness.

## Conclusions

Evidence (not just hope or desperation) is critical to ensure good effective medicines can be made available to patients – and bad, ineffective ones are kept away from them. '...even an

**Table 1.** 'Causality' viewpoints (after Hill [18]) and how they might relate to evaluating evidence of new therapies from uncontrolled trials

| | |
|---|---|
| Strength of association | Bias in uncontrolled studies is always important to consider. Large studies (controlled or not) can be deceptive – their size does not automatically imply reliable conclusions. The well-known Scottish Lanarkshire milk experiment [21] randomised 20,000 children but failed because of failures in the randomisation. Nor do large trials guarantee any degree of 'representativeness'. The Serevent study of Castle et al. [22] recruited over 25,000 patients throughout the United Kingdom. The authors comment 'Because of the large numbers we could compare our results with events related to asthma throughout the UK'. They were misled; large samples are not necessarily representative. |
| Consistency | Again, bias can be deceptive but similar biases can sometimes be less plausible when several independent sites and independent researchers observe similar effects. |
| Specificity | Drugs (or biologics) that seem to cure multiple diseases may be less convincing than those that have very specific effects. |
| Temporality | Temporality (and whether effects happen quickly or slowly) is likely to be context and indication-dependent. Immediate and large effects, seen consistently, are likely to be highly persuasive. (The phase I trial of TGN1412 in London in 2006, although a randomised trial, need not have been so in order for the severe adverse reactions experienced by the healthy volunteers to be convincingly attributed to study drug [23].) |
| Biological gradient | This, in the context of drug development, equates to a dose-finding study; this would not constitute an uncontrolled study. |
| Plausibility | This is in danger of being akin to 'hope'. It is all too easy to develop arguments why a new treatment might work but patients deserve better than theoretical argument and speculation. |
| Coherence | Coherence is linked to plausibility and consistency. Consistent results, seen across various measures and studies all contribute to plausibility of cause and effect. |
| Experiment | This is not relevant in the context of uncontrolled studies – but does, of course, represent one of the highest levels of evidence: that of controlled trials. |
| Analogy | Although this has similarities to 'plausibility' (many of the plausibility arguments will have come from analogy), it is slightly more data and evidence-based. |

opinion held with strong conviction is not a sufficient basis for ethical action; passionate opinion does not make an incorrect opinion into a correct one' [2, 20].

The randomised, double-blind, controlled clinical trial is widely accepted as the gold standard for evaluating therapies to get that evidence. However, its robustness and conservativeness may sometimes lead to inefficiencies. Inefficient research in very rare conditions can be stifling. Inefficient research in serious and life-threatening conditions might be argued to be unethical. Unfortunately, and paradoxically, it is often only data from concurrent, randomised controls that allow us to know whether the control patients were, in fact, necessary.

Despite this, researchers faced with difficult problems of evaluating therapies, particularly in very rare conditions, should consider all options. In many situations, the randomised controlled trial will be necessary – but, at least in some situations, it is likely that it will not. Similarly, critics (journal editors, regulators, prescribers, payers, even patients) should be sufficiently open-minded to consider such evidence, when appropriate.

## References


1 Freireich EJ: Invited remarks on Levine RJ, Lebacqz KL (eds): Ethical Considerations in Clinical Trials. Clin Pharm Ther 1979;25:728–746.
2 Royall RM: Ethics and statistics in randomized clinical trials. Statist Sci 1991; 6:52–88.
3 Eng CM, Guffon N, Wilcox WR, Germain DP, Lee P, Waldek S, Caplan L, Linthorst GE, Desnick RJ: Safety and efficacy of recombinant human α-galactosidase A replacement therapy in Fabry's disease. NEJM 2001;345:9–16.
4 Cuervo LG, Clarke M: Balancing benefits and harms in health care (editorial). BMJ 2003;327:65–66.
5 Braiteh F, Kurzrock R: Uncommon tumors and exceptional therapies: paradox or paradigm? Mol Cancer Ther 2007;6:1175–1179.
6 UK Collaborative ECMO Trial Group: UK collaborative randomised trial of neonatal extracorporeal membrane oxygenation. Lancet 1996;348:75–82.
7 Halpern SD, Karlawish JHT, Berlin JA: The continuing unethical conduct of underpowered clinical trials. JAMA 2002;288:358–362.
8 MacRae KD: The value of small clinical trials. Recent Res Canc Res 1988;111: 191–194.
9 Matthews JNS: Small clinical trials: are they all bad? Statist Med 1995;14:115–126.
10 GovTrack.us. United States Senate Bill S.1956 – 109th Congress: To amend the Federal Food, Drug and Cosmetic Act to create a new three-tiered approval system for drugs, biological products, and devices that is responsive to the needs of seriously ill patients, and for other purposes. Available form http://www.govtrack.us/congress/bill.xpd?bill = s109–1956 (accessed Dec 9, 2008).
11 Chalmers TC: When should randomisation begin? Lancet 1968;i:858.
12 Chalmers TC: Randomization of the first patient: Med Clin N Am 1975;59:1035–1038.
13 Chalmers TC: Randomize the first patient! N Engl J Med 1977;296:107.
14 Kola I, Landis J: Can the pharmaceutical industry reduce attrition rates? Nat Rev Drug Disc 2004;3:711–715.
15 DiMasi JA: Risks in new drug development: approval success rates for investigational drugs. Clin Pharm Ther 2001; 69:297–307.
16 Spodick DH: Randomize the first patient: scientific, ethical, and behavioral bases. Am J Cardiol 1983;51:916–917.
17 Sackett DL, Wennberg JE: Choosing the best research design for each question. BMJ 1997;315:1636.
18 Hill AB: The environment and disease: association or causation? Proc R Soc Med 1965;58:295–300.
19 Pocock SJ: Randomised clinical trials (letter to the editor). BMJ 1977;1:1661.
20 Freund ME: Surgical research; in Greenwald RA, Ryan MK, Mulvihill JE (eds): Human Subjects Research. New York, Plenum Press, 1982, pp 169–179.
21 Student. The Lanarkshire milk experiment. Biometrika 1931;23:398–406.
22 Castle W, Fuller R, Hall J, Palmer J: Serevent nationwide surveillance study: comparison of salmeterol with salbutamol in asthmatic patients who require regular bronchodilator treatment. BMJ 1993;306:1034–1037.
23 Expert Scientific Group on Phase One Clinical Trials: Final Report. London, The Stationary Office, 2006.



Dr. Simon Day
Roche Products Ltd.
Hexagon Place, Shire Park
Welwyn Garden City, Hertfordshire, AL7 1TW (UK)
Tel. +44 1707 366409, Fax +44 1707 383145, E-Mail simon.day@Roche.com

Rose K, van den Anker JN (eds): Guide to Paediatric Drug Development and Clinical Research.
Basel, Karger, 2010, pp 117–127

# Paediatric Formulations

C. Tuleu[a] · D. Solomonidou[b] · J. Breitkreutz[c]

[a]Centre for Paediatric Pharmacy Research, The School of Pharmacy, University of London, London, UK; [b]Novartis Pharma AG,
Novartis Campus, Basel, Switzerland; [c]Heinrich-Heine-University Düsseldorf, Institute of Pharmaceutics and Biopharmaceutics,
Düsseldorf, Germany

An appropriate drug formulation is the basis of an efficient drug therapy for children and it should allow administering medicines to children accurately and safely.

If children refuse to take their medicine or if the formulation concept fails due to a paediatric particularity, the efficacy of the therapy is at risk and medication errors are probable. However, the paediatric population represent a vulnerable group and comprises a wide range of developmental levels, physiological particularities and age related abilities. Moreover, therapeutic outcomes can even be further complicated by the fact that a third contributor (parents, caregivers, nurses) is also involved.

The pharmaceutical companies are not always able to provide a formulation for a single drug substance, comprising all ages, development stages and specificities of children's health state mainly due to the unfavourable physicochemical properties of the compound itself. In addition, only limited knowledge is available on the acceptability of different dosage forms, administration volumes, dosage form size, taste, and, importantly, the acceptability and safety of formulation excipients in relation to the age and development status of the child.

As a consequence, the development of the best suitable drug products for children is a major challenge in industrial drug development. The same issue has to be carefully reflected in sponsor-independent clinical research as inappropriate drug formulations may significantly influence the outcome of the study.

One of the most important issues in the development of medicines for children is the most appropriate dosage form in relation to age. Few studies have been performed to survey the use of different formulations in children. In particular, there are concerns about the age at which young children can safely swallow conventional tablets and capsules and ability of children to swallow oral solids still appears to be based on perception rather than evidence. Whilst this has not often been examined directly in the literature, there is indirect evidence from an examination of prescriptions for different dosage forms in relation to age and anecdotal reports that children as young as 3 years can be trained to manage oral solid dosage forms for chronic illness such as leukaemia and HIV or children with developmental disorder. Suppositories may be prescribed more commonly for children <5 years whilst the prescription of dosage forms such as inhalers and topical treatments remains relatively constant in relation to age through childhood.

## Drug Administration Routes

The oral route of administration is commonly used for dosing medicinal products to children and consequently many medicines should be available in both liquid and solid oral dosage forms. The variety of different oral dosage forms available, such as solutions, syrups, suspensions, powders, granules, effervescent tablets, orodispersible tablets, chewable tablets, chewing gum, mini-tablets, innovative granules, conventional immediate release and modified release tablets and capsules, make this route extremely useful for the administration of medicines to children of a wide age range.

*Swallowability Issues*

Swallowing or deglutition occurs in three phases, controlled by 3 separate neurological mechanisms. The oral phase is voluntary. This phase of chewing and mixing with saliva produces a bolus and inhalation is automatically prevented. When it reaches the posterior wall of the pharynx, the involuntary pharyngeal phase begins as the bolus is forced into the pharynx by the tongue. The airway is closed to prevent the bolus entering the respiratory system and the tongue is retracted to prevent food re-entering the oral cavity. The oesophageal phase is also involuntary and the bolus is moved down the oesophagus by peristalsis and gravity until it reaches the stomach. There are a number of anatomical differences which contribute to young children's difficulty of swallowing solids but the development of feeding and swallowing in infants is the result of complex interactions between the developing nervous system, physiological systems and the environment that begin in the embryologic and foetal periods and

continue to take place from birth, through infancy and into early childhood. Before 4 or 5 months of age, infants possess an extrusion reflex that enables them to swallow only liquids. This is a protective mechanism where the tongue is thrust forward to prevent any non-liquid food or objects from entering the oral cavity. It coincides with the weaning period which is not dependent on only physiological, anatomical and nutritional factors. Moreover, a gag reflex of varying degrees is apparent up until about 7–9 months of age. This normal reflex is independent of swallowing as the two are independently innervated; it is caused by touch over the posterior tongue or pharynx and results in tongue protrusion, head and jaw protrusion and pharyngeal muscles contraction. Nature is performing well here as the first tooth usually appears at around 6 months of age. The complete set of 20 primary teeth (baby teeth) is usually present by the age of 2.5 years.

Hence, from birth (neonates specificity will be discussed later) liquid medicines are the only dosage form option whereas by 6 months of age children can physiologically and anatomically swallow semi-solid formulations of similar consistency (e.g. multi-particulates in soft food or beverages) although grittiness and the risk of chewing has never been investigated. The age at which they can swallow a monolithic dosage form without chewing is discussed later on.

*Peroral Liquid Formulations*

Liquid formulations include solutions, syrups, suspensions and emulsions and are most appropriate for younger children (e.g. birth to 8 years) who are unable to swallow capsules or tablets. The dose volume is a major consideration for the acceptability of a liquid formulation. Typical target dose volumes for paediatric liquid formulations are ≤ 5 ml for children under 5 years and ≤10 ml for children of 5 years and older. However, the more palatable the formulation, the higher the dose volume which will be tolerated. If taste and drug release characteristics are appropriate, solutions are preferred over suspensions due to better oral acceptance and dose uniformity. Furthermore, it is necessary for suspensions that sufficient information on the handling prior to administration is provided, i.e. need to shake the product to ensure correct dosing.

Devices for the delivery of liquid paediatric medicines should allow accurate dose measurement and simple, controlled administration. Household spoons should not be used as dose delivery devices for children's medicines. If a dosing spoon is considered to be appropriate for dose delivery, a 5-ml spoon designed and manufactured to an appropriate international, EU or national standard should be provided by the manufacturer and validated for use with the particular medicinal product. Validated measuring spoons and cups are convenient for toddlers and children who can use them without spilling but it is difficult to control administration if the child is uncooperative.

They are commonly available in a total volume of 10 ml, with and without calibration lines for lower volume, i.e. 5 and 2.5 ml. Measuring spoons and cups can be used for all liquid preparations such as suspensions and solutions. Graduated pipettes and oral syringes are particularly convenient for infants and young children who are not able to use either spoons or cups and allow accurate dose measurement and controlled administration to the buccal cavity for all ages. These dosing devices are recommended for medications with a narrow therapeutic window where accurate dosing is mandatory. Graduated pipettes intended for administration directly into the mouth must not be made of material that could break or cause damage.

Delivery of liquid medicines as a small volume measured as drops may be convenient, particularly for infants and young children. However, the accuracy of dosing depends on several factors, especially the angle at which the dropper bottle is held and the viscosity and density of the preparation.

The device selected should be appropriate to the volumes to be measured, therapeutic index of the active substance, type and taste of formulation and ease of administration in practice. Foaming after reconstitution or in use may affect the accuracy of measurement and appropriate information and warnings should be given.

To avoid the potential for error, graduations on dosing devices should only be stated in ml or fractions of a ml. If markings in other units can be justified (e.g. mg, body weight or body surface area) the device must be labelled for use with that product only.

Design and labelling of the device should enable use and should be evaluated by realistic testing procedures. Compatibility of all components of the device and labelling have to be established, as should resistance to common washing procedures. Appropriate information must be provided to the user.

*Peroral Solid Formulations*

Classical solid drug formulations comprise granules, powders, capsules and tablets. Solid oral dosage forms such as tablets and capsules can offer advantages of greater stability, high content uniformity, and accuracy of dosing and improved portability over liquid formulations. The WHO recommends the use of peroral solid formulations for children, especially in developing countries where the transport costs and the stability of the medicinal product are crucial. Palatability is rarely an issue with film and/or sugar coats used to improve taste. The primary limitation for paediatric use is that solid oral dosage forms can present significant problems for young children and adolescents who have difficulty swallowing. The age at which children can swallow intact tablets or capsules is highly dependent on the individual and the training and support that they receive from healthcare professionals and caregivers. Although pill swallowing 'training sessions' can be successful, modern solid drug preparations like multiple-unit drug carriers or rapidly dissolving formulations seem to be superior for most children.

Fast dissolving drug formulations for administration into the buccal cavity are novel attractive dosage forms for the paediatric use as they combine the major advantages of solid drug formulations, such as improved drug stability, with the easy administration and swallowing. After placing fast dissolving wafers or lyophilisates onto the tongue they dissolve within seconds and release the drug substance. The major limitation for this principle can potentially be the unpleasant taste of the drug substance.

Granules, powders and mini-tablets are mostly designed for the extemporaneous preparation of a liquid or suspension by suspending in water or mixing with food just before the application. Attention should be drawn to the drug stability in the prepared liquid preparation as drugs can rapidly degrade when getting into contact with water and food ingredients. Effervescent or fast-dissolving tablets, and chewable tablets may be considered as alternative dosage forms.

Multiple-unit preparations for paediatric use are small-sized granules, pellets or mini-tablets. With the appropriate administration technique and/or device, dose adaptation of multiple-unit systems is easy, comfortable, less risky and more exact than splitting tablets into pieces or crushing them to a powder. Modification of the release of the drug can be achieved for each unit, e.g. by film-coating. The units are marketed in a multiple-dose container together with a suitable measuring device or as single doses contained in a sachet, stick-pack and capsule or compressed to a tablet. As small-sized units can pass the pylorus in the fastened and full state of the stomach, they are able to minimize variations in bioavailability and accelerate the onset of drug action. Mini-tablets exhibit an improved size uniformity, process robustness/quality control and relative ease to coat. A recent study assessed the acceptability and suitability of 3-mm placebo mini-tablets in 2- to 6-year-olds. In the youngest children, aged 2–4 years, approximately half swallowed the mini-tablets. Above 4 years of age, children were more likely to swallow the mini-tablet than not to swallow it or chew it, irrespective of gender.

Despite the advantages mentioned beforehand, oral drug formulations exhibit some obstacles and drawbacks in paediatric use. General limitations include the lack of complete intestinal drug absorption, varying gastrointestinal transit time, and changing pH conditions along the gastrointestinal tract especially in the younger age groups. Neonates and infants up to 1 year may have pH values of the gastric fluid between 5 and 7 in the fastened state instead of the normal range of pH 1–2 and transit times of several days. Thus, cautious use of enteric-coated formulations is requested in these subpopulations. As the gastrointestinal transit time may substantially vary in neonates and infants (it may be up to one week) the use of sustained release formulations should be carefully considered and must be validated by pharmacokinetic studies.

*Buccal Formulations*

The buccal administration of drugs in children has recently gained increased interest due to novel drug dosage forms such as orodispersible tablets, oral films and lyophilisates and more palatable drug formulations. However, one should be aware that drug absorption after buccal administration is composed of transmucosal drug permeation as well as intestinal absorption after swallowing the drug-containing saliva. Hence, the pharmacokinetic profiles of a drug can vary inter-individually as well as intra-individually. Fundamental limitations associated with this mode of administration are the lack of co-operation of children and their difficulties in coordination. The risk of choking and aspiration depends on the disintegration time of the dosage form and the contemporary administered food or liquid. There are no reports in literature on the aspiration of these novel dosage forms in children yet. As anticipated, taste is one of the major determinants of mucosal contact time and is of particular importance for products especially designed for children.

## Rectal Formulations

The rectal route of administration can be used to achieve either local (e.g. laxative, anti-inflammatory) or systemic (e.g. antipyretic, analgesic, antinauseant, anticonvulsive, sedative) effects.

In paediatric, as in adult therapy, rectal dosage forms may be indicated for a number of reasons:
- The patient cannot take medications orally or the oral route is contraindicated, for example due to nausea and vomiting.
- The oral dosage form is rejected because of palatability issues.
- Immediate systemic effects are required, for example to manage repetitive epileptic seizures.
- Local effects are required, for example laxative or anti-inflammatory preparations.

However, when administering rectal preparations to paediatric patients, there is a danger of the dosage forms being expelled prematurely. In addition, concordance and compliance may be lower than for oral dosage forms, as the rectal route of administration is poorly accepted by patients and caregivers depending on age, countries and cultures. Furthermore, the bioavailability of most drugs is variable and limited after rectal administration. The rectal absorption site shows a minor absorption area, a lack of active drug transporters and a very limited fluid volume for dissolving the drug.

## Nasal Formulations

Whereas nasal preparations like drops or ointments have been widely used for years for local treatment, the nasal route provides direct access to the systemic circulation without first-pass metabolism. Administration is not easy especially with uncooperative children but the small volumes involved, rapidity of execution and feasibility at home has made it more attractive particularly for a no-needle approach to acute illnesses and/or for peptide-like drugs. The use of preservatives in nasal multiple-dose containers that may be toxic for small children has meanwhile been resolved. Due to recent progress in packaging materials and the development of novel drug delivery systems, the use of preservatives is no longer required. Aerosols with an appropriate device can avoid swallowing and dose delivery is more precise. Drugs such as benzodiazepines, fentanyl, diamorphine and ketamine have been used successfully via this route.

## Injectable Formulations

For neonates, infants, and seriously ill children the parenteral route of administration is still a perceivable alternative. The medication may be administered either intravenously, intra-muscularly, or subcutaneously. Intramuscular injections are generally painful for children so the intravenous route may be preferred if several regular injections are required. Many active substances for injection will be presented as lyophilised powders to be reconstituted before administration. Most doses for neonates, infants, and toddlers will require withdrawal of a dose volume which is less than the total volume after reconstitution. The facility to accurately measure small volumes of injections intended for newborns and young children is of particular importance. Concentrations of active substances should be such that the dosage volumes required can be measured with standard syringes and without further dilution. If dilution is required after measurement and prior to administration it must be remembered that a significant extra quantity of active drug may be contained in the hub of the syringe so appropriate instructions must be given. Failure to dilute very small volumes prior to intravenous administration or to flush them into the system may result in delays in delivering the drug or failure to deliver the whole quantity because of loss within administration apparatus.

The osmolarity of the preparation is a critical parameter. Hyperosmolar injections and extremes of pH may irritate small peripheral veins and produce thrombophlebitis and extravasation. Hypo-osmolar injections may induce haemolysis. The clinical need to reduce the fluid uptake, plasticizer desorption (e.g. phthalates) from and drug migration into the containers and catheters should also be thoroughly investigated as well as the punctuation pain or needle phobia of the child. Various needle-free injectors, spring-powered or gas driven, have been recently developed to overcome the needle phobia. However, even the administration with needle-free injectors may be painful. Additional obstacles are the more difficult handling, development and production costs by far higher than for common syringes and targeting the drug efficiently and safely into different tissues of the patients.

*Topical, Dermal and Transdermal Formulations*

As in adults, the transdermal route is restricted to a small number of appropriate active substances. Nevertheless, the stratum corneum is thin in neonates. Percutaneous absorption may be increased and systemic effects enhanced through the high body surface area to weight ratio. Moreover, throughout childhood, the varying hydration and perfusion status of the skin is a major problem that can affect drug permeation, e.g. the use of scopolamine transdermal patches had to be restricted to elderly children due to hallucinogenic reactions caused by unexpected elevated plasma concentrations. Most of the patches licensed for children are for older children (>12 years). However, some dermal patches for local and systemic pain relief are successfully used in younger children. More

recently, a methylphenidate patch for children from 6 years of age affected by ADHD and a fentanyl patch for analgesia for children from 2 years on entered the market.

*Inhalation Products*

Inhalation is a suitable way to administer active substances to the lung. It is the preferred route of administration for patients with asthma. Other diseases such as infection in cystic fibrosis can also be treated locally by inhalation. In the future, inhalation might become more important for the application of active substances for systemic treatment.

Advantages of the inhalation route over the oral route of administration include the avoidance of the hepatic first-pass metabolism. Inhalation might be an alternative route to parenteral application for systemic treatment, e.g. with peptides and proteins. Compared to the parenteral route, pain during application can be avoided.

The fraction delivered to the lung depends on several factors. One important factor is the ability of the patient to use the device correctly. Dependent on their age children will have more or less difficulties with some of the devices. Problems with the coordination of the inhalation determine the effectiveness of getting the drug into the lung. Furthermore, the low inspiration volume and the fast breathing of paediatric patients often limit the proper use of drug dosage forms for inhalation. Often the disposition of the drug in the lung is inferior compared to adolescents and adults. Appropriate inhalational devices are rare, but electronic nebulizers, facemasks and spacers may improve the uniformity of the inhaled dose.

## Manipulation of Adult Dosage Forms

The manipulation of adult medicines for paediatric use should be the last resort, but at the same time it is recognised as an unavoidable and necessary operation in many cases in order to facilitate clinical investigations in paediatric population or the treatment of children in an unlicensed or off-label manner. This section should be read in conjunction with the risks associated with the manipulation of adult medicines.

The following list of manipulations is not exhaustive, it serves chiefly to highlight practices of manipulating licensed products.

*Crushing Tablets*

The objective here is to reduce the monolithic tablet to a fine powder in which the active substance is assumed to be uniformly distributed, and which is amenable to dose reduction or to mixing in food or drink to facilitate ingestion. In the simplest situation a mortar and pestle might be used. A division of the powder might even be made by visual inspection in a domiciliary environment (obviously associated with a high risk of dosage error), or by weight, in proportion to the intended dose to be given. There is also the added risk of segregation of the active substance in the bulk powder caused by prolonged handling and vibration. In a hospital pharmacy environment, manipulations that may increase the homogeneity of the resulting 'bulk' powder might be as follows:

- Milling of the tablets in a small laboratory hammer mill. Changes in particle size may influence bioavailability. Temperature rises may increase potential for chemical degradation or solid-state transitions, particularly in the case of steroids.
- An added manipulation which frequently used in the hospital environment is the blending of powdered tablets with a lactose diluent, subsequently filled into powder papers (sachets) or hard gelatin capsules by hand or using a hand-filling machine to facilitate the preparation of batches of up to 100 or so. This manipulation requires technical skill in validation and operation.

- There is a danger that blending with lactose may be applied as a default operation when this is not relevant. For example, active substances which are primary amines (e.g. amlodipine) are more appropriately formulated to avoid lactose because of the well-known interaction and instability in the presence of such reducing sugars.
- There is also the risk that modified release tablets may be inadvertently crushed or manipulated in this way, so that their special advantageous properties are lost.

*Splitting Tablets into Segments*

From a practical point of view this seems a simple operation where the tablets are scored to facilitate such a manipulation. It relies on the assumption that the active substance will be uniformly distributed throughout the volume of the tablet. However, the potential for dosage error is more apparent with small tablets and low dosage tablets (i.e. potent drugs where the active content may be in the sub-milligram range), and increases if the tablets are not scored even when using devices for containing and cutting tablets available and used in healthcare or domiciliary settings.

New tablet geometries like the Snap-Tab$^{TM}$ principle may improve the splitting of tablets and reveal more uniform segments than conventional tablets with a breaking notch.

Some tablets should not be manipulated in this way, for example, enteric coated tablets, layered tablets (the matrix is not homogeneous) and many modified-release dosage forms; however it may be possible to manipulate some matrix forms. There are some modern techniques like drug macrocrystals, drug embeddings in hydrocolloids or pellet-containing tablets that enable the splitting of monolithic preparations into pieces without compromising the principle of modified release.

*Opening Capsules*

This is a refinement on crushing tablets, in that the manufacturer has already established a powder matrix. As in the case of crushed tablets (see above), the capsule contents might be divided by visual inspection or weight with the attendant risks, or dispersed into drink/food to facilitate ingestion. Ideally compatibility with possible/preferred administration vehicles should and would have been investigated by the originator. Modified release preparations of coated particles packed in capsules can usually be opened and dispersed in food or drink. The contents of capsules may be manipulated into powder papers or smaller capsules as above.

*Cutting Suppositories*

Again, this assumes a uniform distribution of the active substance in the suppository matrix.

Accurate adjustment of dosage is difficult in this case, since very few suppositories are presented in a convenient shape facilitating halving by simple visual inspection. Cutting along a plane of symmetry (i.e. vertically rather than horizontally) would be an obvious solution and carries less risk of dosage error but the resulting shape may not be optimal for rectal insertion. Horizontal truncation of an asymmetric or bullet shape or rounded truncated cone carries the highest risk of dose error.

*Injectable Solutions Administered by Other Routes*

Using injections for oral administration is expensive, but in general this manipulation has the least potential for dosage error since many injections are dilute aqueous solutions, non-viscous, and a dosage reduction can be obtained if necessary with a small syringe, possibly after further dilution. Powders for injection (i.e. lyophilisates) may be taken up in a suitable diluent in the normal way, prior to dose reduction.

For oral administration, unpleasant taste could be a problem and will have to be considered unless nasogastric tubes are used. However, there are a number of more significant risks.

In the case of preserved or multidose injections these may contain benzyl alcohol, propylene glycol, or other substances, or have a pH or osmolality potentially harmful to neonates or children.

Also, the stability of injection solutions may be compromised on dilution, and in the absence of reliable technical information from the original manufacturer, it should not be assumed that the stability profile of the original product will be duplicated on dilution.

Injections have sometimes been given by the pulmonary route following nebulisation. Ignorance of the precise composition of the parent (adult) formulation could pose a significant safety risk in the case of injections stabilised with sulphite-based antioxidants which may provoke bronchoconstriction.


**Neonates Specificity: Administration Routes, Dosage Forms and Excipients**

Intravenous use (commonly via peripheral, umbilical vein or 'long' peripheral lines that can be considered central veins) is frequently used in clinically unstable term and preterm neonates. Neonates may only have a small number of IV lines to administer all medicines as well as blood products, fluid maintenance and total parenteral nutrition (TPN). This may lead to compatibility issues and should be anticipated. Moreover, environmental conditions of the neonatal unit (temperature, humidity and phototherapy) may affect the stability of the medicine and should also be investigated when necessary. The use of inappropriate formulations or strengths requiring complex calculations and measurement of very small volumes or multiple dilutions commonly leads to medication errors in neonatal practice. Formulations must allow accurate measurement and administration. Moreover because of the low doses involved, adsorption to administration sets can lead to erratic dosing which may be clinically relevant. Similarly, displacement values of dry powder formulations should be taken into consideration when dosing is critical, in order to calculate appropriate volume of reconstitution and dosing. Fluid and electrolyte balance must be carefully taken into consideration (e.g. when sodium chloride is used to flush lines it may cause hypernatraemia). Isotonic solutions are preferred for better local tolerance. Special attention should be put on excipients as they may be toxic in neonates because of immature metabolism and elimination. Although not the predominant route, this is especially true with oral liquid dosage forms as they contain more excipients in type and in quantity. Preservative free sterile single use oral dosage forms is a safe approach. Interferences with enteral feeding (tubes, sucking, timing, total daily fluid intake, interaction with common formula/breast milk) have to be considered as well as pharmaceutical properties such as osmolarity, viscosity, particle size etc as the size of the tubes are small, e.g. 6 F/8 F.

Intramuscular administration, particularly in the newborn, is erratic and varies considerably especially in the first few weeks of life. This is mainly due to underdevelopment and variation in muscle blood flow. Another reason to avoid IM is that it is a very painful way to administer a drug and causes tissue damage.

In neonates, skin maturity, the higher body surface area to body mass ratio, and the more moisturized barrier facilitate skin permeation and hence systemic exposure which can increase toxicity when topical preparations are applied. Neonates even have to be protected from dermal contact with antiseptics to avoid intoxications.

Other routes of drug administration such as pulmonary, nasal or rectal drug delivery should be carefully chosen in neonates. The bioavailability of the drug may highly vary both inter- and intra-individually.

## Enabling Formulations for Clinical Trials and for the Future

In Europe under the new paediatric regulation, a paediatric investigation plan needs to be agreed on no later than by completion of the relevant human pharmacokinetic studies in adults (phase I). At this early stage of the drug development process, only very limited data are likely to be available to guide paediatric formulation development. Even final paediatric dosing may not be defined by then. In order not to delay clinical trials and expedite the overall development of the medicinal product, an 'enabling' formulation may play an important contribution. This formulation should be 'industry verified', i.e. produced under industry control using GMP processes, standards and quality assurance. Any additional manipulations at the time of dispensing or administration should also be industry verified (including stability, dose uniformity and bio-performance assessment), so that a robust product of reproducible bioavailability is delivered to the patient. These enabling formulations may be 'bridged' to a more elegant or final commercial preparation at a later stage by undertaking appropriate relative bioavailability studies, but saving another clinical development.

Development of ideal paediatric formulations can be associated with considerable challenges. Platform technologies with universal capabilities such as taste masking or modifying drug release by encapsulation or complexation may reduce development times and costs for a series of different molecules. The development of 'flexible' dosage forms that can take into account the dose variation and the preference of the paediatric patients at the point of administration may considerably simplify and accelerate the formulation development process as well as it may improve compliance and therapeutic outcome. Nevertheless, the employed techniques should not make the medicine too attractive in order to prevent accidental intoxication. There are some commercially available platforms such the Dose Sipping Technology® with a micropellet-loaded straw, the Parvulet® technology with a developing gel with coated microparticles on a spoon or molecular micro-incorporation based upon hydrophobic lipid matrices Oralance® technology. However, the proof of cost effectiveness versus treatment or compliance improvement needs to be established to justify the potentially higher costs. More guidance and evidence should be available in the future to improve and guarantee the quality of 'enabling formulations' in pharmaceutical practice.

## Conclusion

The potential impact of the formulation of a medicine is often underestimated. A survey on recent clinical trials in children clearly demonstrated that despite the recommendation of the ICH Steering Committee on the use of appropriate formulations in paediatric drug trials, detailed information on drug formulation and administration was not adequately provided in highly cited peer-reviewed journals, even where the medicines were unlicensed and had to be manipulated before administration. It is unacceptable as the problems resulting from a lack of suitably designed formulations for children can include the child not taking the medicine, inaccurate dosing with increased risk of adverse reactions by overdosing, ineffective treatment by underdosing and the use of extemporaneous formulations for children, which may exhibit poor or inconsistent bioavailability, low quality and safety. This can impair the reliability of the whole study, its validity and therefore the implementation of the treatment in clinical practice after complex, expensive and awaited clinical trials.

It is expected that now, with the appropriate attention and the speed of technical advances in pharmaceutical technology, strong progress in developing medicines adapted for children will take place over the coming years.


## References

1 Committee for Medicinal Products for Human Use (CHMP): Reflection paper: formulations of choice for the paediatric population. EMA/CHMP/PEG/194810/2005

2 Yeung WV, Wong IC: When do children convert from liquid antiretroviral to solid formulations? Pharm World Sci 2005;27:399–402.

3 Rogers B, Arvedson J: Assessment of infant oral sensorimotor and swallowing function. Ment Retard Dev Disab Res Rev 2005;11:74–82.

4 Delaney AL, Arvedson JC: Development of swallowing and feeding: prenatal through first year of life. Dev Disab Res Rev 2008;14:105–117.

5 Bowles A, Keane J, Ernest T, Clapham D, Tuleu C: On the specific aspects of gastro-intestinal transit in children. The Open Drug Delivery Journal. In press January 2010.

6 Ansel HC, Allen LV, Popovitch NG: Pharmaceutical Dosage Forms and Drug Delivery Systems, ed 7. Baltimore, Lippincott Williams & Wilkins, 1999.

7 Schirm E, Tobi H, de Vries TW, Choonara I, de Jong-van den Berg LTW: Lack of appropriate formulations of medicines for children in the community. Acta Paediatr 2003;92:1486–1489.

8 Committee on Drugs: Inaccuracies in administering liquid medication. Pediatrics 1975;56:327–328.

9 Litovitz T: Implication of dispensing cups in dosing errors and pediatric poisonings: a report from the American Association of Poison Control Centers. Ann Pharmac 1992;26:917–918.

10 McKenzie M: Administration of oral medications to infants and young children. US Pharmacist 1981;55–65.

11 Deeks T, Nash S: Accuracy of oral liquid syringes. Pharm J 1983;231:462.

12 Monk PM, Ball PA: The accuracy of a paediatric dosing device. Aust J Hosp Pharmacy 1999;27:323–324.

13 Pugh J, Pugh CH: Accuracy of measurement of 2.5 ml dose by oral syringe and spoon. Pharm J 1994;253:168–169.

14 Griessmann K, Breitkreutz J, Schubert-Zsilavecz M, Abdel Tawab M: Dosing accuracy of measuring devices provided with antibiotic oral suspensions. Paediatr Perinat Drug Ther 2007;8:61–70.

15 World Health Organisation: Report of the Informal Expert Meeting on Dosage Forms of Medicines for Children, 2008. http://www.who.int/selection_medicines/committees/expert/17/application/paediatric/Dosage_form_report-DEC2008.pdf

16 Krause J, Breitkreutz J: Improving drug delivery in pediatric medicine. Pharm Med 2008;22:41–50.


                                      

17 Thomson SA, Tuleu C, Wong ICK, Keady S, Pitt K, Sutcliff A: Assessing the acceptability of mini-tablets for use in children aged 2–6 years old. Pediatrics 2009;123: e235–e238.

18 McElnay JC, Hughes CM: Drug delivery – buccal route. E-EPT 2002;1:800–810.

19 Bunn G: Administration of oral liquids. Pharm J 1983;231:168–169.

20 Goldman RD: Intranasal drug delivery for children with acute illness. Curr Drug Ther 2006;1:127–130.

21 Reis EC, Roth EK, Syphan JL, Tarbell SE, Holbkov R: Effective pain reduction for multiple immunization injections in young infants. Arch Paediatr Adolesc Med 2003;157:1115–1120.

22 Reis EC, Holubkov R: Vapocoolant spray is equally effective as EMLA cream in reducing immunization pain in school-age children. Pediatrics 1997;100:E5.

23 Cassidy KL, Reid GJ, McGrath PJ, Smith DJ, Brown TL, Finley GA: A randomised double-blind, placebo-controlled trial of the EMLA patch for the reduction of pain associated with intramuscular injection in four to six-year-old children. Acta Paediatr 2001;90:1329–1336.

24 Phelps SJ, Helms RA: Risk factors affecting infiltration of peripheral venous lines in infants. J Pediatr 1987;111:384–389.

25 Phelps SJ (ed): Teddy Bear Book, Pediatric Injectable Drugs, ed 6. Bethesda, American Society of Health-Systems Pharmacists, 2002.

26 Anonymous: Paediatric Injectable Therapy Guidelines. Liverpool, Royal Liverpool Children's NHS Trust, 2000.

27 Standing JF, Khaki ZF, Wong IC: Poor formulation information in published pediatric drug trials. Pediatrics 2005; 116:e559–e562.

28 Whittaker A, Currie AE, Turner MA, Field DJ, Mulla H, Pandya HC: Toxic additives in medication for preterm infants. Arch Dis Child Fetal Neonatal Ed 2009;94:F236–F240.

29 European Medicines Agency, Committee for Medicinal Products for Human Use (CHMP) and Paediatric Committee (PDCO): Guideline on the investigation of medicinal products in the term and preterm neonate. EMA/536810/2008. 2009:1–21.

30 Breitkreutz J: European perspectives on pediatric formulations. Clin Ther 2008; 30:2146–2154.

31 Hempenstall J, Tuleu C: Formulating better medicines for children. Int J Pharm 2009;379:143–145.

32 Cram A, Breitkreutz J, Desset-Brèthes S, Nunn T, Tuleu C: Challenges of developing palatable oral paediatric formulations. Int J Pharm. 2009;365:1–3.



Dr. Catherine Tuleu
Centre for Paediatric Pharmacy Research, School of Pharmacy, University of London
29–39 Brunswick Square
London WC1N 1AX (UK)
Tel. +44 2077535857, Fax +44 2077535942, E-Mail catherine.tuleu@pharmacy.ac.uk

Rose K, van den Anker JN (eds): Guide to Paediatric Drug Development and Clinical Research.
Basel, Karger, 2010, pp 128–130

# The Future of Oral Paediatric Formulations

Daniel Bar-Shalom

Department of Pharmaceutics and Analytical Chemistry, Faculty of Pharmaceutical Sciences, University of Copenhagen,
Copenhagen, Denmark

*'It is difficult to predict, in particular the future'
– Robert Storm Petersen (1882–1949). This chapter, dealing with the future, is nothing more than
an attempt to analyze the obstacles and propose
ways to overcome them to the best of the author's
knowledge and imagination. 'The best way to
predict the future is to create it' – Peter Drucker
(1909–2005).*

The US Food and Drug Administration, FDA,
in its *Guidance* on Drug *Registration* lists more
than 100 entries under *Routes of Administration*
and yet the position of The Oral Route of
Administration as the most important one remains unquestioned. This is true for the paediatric population as well.

Animals (including humans) obtain the energy
needed to sustain life from food but they need to
shield themselves from the environment by barriers, the epithelia. Therefore, 'legal' routes have developed to overcome this incongruity. Mammals
have lungs for the exchange of gases and the al-
imentary tract for the intake of food. It follows
that the oral route is the 'natural' gate for foreign
substances and that explains its popularity as the
preferred route for medicines. Conversely, mechanisms have evolved to reject potentially harmful substances involving all senses, primarily taste
and smell but all five are involved (and, let us re-
member, drugs are poisons).

The control over the swallowing reflex is transferred back and forth between the voluntary and
the involuntary nervous systems many times before the bolus finally passes the throat. An adult
may overcome the innate reluctance to swallow a
bitter pill by forcing repeated swallows, small children (and cats and dogs for that matter) cannot
make that 'educated decision'. The senses of smell
and taste involve different receptors with different
binding coefficients, taste and smell are the integration of the action of the individual components
on individual receptors. The binding coefficients
of different components to different receptors are
specific and vary from case to case. In other words,
the perception of taste and smell changes over
time. Bitter taste usually 'lingers' longer than other
tastes ('aftertaste'). This may explain why 'masking'
a taste by adding other tastes is very difficult (if not
impossible). Arguably, the only solution may be
encapsulation to render the taste imperceptible.

It is not only the taste and smell that matters,
humans are 'creatures of habits' and when it comes
to food, children even more so. It is difficult to introduce children to novel foods and the younger
the child, the worse. Neonates-infants up to the
age of 6 months are used to suck more or less thick
liquids, from 6 months to 5 years of age, the semi-
solid form is the most accepted consistency. Some
children requiring chronic drug administration

might be trained to swallow pills or capsules at a very young age but even then the occasional user remains a problem.

At the beginning of this century, the typical paediatric oral product is an overly sweet, intensely flavoured liquid, the syrup. The syrup as a concept suffers from the fact that children older than 6 months are not used to taking liquids with a spoon and from the above mentioned taste and smell issues.

To make matters worse, there is a clear dichotomy of needs: 'Healthy' children occasionally need medicine, often antibiotics and maybe an antipyretic and cough medicine. Fixed-dose formulations are fine here. Other children may need chronic medication as in asthma, allergy and other disorders typically treated with one or two agents where fixed doses are appropriate. In contrast, a significant minority of children require individualized doses of multiple agents, notably cardiovascular and neoplastic disorders (and complicated asthma).

An overlooked factor in this context is cost. The vast majority of drugs dispensed to children are generics, out of patent drugs and, perversely, the poorer the population the more the children require (and would benefit from) medicines. The obvious way out of this is either to find cheap and effective solutions or give the industry incentives to introduce better formulations.


## Emerging Concepts

Prompted by legislation and by consumer demand for better dosage forms for the paediatric population, the pharmaceutical industry is actively trying to improve the situation. Creativity is beginning to show its impact.


## ElixSure

Liquids are not well accepted by children older than 6 months old, gels are better accepted but difficult to measure. ElixSure (Taro Pharmaceutical Industries, Israel) is a very thixotropic gel. When vigorously shaken, its viscosity decreases, allowing pouring and measuring. After a few seconds on the spoon, the viscosity increases to that of a gel making it more acceptable. At the time of this writing, ElixSure is employed as a vehicle where the medication is dissolved and the taste masked by sweeteners and flavours.


## SIP Technology

In the SIP Technology (Grünenthal Group, Germany), the drinking straw contains the already premeasured dose as dry medication in the form of coated taste-masked granules. When the patient sucks a beverage of choice through it, he/she takes the medicine almost without noticing.


## Parvulet

The Parvulet technology (Egalet a/s, Denmark) affords a microencapsulated drug mixed with a granulate, the mixture is typically glued as a thin layer to a spoon. Once the spoon is filled with water, the granulate swells within seconds into a pudding-like mass which is mildly flavoured and sweetened. The microencapsulate is dispersed and, being under 200 µm in size, undetectable to the sense of touch (in the mouth). Losan Pharma, Germany, has developed a similar concept where the swelling material is coated on the drug rather than as a separated granulate.


## Automated Magisterial Formulation Device for Paediatric Use

As mentioned above, there is a need for a dosage form for individualized, multiple agent therapy. Researchers at the Faculty of Pharmaceutical Sciences, University of Copenhagen, Denmark, have reasoned that, since there is a need for encapsulation for taste masking, the encapsulation can be used to prevent physico-chemical interactions between substances present in the same dosage unit and that that, coupled with a dispensing robot to ensure accuracy, may address the needs of children requiring combinations of drugs.

## Conclusion

After many years of relative stagnation, there seems to be a flurry of activity in this neglected field. It is natural to assume that the more the oral dosage form resembles children's food, the more acceptable it will be to children. The food industry has a large as yet untapped pool of knowledge and solutions which can provide valuable inspiration. *The* universal solution may be readily available, or *the* universal solution may not exist at all, and different approaches might be developed for different challenges. As usual, it is nice to speculate about the future but impossible to predict it. We can, however, be sure that cost-consciousness will play an increasing role in the assessment of new technical approaches.

Daniel Bar-Shalom, Associate Professor
Department of Pharmaceutics and Analytical Chemistry, Faculty of Pharmaceutical Sciences
University of Copenhagen, Universitetsparken 2
DK–2100 Copenhagen Ø (Denmark)
Tel. +45 35 33 63 51, Fax +45 35 33 60 01, E-Mail dbs@farma.ku.dk

Rose K, van den Anker JN (eds): Guide to Paediatric Drug Development and Clinical Research.
Basel, Karger, 2010, pp 131–137

# Paediatric Pharmacovigilance in Clinical Research and Drug Development

Dirk Mentzer[a] · Simon Day[b]

[a]Paul-Ehrlich-Institut, Langen, Germany; [b]Roche Products Ltd., Welwyn Garden City, UK

The paediatric population comprises a large spectrum of different physiologies reflecting the enormously dynamic period starting with the foetal and embryonic phase, through birth and infancy, up to puberty and adolescence. This makes children very vulnerable to adverse drug reactions (ADRs).

A large number of diseases occurring in the growing and maturating paediatric subgroups are not seen in the adult population and yet treatment with medicines in children should be based on equal specific pharmacological principles. Hence, as well as research and drug development, the safety monitoring of medicine used in children is very important so that children can receive the same high quality standards of drug treatment and monitoring as do adults. Once a medicine becomes available on the market for adults, it is possible to use it in children in an 'off-label' way. Such medicines may even be recommended in established paediatric treatment guidelines. Thus, the use of unlicensed and off-label medicines for children has been a common practice for decades but it does not based on the same standards of evidence of efficacy and safety of medicines as for adults. This has resulted from a common practice: that systematic drug development, like conducting clinical trials in the paediatric population, was rarely performed. Consequently, children are regularly treated with medicines which were neither studied nor licensed for this age group [1].

An additional difficulty is that a number of distinct age groups, each of which is of relevance within the target paediatric population, have to be considered for each drug being developed. Taking these points into consideration, the International Conference on Harmonisation (ICH) has agreed to a classification of the paediatric population [2, 3].

The lack of information from systematic drug development and clinical trials has been claimed to be responsible for some complications and difficulties following treatment in the paediatric population. In most cases it has been related to missing information on the right dose and appropriate formulation [4]. These deficiencies need to be reflected according to each of the different age subpopulations when addressing different pharmacological and pathophysiological specialties of the paediatric population in order to strive towards safer medicines for children.

Most importantly, the age related physiological aspects should not only be considered when conducting clinical trials in the paediatric population, but they are also very important for the monitoring of the safety aspect of the product once used in children [5, 6].

Medicines of major clinical importance, even essential medicines, are not readily tested and labelled in children, especially not in the very young child. Conducting, analysing, and interpreting clinical trials within the paediatric population may at times be constrained by the low prevalence of the disease and varying degrees of phenotype (e.g. neurometabolic disease) particularly if there is little knowledge about the validity of laboratory parameters and the value of diagnostic and clinical endpoints for measuring benefit, which also could be essential to define potential risks. Today's standards of clinical drug development required sponsors to conduct large clinical trials but for paediatric development, clinical trials enrolling several hundred patients may not be practical or possible. However, the implementation of paediatric clinical trials may be essential, especially pharmacokinetic and pharmacodynamic studies. In this respect, efficacy and safety studies in the target population may also be necessary if information from adult studies cannot be extrapolated for this purpose.

**Safety and Age Appropriate Formulation**

The lack of reliable pharmacokinetic and pharmacodynamic data in paediatric populations is associated with particular problems commonly demonstrated in safety concerns seen with off-label use. Incorrect dosing, under- as well as over-dosing, and consequently the use of products with improvised formulations of less well controlled quality or inappropriate drug concentration are known to be responsible for adverse drug reactions [7, 8]. Where unlicensed and off-label paediatric use is common, it is important for both the marketing authorisation holder and the regulatory authorities to monitor for any consequential safety concerns and to take appropriate measures to address them in, for example, periodic safety update reports (PSURs).

Since the implementation of the EU Paediatric Regulation 1901/2006 (EU) in January 2007, the approach to clinical development of medicines for children has changed significantly. The assessment of safety of medicines in the paediatric population has been specifically addressed in this regulation [9].

**Efficacy, Pharmacodynamics and Pharmacokinetics in Paediatric Pharmacovigilance**

The much higher extracellular fluid volume, especially in premature babies as compared to full-term infants, older infants or adults is an important example of the need for thorough investigation of the pharmacokinetics of drugs. Conversely, fat content is lowest in premature babies, higher in neonates and still higher in infants so this has to be considered when applying doses on a mg/kg body weight basis to achieve plasma concentrations similar to those of adults. An initial loading dose (for example) may need to be included in the treatment regimen. The dosage interval may need to be increased and the total dose decreased based on hepatic and renal function. For medicines that are cleared by the liver, they may have a longer plasma half-life and thus a longer time to reach steady state. Similarly, for medicines that are entirely eliminated through the kidney, the greater the prematurity, the less able are the kidneys to excrete drug substance and therefore the longer will be the half-life. All such relevant information should be obtained to reduce the risk of adverse drug reactions in the paediatric population.

All available efficacy data (which will typically have been evaluated during drug development using adult subjects) need to be reviewed and the available pharmacological evidence for the drug should be re-assessed focusing on the feasibility for extrapolation into the paediatric population. For the majority of drugs this extrapolation may be possible, at least for some paediatric subpopulations but – in contrast – the extrapolation of the safety data will likely be very much more difficult as the growing and maturing organs of children may react very differently.

## Pre-Authorization Paediatric Pharmacovigilance

For most medicines (for adults as well as for the paediatric population) it is almost impossible to fully investigate rare adverse reactions prior to authorisation, as to do so would necessitate exposing a very large number of subjects to the medicinal product [10]. Therefore, pharmacovigilance measures should be assessed at all stages of a product's life cycle. The major concern is for serious adverse reactions, which are often rare, and will generally not be observed in the paediatric clinical trial programme, particularly if there is a latent period before onset or a trigger such as a change in growth or development. An additional constraint is that some serious ADRs may only be diagnosed in a distinct age subgroup of the paediatric population (e.g. febrile convulsion, growth retardation).

In the case of products rarely used in the paediatric population, methods for detecting new safety signals with extensively used drugs may be much less effective. A different, more proactive, approach is needed to conduct pharmacovigilance for these types of low usage products. The use of disease databases and registries as well as active surveillance systems and enhanced reporting may be helpful to increase background information and event rates. Furthermore, specialist networks and paediatric clinical trial networks may be equally useful in this context [11, 12].

Given these limitations every opportunity should be taken to maximise the information obtained following the occurrence of an ADR during the paediatric development programme. Clinical trial protocols should set out, by category of ADR, the actions to be taken and their timing, if an ADR occurs. For example, if a serious ADR is suspected, a blood, saliva or urine sample (as appropriate) should be taken as soon as possible after the suspected event. Preferably the samples should be frozen for drug and metabolite measurement. For post-authorisation safety studies similar provisions might be appropriate, but then it needs to be understood that including such a provision in a trial protocol would disqualify it from having a non-interventional status.

Special consideration should be given to the need for long-term follow-up, for example through treatment registries, including possible effects on skeletal, neurological, behavioural, sexual and immune maturation and development. Open questions concerning long-term safety may be answered by results from additional animal studies, such as juvenile animal toxicology studies. Mutagenicity and carcinogenicity data are also important and may need further scientific investigation through juvenile animal studies [13]. However, the predictive value of such studies in terms of subsequent effects in the paediatric population is currently unknown.

## Post-Marketing Paediatric Pharmacovigilance

Childhood diseases and disorders may be qualitatively and quantitatively different from their adult counterparts. This may affect either the benefit or the risk of therapies, or both, with a resulting impact on the risk/benefit balance in the paediatric population. With regard to the collection of safety data in the paediatric population, extrapolation from data in adults is not always possible because some ADRs may only be seen in the paediatric population because of age, the maturation of organ systems (e.g. skin, airways, kidney, liver, blood-brain barrier), metabolism, growth and development. As these ADRs may be only relevant for some paediatric age groups, it is necessary that specific pharmacovigilance plans, strategies and activities should be tailored accordingly. Additional constraints for the collection of ADRs may be because children are less experienced in communicating ADRs clearly to their carers/health care professionals or may not even be aware of the adverse reactions and therefore need an enhanced pharmacovigilance approach.

In this population the susceptibility to adverse drug reactions may change throughout the patient's lifetime according to age and the stage of growth and development when treatment is initiated. This applies especially for chronic conditions, which may require long-term or even lifelong treatment. In this respect, ADRs related to the central nervous system are often of critical importance.

Given these difficulties, every opportunity should be taken to increase the information from ADR monitoring and communicate this information to the medical community and the general public. Several methods have been used to encourage and facilitate reporting by healthcare professionals in different situations, such as in-hospital settings for new products or for limited time periods. Such methods include on-line reporting of adverse events and systematic enhanced reporting of adverse events based on predefined criteria. Whilst these methods have been shown to improve, reporting the limitations of passive surveillance, especially selective reporting, is well known [11, 12]. Hence although spontaneously reported ADRs remain one of the most important sources of detecting safety signals or issues in the post-authorization period, it is still expected to be of only limited value monitoring in paediatric medicine safety, unless the notorious under-reporting among health professionals – including paediatricians – can be overcome.

Active surveillance, in contrast to passive surveillance, seeks to ascertain completely the number of adverse events via a continuous pre-organised process. An example of active surveillance is the follow-up of patients treated with a particular drug through a risk management program. In general, it is more feasible to get comprehensive data on individual ADR reports through an active surveillance system than through a passive reporting system. Elaborating surrogate parameters and indicator symptoms for adverse reactions is useful to establish specific case definitions for adverse drug reactions in children [14].

Different categories of adverse effects may need different methods for detection. Routine pharmacovigilance is predominantly based on spontaneous reporting, but other methods may be considered depending on the estimated frequency of the expected ADRs (table 1) [15].

To provide evidence-based evaluation of the relative frequency of adverse drug reactions or of the incidence associated with disease in relation to drug administration, pharmaco-epidemiological studies should be performed to validate safety signals. To establish a causal association between treatment and adverse drug reaction, cohort or case-control studies may be considered; these have been established in adult post-marketing safety studies. Epidemiological studies using patient databases have been helpful for collecting information regarding the natural (background) incidence of a specific event in the general population and may be useful for increasing knowledge of particular safety issues [16]. In the case of lifelong treatment for chronic diseases, the patient may have an increased risk of medicine toxicity and adverse reactions. In cases where the safety issue is predictable, for example based on preclinical findings, long-term follow-up registries or long-term cohort studies should be considered.

**Signal Detection**

By definition a drug safety signal may arise from a previously unrecognised safety issue, a change in the frequency or severity of a known safety issue or identification of a new at risk group. These aspects are all relevant in the paediatric population and both the Marketing Authorisation Holder and the regulatory authorities are responsible to

| Methods | Frequency of reaction | | | | | |
|---|---|---|---|---|---|---|
| | >1/10–1/100 | 1/100–1/1,000 | 1/1,000–1/5,000 | 1/5,000–1/10,000 | 1/10,000–1/50,000 | <1/50,000 |
| Spontaneous reporting (international) | + | ++ | ++ | ++ | ++ | +/– |
| Intensified monitoring | + | ++ | ++ | + | – | – |
| Prescription event monitoring | + | ++ | ++ | + | – | – |
| Case-control studies | – | + | ++ | ++ | – | – |
| Post-marketing surveillance studies | + | ++ | + | – | – | – |
| Large data resources (+ record linkage) | – | ++ | ++ | + | + | – |
| Clinical trials | ++ | + | – | – | – | – |

– = No relevance; + = possible supportive; ++ = supportive.

assure that systems and processes are in place to identify these kinds of signals.

Signal detection and data mining in the paediatric population are dependent on using appropriate detection methods used and these need to be effective for small populations and low numbers of possible cases. Enhanced data capture techniques can increase the completeness and quality of the information obtained [17, 18].

Signal detection should include appropriate stratification for the data collected based on specific needs (for example by age group or specific populations like vaccinees), as this can be helpful to increase the ability to detect signals from spontaneous databases. However, signal detection is an evolving field and the most up-to-date and suitable statistical methods should be considered based on the content of data and the size of database used [19].

The review and interpretation of results coming from signal detection analyses should be at a high and cautious level of suspicion and should have an emphasis on follow-up to obtain essential information before coming to a final conclusion. Even one case report may be enough to trigger further investigation or risk minimisation measures.

## Risk Management Plans

Data for paediatric pharmacovigilance assessments are expected to be rather limited before marketing authorization as there are limitations in pre-authorization clinical trials of medicines for paediatric use. However, the benefit-risk assessment for a medicinal therapy in any population is essential and the indication of the treatment is not appropriate without any safety data and knowledge [2]. Based on this knowledge, the application for a marketing authorisation in the EU community has to provide a Risk Management Plan (EU-RMP) as a part of the application dossier. The EU-RMP describes the available safety database, addressing the safety specification and the Pharmacovigilance Plan. The Pharmacovigilance Plan should include a paediatric section and, where appropriate, specific paediatric risk minimisation activities should be included in a risk minimisation plan. The specific paediatric proposals should be based on relevant epidemiological data regarding the prevalence of disease in the appropriate paediatric age groups. These data may come only from preclinical studies/juvenile animal studies and if appropriate these findings should be described in the safety specification, defining them as a potential risk.

The safety specification and pharmacovigilance plan should highlight areas where data are lacking (for example, where safety in the paediatric population has not been demonstrated). This should reflect duration of use and patient numbers ('exposure'), both overall and in the different age categories and indications studied. The document should highlight potential risks of using the medicine in the paediatric population and suggest both post-authorisation safety data collection mechanisms (possibly post-authorisation safety studies, or registries) and risk minimisation strategies.

## Risk Minimisation Measures

A risk minimisation plan should be in place whenever there is suggestion of a concern or potential safety concern, independent from the age related population, or where data are limited, or for other reasons identified by regulators. There should be particular emphasis on off-label use, medication errors and reports of poisoning.

Special consideration should be given to the need for long-term follow-up, for example through treatment registries, including possible effects on skeletal, neural, behavioural, sexual and immune maturation and development. Specific proposals for prospective monitoring will depend on the size of the target population and expected incidence of ADRs (if available).

If important safety information relating to off-label use becomes available, this should be included in the Summary of Product Characteristics as a standard risk minimisation measure. The reasons for a relative or absolute contraindication should also be presented in the product information so that a prescriber (and parent/carer or patient) is informed of the risk assessment of off-label use.

## Conclusion

Since the introduction of the EU paediatric regulation in January 2007, the development and the life cycle of a drug in the pre- and post-authorisation periods has change significantly. Pharmacovigilance science has traditionally been a discipline focussed on the post-marketing or post-authorisation period, albeit with due attention directed towards pre-clinical safety data, clinical trials and adverse events. As the biological sciences have evolved, pharmacovigilance has slowly shifted toward earlier, proactive consideration of the risks and potential benefits of drugs in the pre- and post-approval stages of drug development, leading to a maturing of drug safety guarded by an agreed risk management plan.

The development of drugs for the paediatric population has changed the awareness that both safety and efficacy need to be thoroughly investigated for safe treatment of children. In conjunction with the knowledge about efficacy, pharmacokinetics, pharmacodynamics and the age-appropriate formulation for the concerned drug, the impact on the objective of making available safe medicines for children will steadily improve. Under the umbrella of the proposal for safer medicines for children a joint effort is needed to carry out clinical research and appropriate drug development. Therefore, clinical trials in children need strong support from a number of stakeholders such as clinical trial networks, paediatric societies, the pharmaceutical industry and regulatory authorities.

# References


1 Kimland E, Bergman U, Lindemalm S, Bottiger Y: Drug related problems and off-label drug treatment in children as seen at a drug information centre. Eur J Pediatr 2006;166:527–532.
2 Hartford CG, Petchel KS, Mickail H, Perez-Gutthann S, McHale M, Grana JM, Marquez P: Pharmacovigilance during the pre-approval phases: an evolving pharmaceutical industry model in response to ICH E2E, CIOMS VI, FDA and EMA/CHMP risk-management guidelines. Drug Saf 2006;29:657–673.
3 International Conference on Harmonisation (ICH), 2000: Topic E 11: Clinical Investigation of Medicinal Products in the Paediatric Population. http://www.europa.ema.eu./pdfs/human/ich/271199EN.pdf
4 Nunn T, Williams J: Formulation of medicines for children. Br J Clin Pharmacol 2005;59:674–676.
5 Kearns GL, Abdel-Rahman SM, Alander SW, Blowey DL, Leeder JS, Kauffman RE: Developmental pharmacology – drug disposition, action, and therapy in infants and children. N Engl J Med 2003;349:1157–1167.
6 World Health Organization Guideline published in 2007, Promoting safety of medicines for children. www.who.int/medicines/publications/essentialmedicines/Promotion_safe_med_childrens.pdf
7 Turner S, Nunn AJ, Fielding K, Choonara I: Adverse drug reactions to unlicensed and off label drugs on paediatric wards: a prospective study. Acta Paediatr 1999;88:965–968.
8 Hören B, Montastruc JL, Lapeyre-Mestre M: Adverse drug reactions and off-label drug use in paediatric outpatients. Br J Clin Pharmacol 2002;54:665–670.
9 Regulation (EC) No 1901/2006 of the European Parliament and of the Council of 27 December 2006 on medicinal products for paediatric use. http://www.ema.europa.eu/htms/human/paediatrics/regulation.htm
10 Impicciatore P, Choonara I, Clarkson A, Provasi D, Pandolfini C, Bonati M: Incidence of adverse drug reactions in paediatric in/out-patients: a systematic review and meta-analysis of prospective studies. Br J Clin Pharmacol 2001;52:77–83.
11 Haffner S, von Laue N, Wirth S, Thürmann PA: Detecting adverse drug reactions on paediatric wards: intensified surveillance versus computerised screening of laboratory values. Drug Saf 2005;28:453–464.
12 Neubert A, Dormann H, Weiss J, et al: Are computerised monitoring systems of value to improve pharmacovigilance in paediatric patients? Eur J Clin Pharmacol 2006;62:959–965.
13 Guideline on the need for non-clinical testing in juvenile animals of pharmaceuticals for paediatric indication (EMA/CHMP/SWP/169215/2005), published 24.01.2008.
14 Wong I, Murray ML: The potential of UK clinical databases in enhancing paediatric medication research. Br J Clin Pharmacol 2005;59:750–755.
15 Meyboom RH, Egberts AC, Edwards IR, Hekster YA, de Koning FH, Gribnau FW: Principles of signal detection in pharmacovigilance. Drug Saf 1997;16:355–365.
16 Garcia Rodriguez LA, Perez Gutthann S: Use of the UK General Practice Research Database for Pharmacoepidemiology. Br J Clin Pharmacol 1998;45:419–425.
17 Bate A, Lindquist M, Edwards IR: A Bayesian neural network method for adverse drug reaction signal generation. Eur J Clin Pharmacology 1998;54:315–321.
18 Evans SJW, Waller PC, Davis S: Use of proportional reporting ratios (PRRs) for signal generation from spontaneous adverse drug reaction reports. Pharmacoepidemiol Drug Saf 2001;10:483–486.
19 Evans SJW: Stratification for spontaneous report databases. Drug Saf 2008;31:1049–1053.



Dr. med. Dirk Mentzer
Paul-Ehrlich-Institut
Paul Ehrlich Strasse 51–59
DE–63225 Langen (Germany)
Tel. +49 6103 771011, E-Mail mendi@pei.de

Rose K, van den Anker JN (eds): Guide to Paediatric Drug Development and Clinical Research.
Basel, Karger, 2010, pp 138–143

# Role of Non-Clinical Safety Assessment in Paediatric Drug Development

Luc M. De Schaepdrijver

Global Preclinical Development, Johnson and Johnson Pharmaceutical Research and Development, Beerse, Belgium

Safety data from non-clinical studies have basically the same objective with regard to supporting drug development in both paediatric and adult populations. The goals of these investigations are to identify potential target organs for toxicity and characterize the absorption, distribution, metabolism and excretion (ADME) and toxicokinetics in animals. In addition, an understanding of the dose-response relationship and of the reversibility for any identified targets, and respective safety margins relative to human exposure are assessed.

With the new regulatory environment [1–3] an increasing number of juvenile animal (including all age groups from neonatal to adolescents) toxicity studies have being conducted over the past 5–10 years to support the development of pharmaceutical or biotechnology products for paediatric use. Much like the situation for adult animal toxicity testing, juvenile animals offer the potential benefit of flagging possible safety concerns or identifying biomarkers for clinical evaluation. When considering non-clinical support of paediatrics an additional level of complexity is involved, as evaluation of the human relevance not only involves consideration of cross-species applicability of findings but also of comparative postnatal developmental stages of different organ systems. A general guide for comparative age categories between different animal species and humans with regard to central nervous system and reproductive organ development is presented in figure 1 [4].

The main objective of juvenile animal studies is to determine potential toxicities unique to immature animals, and if particular stages of postnatal development might be more sensitive or whether there are any late stage consequences when the animal matures into adulthood. In addition, these studies may assess a specific concern, reversibility, aggravation of expected findings or establish safety margins sufficient to support dosing in human paediatric populations. They may also identify age groups in which the drug should not be used or where special warnings are needed.

## Regulatory Guidance of Non-Clinical Safety Evaluations of Paediatric Drug Products

The ICH M3 guidance [3] states that 'when paediatric patients are included in clinical trials, safety data from previous adult human experience would usually represent the most relevant information and should generally be available before initiation of paediatric clinical trials'. The basic non-clinical package required to support entry into a paediatric population should include: results from repeated-

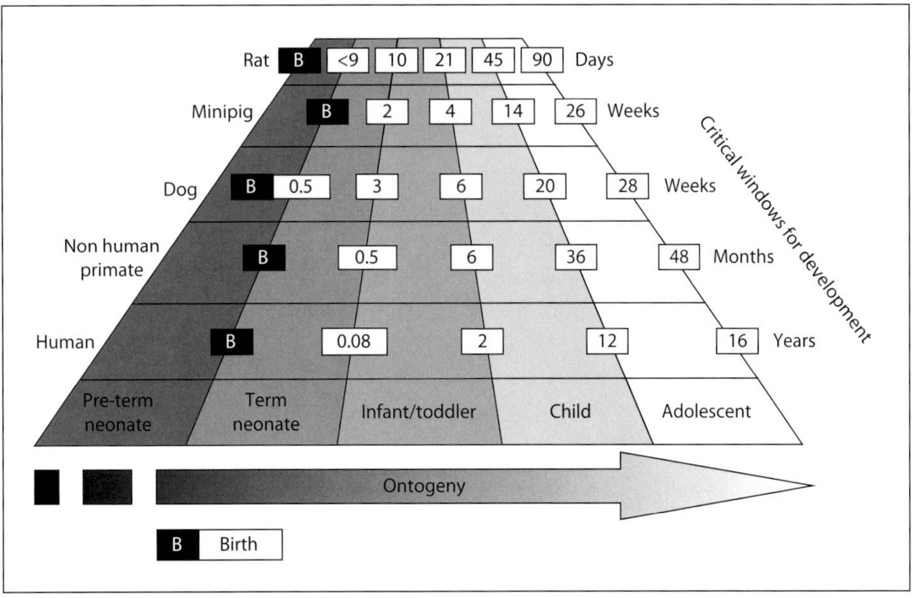

**Fig. 1.** Comparative age categories across species based on CNS and reproductive development. Estimates are based on combined general developmental events occurring in both sexes, and represent only the overall schedule for CNS and reproductive development in these species. Note that the end age of the comparative category to human infant/toddler corresponds roughly to the usual age at weaning for laboratory species. From Buelke-Sam [4], with permission.

dose toxicity studies of appropriate duration in adult animals both in an adult rodent and non-rodent species, the core safety pharmacology package, and the standard battery of genotoxicity test. Reproduction toxicity studies relevant to the age and gender of the paediatric patient populations of interest can also provide important information on direct toxic or developmental risks (e.g. fertility and pre- and post-natal developmental studies). Carcinogenicity studies may be required depending on the length of exposure in clinical. The ICH M3 guidance also states that 'the conduct of any juvenile animal toxicity studies should be considered only when previous animal data and human safety data, including effects from other drugs of the pharmacological class, are judged to be insufficient to support paediatric studies'. ICH M3 highlights that 'the appropriateness of obtaining juvenile animal study results before initiation of short-duration

multiple-dose efficacy and safety trials should be considered taking into consideration the therapeutic indication, age of the paediatric population, and safety data from adult animal and human exposure'. The age of the trial subjects in relation to the duration of the clinical study (i.e. the fraction of a developmental period of concern during which clinical study participants are exposed) being among the most important considerations. Serious irreversible adverse effects are of the utmost concern to the health authorities, e.g. those affecting organ systems with a long susceptible developmental period such as central nervous system (CNS), skeletal, reproductive and immune systems. Clearly, for a target organ with limited repair capacity, any longterm consequences of early insult during a critical developmental time window could be devastating. A conservative approach when making a risk-benefit analysis is thus warranted.

**Table 1.** Key considerations impacting the need and design of juvenile animal toxicity studies

Lowest age of study participants to be included in the clinical paediatric program (e.g. neonates, or >6 years old)
Duration of treatment (e.g. acute vs. chronic)
Pharmacology (mode of action)
Known adult target organs in adult clinical program
Known adult target organs in adult animal toxicity assessments
Identified reproductive toxicity (e.g. from pre- and post-natal toxicity study)
Pharmacokinetic and metabolism data in adult animals and humans
Species sensitivity and selection (e.g. mostly rat, dog, other species)
Route of administration
Unique formulation requirements with novel excipients
Class history of effects on developing systems

Both the US FDA [1] and the European EMA [2] have issued a guidance regarding nonclinical safety evaluation of paediatric drug products. Both documents provide valuable information regarding the role, study design and conduct, as well as potential timing of studies relative to clinical paediatric testing. Both conclude that the requirement and design should be on a case-by-case basis and only after careful consideration of all available data, the indication and the age and duration of treatment of the intended paediatric population. If a study is warranted, one relevant species, preferably a rodent, is generally considered adequate. A study in a non-rodent species – as single or as additional, i.e. second species – may be appropriate when scientifically justified. The EMA guidance emphasizes that juvenile animal studies may be useful 'to investigate findings that cannot be adequately, ethically and safely assessed in paediatric clinical trials'.

**Key Considerations Determining the Need/ Design of a Juvenile Animal Toxicity Study**

There are a number of factors that impact the design of toxicological assessment in juvenile animals and for clarity, a list of key factors is presented in table 1. All those factors determine the relevant species, the appropriate age of animals at the onset of dosing, and assessments to be performed. The ultimate goal is to treat corresponding growth phases in the animal species reflecting the temporal developmental differences versus the human. Technical considerations of the route of exposure and obtaining biological samples for toxicokinetics and clinical pathology evaluations need also to be considered. It is obvious that any knowledge obtained on an investigational drug from adult clinical and non-clinical studies also shape the assessments in juvenile animals.

A good knowledge on comparative postnatal development in animal models and humans is essential in selecting the appropriate species and study endpoints. In this perspective we refer to a series of mini-reviews covering the heart [5], lung [6], kidney [7], central nervous system (CNS) [8, 9], immune system [10], male [11] and female [12] reproductive system, the bone and postnatal growth [13]. These papers review the current knowledge of functional and/or physiological postnatal development identifying stage marks for organ system development and key physiological developmental landmarks.

In an ILSI/HESI (International Life Science Institute/Health and Environmental Sciences

Institute) workshop in 2003 which brought together academia, industry and regulatory agencies from US, EU and Japan there was clear agreement on the following [14]:

1  Whether or not juvenile animal studies should be conducted needs to be considered on a case-by-case basis.
2  Testing in a single species is generally sufficient. The rat was preferred, however, consideration of other species should be made when the rat is clearly not appropriate.
3  Studies should include a toxicokinetic or pharmacokinetic assessment.
4  Study designs including endpoints and study duration need to be based on the individual case.

Extensive adult experience might not be available before paediatric exposures (e.g. for paediatric-specific indications). In these cases, non-clinical safety/ADME data in juvenile animals carry great weight in the overall assessment of a therapeutics' paediatric safety profile.

## Conduct of a Juvenile Animal Toxicity Study

Testing in juvenile animals (in which there is direct dosing of the offspring) is intended to fill the gap between the pre- and postnatal developmental toxicity studies (in which there is an uncontrolled and generally unquantified exposure of the pup, either in utero or via mother's milk) and the adult toxicity studies [15, 16]. Also, upon initial dosing young animals may still be with their mothers and important considerations in designing any juvenile toxicity study need to take into account the potential effects on mother/offspring interactions. Juvenile animal studies are designed either to perform a first tier general screening or to assess specific concerns/aspects of function or development of a particular target organ(s). In the latter case, they have been much more informative since they are designed case-by-case to address a specific scientific question [15, 16]. With respect to the general screen approach, calling for a comprehensive 'standard design', these juvenile studies represent a marriage of repeat dose study design with parameters routinely found in the pre- and post-natal (PPN) reproductive study. So the routine toxicology parameters comprises of: in life monitoring of the animals including daily examination for signs of reaction to treatment, body weight and food consumption assessment, ophthalmoscopy, laboratory investigations (haematology, biochemistry and urinalysis, and immune function), gross and histopathological examinations of selected tissues and organ weights. In addition, the developmental parameters assessed in the PPN studies: physical and sexual developmental milestones, reflex ontogeny, general growth and development, effects on behaviour, learning and memory, and reproductive performance.

The conduct of a preliminary (dose-range-finding) study to assess tolerability and exposure in the juvenile animals is highly recommended before embarking in a comprehensive regulatory study.

## Experiences with Juvenile Animal Studies

The most common differences in sensitivity are often related to differing pharmacokinetics as a function of age. Toxicokinetic assessments often show higher systemic exposures in the immature animal versus the adult animal resulting in greater sensitivity of the former for the same dose level. A well-known example is oseltamivir (Tamiflu®) [17] which currently has a contra-indication in the label in children of less than 1 year of age because of uncertainties regarding the rate of development of the human blood-brain barrier and the unknown clinical significance of animal toxicology data for the paediatric population. The role of exposure differences is also illustrated in the following example with drug X [18]. In repeat dose toxicity studies no mortality or significant toxicity was recorded at dose levels up to 1,000 mg/kg/day in the adult rat. In the initial juvenile rat study the drug was administered to pups from days 12–25 of age at dose levels of 40, 200, 500 and 1,000 mg/kg/day. All these dose levels were associated with clinical signs and mortality after dosing on day 12. At 500 and 1,000 mg/kg, 50% deaths were observed within 24 h of the first dose. There were, however, no effects observed on the surviving pups. When a single dose of 1,000 mg/kg was administered to naïve rats on day 26, no clinical findings or mortality were observed. Following further toxicokinetic assessments, it became clear that exposure to the drug was both dose and age dependent with appreciably high plasma exposure at day 12 and showing a marked drop to adult levels between days 12 and 26. This was probably due to the maturation of the cytochrome P450 liver enzymes involved in the elimination of the drug. Rats at day 12 of age have limited metabolic capacity relative to older animals, exposures on day 26 were comparable to those obtained in adult rats. Although extensive studies were subsequently performed in juvenile animals, the toxicity observed was no different to that observed in the adult rat at comparable systemic exposures, only that these exposures were achieved at appreciably lower dose levels in the juvenile animals.

To understand the relevance of juvenile animal toxicity testing, a number of factors must be taken into consideration. These include, but are not limited to, the timing of development of specific organ systems in each species relative to human. Additionally, ontogeny of metabolism enzymes and transport proteins and their corresponding development in humans has a key role in the design and interpretation of findings from toxicology studies in juvenile animals [19].

**What Is the Value of Juvenile Animal Studies?**

An understanding of the clinical relevance of findings in juvenile animals has been demonstrated in a few cases but mostly the potential impact of findings on paediatric development programs is unclear and viewed skeptically due to insufficient understanding of the animal models used [20, 21].

Conduct of juvenile animal toxicity studies without a justified rationale (based on weight-of-evidence from accumulated data) rarely yields meaningful data for the assessment of paediatric safety. However, when a clear or scientifically based potential safety concern exists, juvenile animal studies might be valuable adjunct studies to address specific concerns or fill a data gap.

It is fair to say that up to now the pharmaceutical industry has not broadly succeeded in demonstrating added value of juvenile animal studies. Regulators have not maintained a consistent approach or clarity when requesting these studies. The case-by-case (thinking) approach has come under considerable pressure. Instead, a general screen or 'standard design' approach is now commonly being used in order to comply with the most stringent regulatory guidelines [18].

Recently initiatives were taken to investigate the value of juvenile animal toxicity studies. An exploratory survey [22] was conducted to investigate what we have learned from those studies in terms of novel toxicity and study design parameters. A new ILSI/HESI project is ongoing with the primary objective of assessing the clinical relevance of any potential findings from these juvenile animal studies. Based on data gathering from industry and FDA/EMA on juvenile animal toxicity studies conducted (e.g. study types, species used, purpose, design, outcomes,...), the impact on clinical development and label information is assessed. At present there are only a small number of drug labels that have added juvenile toxicity data (e.g. Strattera®, Tamiflu®, Neumega®). It appears that the data are added, not by default, but only if the information is relevant to safety.

In conclusion, the non-clinical science of toxicology and ADME plays an important role in paediatric drug development. Animal data can provide an initial flag of potential target organs that should result in greater scrutiny during paediatric clinical programs. It is too early to fully understand the impact of the juvenile animal data to the risk assessment for pharmaceuticals. Clearly, this is an area that requires greater understanding and research.

## Acknowledgements

Graham Bailey, Johnson and Johnson Pharmaceutical Research and Development, Beerse, Belgium; Georg Schmitt, F. Hoffmann-La Roche Ltd., Pharma Research and Development, Basel, Switzerland.

## References


1 US FDA, Center for Drug Evaluation and Research: Guidance for Industry, Nonclinical Safety Evaluation of Pediatic Drug Products. Rockville, US Department of Health and Human Services, 2006.

2 European Medicines Evaluation Agency (EMA), Committee for Human Medicinal Products (CHMP): Guideline on the Need for Non-clinical Testing in Juvenile Animals on Human Pharmaceuticals for Pediatric Indications, Draft, September 2005.

3 ICH Harmonized Tripartite Guideline: Guidance on the Non-Clinical Safety Studies for the Conduct of Human Clinical Trials and Marketing Authorization for Pharmaceuticals M3 (R2), June, 2009.

4 Buelke-Sam J: Comparative schedules of development in rats and humans: implications for developmental neurotoxicity testing. Annual Meeting of the Society of Toxicology, Salt Lake City, 2003.

5 Hew KW, Keller KA: Postnatal anatomical and functional development of the heart: a species comparison. Birth Defects Res [B] 2003;68:309–320.

6 Zoetis T, Hurtt ME: Species comparison of lung development. Birth Defects Res [B] 2003;68:121–124.

7 Zoetis T, Hurtt ME: Species comparison of anatomical and functional renal development. Birth Defects Res [B] 2003;68:111–120.

8 Wood SL, Beyer BK, Cappon GD: Species comparison of postnatal CNS development: functional measures. Birth Defects Res [B] 2003;68:391–407.

9 Watson RE, DeSesso JM, Hurtt ME, et al: Postnatal growth and morphological development of the brain: a species comparison. Birth Defects Res [B] 2006;77:471–484.

10 Holsapple MP, West LJ, Landreth KS: Species comparison of anatomical and functional immune system development. Birth Defects Res [B] 2003;68: 321–334.

11 Marty MS, Chapin RE, Parks LG, et al: Development and maturation of the male reproductive system. Birth Defects Res [B] 2003;68:125–136.

12 Beckman DA, Feuston M: Landmarks in the development of the female reproductive system. Birth Defects Res [B] 2003;68:137–143.

13 Zoetis T, Tassinari MS, Bagi C, Walthall K, et al: Species comparison of postnatal bone growth and development. Birth Defects Res [B] 2003;68:86–110.

14 Hurtt ME, Daston G, Davis-Bruno K, et al: Juvenile animal studies: testing strategy and design. Birth Defects Res [B] 2004;71:281–288.

15 De Schaepdrijver LM, Bailey GP, et al: Preclinical juvenile toxicity assessments and study designs; in Mulberg AE, Silber SS, van den Anker JN: Pediatric Drug Development: Concepts and Applications. Hoboken, Wiley, 2009.

16 Beck MJ, Padgett EL, Bowman CJ, et al: Nonclinical juvenile toxicity testing; in Hood RD (eds): Developmental and Reproductive Toxicology: A Practical Approach. Boca Raton, CRC Press, Taylor & Francis Group, 2006.

17 Freichel C, Prinssen E, Hoffmann G, Gand L, Beck M, Weiser T, Breidenbach A: Oseltamivir is devoid of specific behavioral and other central nervous system effects in juvenile rats at supratherapeutic oral doses. Int J Virol 2009;ISSN 1816–4900, 11 pp.

18 De Schaepdrijver LM, Rouan MC, Raoof A, Bailey GP, De Zwart L, Monbaliu J, Coogan TP, Lammens L, Coussement W: Real life toxicity case studies: the good, the bad and the ugly. Reprod Toxicol 2008;26:54–55.

19 De Zwart L, Scholten M, Monbaliu JG, Annaert PP, Van Houdt J, Van den Wijngaert I, De Schaepdrijver LM, Bailey GP, Coogan TP, Coussement WC, Mannens GS: The ontogeny of drug metabolizing enzymes and transporters in the rat. Reprod Toxicol 2008;26:220–230.

20 Brent RL: Utilization of juvenile animal studies to determine the human effects and risks of environmental toxicants during postnatal developmental stages. Birth Defects Res [B] 2004;71:303–320.

21 Baldrick P: Developing drugs for paediatric use: a role for juvenile animal studies? Regul Toxicol Pharmacol 2004;39:381–389.

22 Bailey GP, Dirk Marien: What have we learned from pre-clinical juvenile toxicity studies? Reprod Toxicol 2009;28:226–229.



Luc M. De Schaepdrijver, DVM, PhD, MSc
Global Preclinical Development, Johnson and Johnson Pharmaceutical Research and Development
Turnhoutseweg 30
BE–2340 Beerse (Belgium)
Tel. +32 14605062, Fax +32 14606130, E-Mail ldschaep@its.jnj.com

Rose K, van den Anker JN (eds): Guide to Paediatric Drug Development and Clinical Research.
Basel, Karger, 2010, pp 144–154

# Paediatric Critical Care

Brahm Goldstein[a] · Robert M. Nelson[b] · Simon Nadel[c]

[a]Ikaria, Inc., Clinton, N.J., University of Medicine and Dentistry of New Jersey and Robert Wood Johnson Medical School, New Brunswick, N.J., and [b]Office of Paediatric Therapeutics, Office of the Commissioner, United States Food and Drug Administration, Silver Spring, Md., USA; [c]Paediatric Intensive Care, Imperial College Healthcare NHS Trust, St. Mary's Campus, London, UK

The history of drug development for children is well documented elsewhere in this textbook. While this has been a long and difficult road for many decades, since the FDA Modernization Act (FDAMA) became law in 1997 [1], there are new initiatives and regulations that are now showing significant results in the United States, Europe and the rest of the world for developing both new drugs and obtaining important safety and efficacy information about existing drugs [1, 2].

However, there are still subpopulations of children that deserve special attention and will require out-of-the-box thinking and novel ideas if we are to progress at a similar pace as for the general paediatric population. Infants, children and adolescents all make up those patients admitted to a paediatric intensive care unit (PICU) and are an important group to consider. Many drugs used everyday in the PICU evolved without adequate study or were adopted from adult, neonatal, or anaesthesia/operating room experiences or trials. Therefore, significant risks remain associated with using these untested drugs.

Paediatric ICU patients encompass all ages and developmental stages. Most range in age from a few weeks old to 18 years. However, it is not unusual to have newborns as well as adults greater than 18 years old with histories of congenital or childhood-onset conditions that make their care difficult for adult health care providers who are not experienced with such diseases and their treatment. Some of most common diagnoses in patients admitted to the PICU include respiratory distress or failure, shock, trauma, sepsis, hypovolaemia, renal or hepatic failure, or an acute postoperative state that encompasses many of the preceding conditions. Furthermore, the absolute number of cases of these diseases occurs in only a small fraction of single PICU population. This means that expensive and difficult to perform multicenter studies are required to reach satisfactory conclusions.

Thus, given the very broad age, developmental, and disease ranges that is the norm for a PICU patient coupled with the relative infrequency of any specific disease and the difficulties and costs in carrying out multicenter clinical drug trials, it is not hard to understand why drug development for this diverse population poses such a challenge. Nonetheless, it is clear that such research is needed in order to provide the solid data that can inform effective paediatric critical care practice.

**The PICU Clinical Research Team**

The research team in most PICUs is comprised of the principal investigator, a study coordinator, one or more sub-investigators, and other members of the PICU medical staff including nurses, respiratory therapists, and clinical or research pharmacists. Bringing such a multi-disciplinary approach to a clinical trial is very important, especially so in the PICU. Close communication from study inception through the end of enrollment is vital to ensure success. The 24×7 status of PICU activity often dictates that enrollment into a clinical trial be open around the clock. This demands coordination between the PI and sub-investigators (usually all paediatric critical care physicians but may include paediatric surgeons and sub-specialists) who need to understand the intricacies of the study protocol including inclusion and exclusion criteria and study procedures. Additionally, cooperation between the study coordinator and bedside nurses and other PICU clinical personnel is vital for obtaining study related samples and recording clinical data required by the protocol. Finally, the research pharmacist must be able to prepare the study drug for administration in a timely fashion.

**CONSORT Statements and Registration of Clinical Trails**

Each PICU clinical research team member needs to be familiar with the CONSORT guidelines [3]. CONSORT stands for Consolidated Standards of Reporting Trials. The guidelines include various initiatives developed by the CONSORT Group to address problems due to inadequate reporting of randomized controlled trials (RCT). The CONSORT Statement is an evidence-based, minimum set of recommendations for reporting RCTs and standardizes the way authors prepare study reports [3]. The end result is an improved method for reporting of a RCT that allow straightforward

and transparent understanding trial design, conduct, analysis and interpretation of results [3]. The CONSORT Statement is a 22-item checklist and a flow diagram that focus on reporting how the trial was designed, analyzed, and interpreted; how subjects progressed through the trial; and is available in multiple languages for use [4].

Also as a result of FDAMA, the US National Institutes of Health (NIH), through the National Library of Medicine (NLM), developed the ClinicalTrials.gov web site in along with the U.S. Food and Drug Administration (FDA) in 1997 [5]. ClinicalTrials.gov provides current information for locating federally and privately supported clinical trials for a wide range of diseases and conditions [5]. ClinicalTrials.gov currently contains >70,000 trials sponsored by the National Institutes of Health, other federal agencies, and private industry that have been conducted in over 160 countries [5].

For trial results to be published in many leading journals, studies need to conform to CONSORT guidelines. Clinical trials of drugs and biologics subject to FDA regulation, including controlled, clinical investigations (except phase I) are required to be listed on ClinicalTrails.gov [1]. Similarly, trials of medical devices that include health outcomes studies of a product subject to FDA regulation (except small feasibility studies) are also required to be listed [1].

**Development of Drugs for Use in the PICU – Application of Preclinical and Adult Trials**

Successful translation of promising research obtained from preclinical models to the clinical arena is always a difficult and challenging proposition. Performing strictly controlled in vitro and animal experiments is vastly different from the more heterogeneous situation of a clinical trial environment. Add to this already daunting task the aforementioned broad ranges of age, developmental stage, disease factors (e.g. stage, severity, organ involvement), and other variables and the translation from bench to PICU bedside becomes even more difficult.

Nevertheless, there are a growing number of juvenile models that allow for reasonable approximation of a variety of PICU-related diseases such as sepsis, traumatic brain injury, acute lung injury, and others. Furthermore, while the PICU population is often heterogeneous and afflicted by relatively rare diseases, there are some advantages when compared to the adult ICU populations. For example, the confounding factors of old age, co-morbidities such as smoking, atherosclerosis, alcohol and drug consumptions, and others make studying a disease in previously healthy children somewhat simplified and may also make information learned from experimental models more relevant.

Examples of this include the trials involving bacterial permeability increasing protein (rBPI$_{21}$) in paediatric patients with meningococcaemia [6, 7]. By limiting enrollment to those patients with a readily diagnosed clear clinical presentation (onset of the petechial rash, fever, and signs of severe infection) and high severity of illness score on PICU admission (the Glasgow Meningococcal Septicaemia Prognostic Score, GMSPS) [8, 9], the clinical trials accomplished most of what the recent recommendations published for improving clinical sepsis trials in adults called for: avoiding mixing patients with sepsis and septic shock, including only patients with undisputable sepsis, and using a validated severity of illness score for eligibility [10, 11].

However, the most common pathway for drug development in critically ill and injured children remains as follow-on studies to larger adult ICU trials. Examples include studies in acute lung injury, sepsis (see below), and traumatic brain injury [12–19].

Interestingly, there is a new pathway that may have significant applicability to drug development in the ICU and especially for small populations such as children. Complex computer models of pathophysiologic disease processes ('in silico' modeling), from the molecular to the organism level, are now possible and have yielded encouraging results to date [20–23].

## Working with Sponsors – Developing a Study Protocol, Investigator Meetings, and Data Safety Monitoring Boards

Most pharmaceutical companies do not have internal expertise in paediatric critical care. Therefore, the most common practice is to convene a medical advisory board when considering the move into clinical trials. Usually, paediatric critical care physicians with particular clinical and/or research expertise in the therapeutic areas under investigation are invited to attend a meeting with company representatives along with internal or external experts in paediatric clinical trial design, biostatistics and regulatory issues. The meeting agenda may be limited to providing advice on current incidence, treatment, and issues related to a specific disease or condition or may also address the design of a study from start to finish.

Investigator meetings are crucial for study success as this is the venue where investigators, sub-investigators, and study coordinators have a chance to meet with the sponsor's medical, operational and regulatory personnel and become familiar with the details of the study protocol and procedures. It is not uncommon at these meetings for two-way interactions to occur which may result in needed final revisions of the trial protocol before the first patient is enrolled.

To ensure subject safety, an external data safety monitoring board (DSMB) or an internal data monitoring committee (DMC) is often formed which has predefined roles and responsibilities in terms of dose escalation, dose expansion, monitoring of adverse events, and assessment of efficacy. Again, as most sponsors do not have internal PICU expertise, it is not unusual for an external paediatric critical care physician with special expertise in the trial's therapeutic area to serve as a consultant or chair of the committee.

## Working with Regulatory Authorities – Selecting a Patient Population, Dosing, Use of Placebo, and Outcome Variables

The equitable selection of subjects based on the principle of justice requires, when scientifically appropriate, the study of adults prior to the study of children when choosing a study population. Although data on dosing (i.e., drug exposure) and safety are necessary given known differences between children and adults, we may be able to extrapolate efficacy based on adequate and well controlled studies in adults if the course of the disease and response to treatment are similar in children [24]. However, the extrapolation of efficacy to critically ill children based on a study of critically ill adults may be difficult given, for example, differing co-morbidities even if the target disease process is similar. This problem of inference from adults to children may be minimized by eliminating population differences through the careful choice of appropriate inclusion and exclusion criteria. Although a narrowly defined study population may reduce risk and may optimize potential benefit by eliminating co-morbid conditions, for example, it also may decrease the ability to generalize the research findings to a broader population of critically ill children.

Determining the appropriate paediatric drug exposure to optimize the balance between risk and potential benefit may depend on information previously obtained from adult studies. Single or multiple dose pharmacokinetic (PK) studies may be designed to target a similar drug exposure that correlated with efficacy in adult trials. In the absence of such data, dose-ranging studies may need to be performed which target selected response criteria such as a physiologic parameter or biomarker. Alternatively, dose ranging may need to be incorporated into the design of an efficacy trial. Paediatric studies of drugs which have proven effective in adults may fail to demonstrate efficacy in children simply because the wrong dose was used in the study [25].

The scientific necessity of a paediatric trial is the first step to ensure that children are enrolled in trials that are scientifically and ethically sound. The second step is to ensure that the study presents an appropriate balance of risk and potential benefit. The administration of an FDA-regulated experimental drug presents greater than minimal risk. An exception might be when two FDA-approved drugs are being compared with both drugs administered according to their labeled indications. In this case, the incremental research risk could be considered minimal as the only difference between research and the administration of either one of two proven effective treatment is randomization [26]. This narrow exception, however, has limited utility for FDA-regulated research in paediatric critical care as there is no provision for waiver of parental permission for minimal risk research under FDA regulations. In the absence of the prospect of direct benefit to the enrolled child, the administration of the experimental drug must present no more than a minor increase over minimal risk and the research must be performed in a paediatric population with an appropriate disease or condition. For example, a single-dose PK study could be performed in children 'at risk' for the infection if there are sufficient data from adult studies to conclude that the risks of such a study are only slightly more than minimal risk [27]. Otherwise, the administration of the experimental drug must offer a sufficient prospect of direct benefit to justify the risks. This may require an initial dose ranging phase of a study designed for efficacy, with the starting dose chosen to approximate the expected effective drug exposure.

The choice of an appropriate control group is essential to ensure the scientific credibility of the clinical trial. If there is no proven effective treatment, it is appropriate to compare the investigational drug with an inactive placebo control.

There may be other circumstances when the use of a placebo control is appropriate even if proven effective treatment exists. For example, the existing treatment may present significant toxicity and/or marginal efficacy such that a placebo control is appropriate. In addition, the use of an active comparator may not be scientifically sound if one cannot assume that the active comparator is effective under the conditions of the trial. For a clinical trial using an active comparator to be sensitive enough to detect whether the experimental drug is effective, certain features of the trial, such as subject population and inclusion and exclusion criteria, must be similar to the previous trial in which the active comparator demonstrated efficacy [28]. Many treatments provided in the PICU have not been demonstrated to be safe and effective for that population. The use of an active comparator which has become 'standard of care' absent sufficient data demonstrating efficacy in the PICU population will not provide any useful information. Under these circumstances, a three-arm study may be warranted. Such a clinical trial would randomize subjects to active comparator, experimental drug, or placebo. With a three-arm study, one would be able to assess whether the active comparator or the experimental drug demonstrated efficacy. One would also have placebo-controlled safety data. However, a three-arm design still raises ethical concerns about the use of a placebo control.

The ethical principle behind the bias against placebo controls is that children should not be placed at a disadvantage by being enrolled in a clinical trial. Often, the concept of equipoise is cited in support of this ethical principle. The concept of equipoise, however, has two meanings. The first meaning is that there must be scientific uncertainty about the hypothesis of a clinical trial, i.e. whether the null hypothesis is not true, which means that there is no difference between the experimental drug and the comparator (whether active control or placebo). This first meaning of equipoise is an absolute requirement for any clinical trial to be justified. The second meaning is that no one should be randomized to treatment that is known to be inferior. It is this second use of the concept of equipoise that generates controversy [24]. When there is known effective treatment available, the risk of placebo administration consists of the risks of the known effective treatment being withheld from those subjects in the placebo arm of the clinical trial. It should be noted that these risks also accrue to the subjects who are randomized to the experimental drug. For paediatric studies to be ethically sound, the risk of being randomized to the placebo control and thus subject to withholding known effective treatment must present no more than a minor increase over minimal risk [24]. This standard is consistent with, but arguably more stringent than, the current 2008 version of the Declaration of Helsinki [29] and the International Conference on Harmonisation (ICH) guidance on choice and control group [28].

A special problem arises within the practice of paediatric critical care medicine when there is a prevalent belief that a drug is effective absent adequate and well-controlled studies. Such a drug may become 'standard of care' in many PICUs, rendering the withholding of such a drug in favor of a placebo control problematic. The administration of study drug as a 'rescue' intervention for a child's deteriorating condition alters the design of a clinical trial from a test of efficacy of the study drug to one of early versus late administration [30]. In the absence of data supporting efficacy, the use of a study drug as a 'rescue' is scientifically and ethically problematic. It should be noted that there are appropriate study designs that use a rescue medication. Clinical trials of paediatric hypertension often use a randomized withdrawal study design, with the administration of rescue medication once a child's blood pressure exceeds a predetermined number. Clinical trials of pain medication will often use rescue medication to be administered at a predetermined interval after the study drug has been given if a child's pain has not been relieved. However, in both these cases, a drug that is known to be effective is being administered.

The choice of an outcome variable should be grounded in the pathophysiology of the disease process that the experimental drug is intended to interrupt or alter. In the absence of a proven surrogate marker, an outcome variable must be a clinically meaningful endpoint. The choice of 'all cause' mortality at an appropriate interval after the experimental intervention offers the advantage of being insensitive to clinician bias. However, if the experimental drug or device is available 'off label,' clinicians may feel obligated to administer the drug or device in order to 'do everything' for a dying child. Although understandable, the result is that the trial will be undermined and potentially worthless [30]. Physiologic endpoints may be an appropriate outcome measure, as is the case with studies of hypertension or sedation. Here, the physiologic endpoint is felt to be sufficiently valuable and potentially (or actually) linked with positive clinical outcomes to serve as an appropriate primary outcome for the clinical trial. The randomized withdrawal design is an effective approach in these situations given that withdrawal from the study in order to deliver known effective treatment can be used as an appropriate endpoint indicating lack of efficacy.

## Issues of Informed Consent and Assent

In addition to scientific necessity and the appropriate balance of risk and potential benefit, parental permission and child assent are an important ethical component of a clinical PICU trial. Often, a child who is admitted to a PICU is not capable of assent given his or her critical clinical condition. This may not always be the case, as in a single-dose PK study of an antibiotic in a child who has a condition which places them at risk for a future infection [27]. Ethicists debate whether the age (i.e. developmental capacity) at which a child should be asked for assent is as low as 6 or 7 years or as high as 14 years. The answer to this question depends to some extent on the relationship between child assent and parental permission. A parent is the one who is responsible for assessing whether the risks and potential benefits of participation in a clinical trial are appropriate for his or her child. A child is only asked to assent after this parental assessment has been made, and the parent has already agreed to permit the researcher to approach the child. From this perspective, the child's assent becomes a simple 'yes' (or no, as the case may be) based on information that is appropriate for the child's developmental level. Child assent should not be understood as requiring the same capacity as adult consent [31–33].

The requirements for parental permission are effectively the same as the requirements for adult informed consent. Concerns are often raised that parents may be incapable of meaningful permission given the duress of a child's critical illness. One approach to this problem is to have the individual who approaches a parent about research participation to be separate from the clinical team. Often, parents may still ask their clinician about his or her views on the research. Hopefully, the clinician can affirm the existence of scientific uncertainty about the safety and efficacy of the experimental drug while remaining neutral about study participation. In the critical care setting, there may be situations where administration of the experimental drug or intervention must be done prior to the possibility of obtaining adequate informed and voluntary parental permission. FDA regulations allow for an exception from informed consent for interventions that offer the prospect of direct benefit and must be administered within a therapeutic window that makes obtaining informed consent not feasible. The requirement for parental permission may be waived under these regulations. The concept of 'deferred consent' is ethically meaningless. In effect, the individual (whether patient or proxy) is simply stating that what was performed without consent was in retrospect acceptable. One would expect that most patients and/or proxies would feel this way if the initial exception from informed consent was appropriate. The requirement for community consultation and public disclosure is an attempt to ascertain whether this expectation is indeed appropriate for any given clinical trial. For clinical trials that are being conducted in the PICU, the requirement for community consultation and public disclosure does not present an obstacle to the performance of important research [34, 35].

## Challenges of Multi-Center Trials and PICU Clinical Research Networks

Critically ill and injured children remain at significant risk for morbidity and mortality from many different diseases including sepsis, acute respiratory failure, trauma, status asthmaticus, status epilepticus, and many others. Unfortunately, the relative rarity of severe paediatric diseases coupled with their relatively low mortality rates make meaningful clinical studies difficult or impossible to perform, including trials of novel therapeutic agents.

Clinicians are failing these children due to the lack of well-defined clinical studies. The paediatric critical care community has developed coordinated networks for collaborative clinical studies to facilitate performance of large RCTs: the Paediatric Acute Lung Injury and Sepsis Investigators (PALISI) and the National Collaborative Paediatric Critical Care Research Network (CPCCRN).

The PALISI Investigators are a collaboration of clinical researchers in more than 79 large paediatric intensive care units across North America [36]. These researchers have joined together to identify optimal supportive, preventive and therapeutic strategies for acute lung injury, sepsis, multiorgan failure, and other acute, life-threatening pulmonary or systemic inflammatory syndromes

that affect infants and children [36]. The PALISI Network's goal is to perform multi-center research studies to better describe disease processes and outcomes in paediatric patients and to evaluate interventions in this population [36]. Study designs include prospective cohort studies, case-control studies, genetic epidemiology and gene expression studies, drug dosing and metabolism studies, and phase I, II, III and IV clinical trials. PALISI network members have the ultimate goal of improving the care and health outcomes of critically ill infants and children. They already have had successes in testing new outcome scoring systems, as well as therapies for respiratory failure and other diseases [37–40].

In April 2004, the National Center for Medical Rehabilitation Research of the National Institute for Child Health and Human Development issued a request for applications to establish the Collaborative Paediatric Critical Care Research Network (CPCCRN) [41]. The CPCCRN provides an infrastructure for collaborative clinical trials and descriptive studies. Six paediatric centers including seven intensive care units and a data-coordinating center were selected through a competitive application process. CPCCRN goals include the support of collaborative multi-center clinical trials otherwise impossible in single institutions and the establishment of a framework for developing the scientific basis for paediatric critical care practice [42].

Beyond the impressive first steps of PALISI and CPCCRN, what is needed is a rethink of paediatric critical illness and injury. A case in point is the sepsis syndrome (also see 'Case Studies'). Sepsis is an important cause of morbidity and mortality in children. Children are less likely than adults to have significant underlying co-morbidity and are a more homogeneous population than are recruited to adult sepsis studies. Lacking such comorbidities, children may be a more suitable population to evaluate newer therapies in a controlled trial setting, once sufficient proof of concept has been established to justify the risks.

Routine therapies should be standardized according to protocol, thus removing unwarranted heterogeneity of therapies between centers. The use of standardized and possibly new therapeutic regimens could thus be assessed in a logical and sequential manner using, for example, a shared data registry. The ultimate goal would be to proceed with evaluation of new therapies in critically ill children in a rational scientific manner, much as new therapies for childhood cancer have been and continue to be evaluated by paediatric oncologists [43]. Only by a radical rethink of the way we evaluate new therapies in critically ill children will we be able to properly assess experimental treatment modalities, thus allowing children with at high risk of morbidity and death to maximally benefit from new drug therapies.

## Case Studies of Clinical Trials in the PICU: Activated Protein C in Severe Sepsis

Drotrecogin alfa (activated) (DrotAA), a recombinant form of human activated protein C, has been approved in over 50 countries for treatment of severe sepsis in adults at high risk of death. Approval was based on a highly significant reduction in 28-day mortality shown in the phase 3 PROWESS (Recombinant Human Protein C Worldwide Evaluation in Severe Sepsis) trial, which excluded patients younger than 18 years [15].

An open-label phase 2 study (called EVAO) in children with severe sepsis indicated that pharmacokinetics and pharmacodynamics of DrotAA are similar to that in adults [44]. Children in the EVAO study had higher rates of cardiovascular dysfunction and two or more organ dysfunctions (93 and 85%, respectively) than did adults in the PROWESS study (72 and 75%, respectively). The most common infection in the EVAO study was that from *Neisseria meningitidis* (26.5%), which was documented in only 1% of PROWESS patients.

As a result of the mortality benefit demonstrated in the PROWESS trial, and before initial approval of DrotAA and the completion of the EVAO trail, ENHANCE (Extended Evaluation of Recombinant Activated Protein C), a global open-label trial in adult and paediatric severe sepsis patients, was initiated to gather additional mortality and safety data in anticipation of the likelihood of a call for the use of DrotAA in children with severe sepsis [14]. The ENHANCE study in paediatric patients was continued pending the design and initiation of the randomized, placebo-controlled RESOLVE trial (Researching Severe Sepsis and Organ Dysfunction in Children: A Global Perspective).

RESOLVE, a phase 3, randomized placebo-controlled trial, was designed to determine the efficacy and safety of DrotAA in children [45]. RESOLVE was the largest randomized placebo-controlled trial performed so far in critically ill children, and the only placebo-controlled study of DrotAA in children. Analysis of results showed that there was no significant difference in morbidity, a composite endpoint of time to complete organ failure resolution (CTFCOFR), or mortality endpoints between patients on DrotAA compared with those on placebo. Nor were there any significant differences between groups in serious adverse events, serious bleeding, or central nervous system (CNS) bleeding.

Given the lower mortality and relative paucity of children available for inclusion in any trial targeting life-threatening illness, there were some key caveats and limitations in the RESOLVE study:

- To maximize the opportunity for a valid outcome, 104 major paediatric centers in 18 countries were enlisted and extensively trained in screening and assessment procedures; only patients deemed to be at the highest risk of mortality or significant morbidity were included; and, the primary outcome variable (CTFCOFR) was selected that was thought to be meaningful to the clinician, patient, and patient's family.

- Because of the huge variability in patients and sites, heterogeneity in patient populations and therapeutic approaches could have influenced the trial's outcome.
- The large number of centers, each enrolling relatively few patients, might have resulted in a 'first patient effect', which could significantly impact a clinical trial result [46]. Although each site underwent extensive education in patient identification, recruitment, and study procedures, most had very limited previous experience with administration and use of DrotAA in children.
- The choice of primary outcome variable may have been inappropriate, although a similar endpoint has been useful in other paediatric studies [47]. Endpoints such as cessation of mechanical ventilation (the definition of respiratory organ resolution) or resolution of cardiovascular failure may also have been influenced by local weaning practices, which were not dictated by the study protocol.
- Differing medical practice in PICUs, within and between countries, might also have affected the reliability of an endpoint such as CTCOFR in multi-center studies.
- Because mortality is a dominant component of the CTCOFR composite endpoint, there would have to be a large difference in mortality, or much faster organ resolution in the interventional group, or both, to create a difference. If there was a reduction in mortality but an associated increase in resource use, the CTCOFR score could have remained similar between groups. However, if mortality was significantly reduced because of a short-term increase in hospital stay, the study's results (albeit formally negative) could have supported use of DrotAA in children.

In future trials, the nuances of composite and clinically unproven endpoints such as CTCOFR use should be carefully considered. The results of RESOLVE differed significantly from those of the PROWESS trial in adults, in which DrotAA significantly reduced mortality compared with placebo [15]. In the PROWESS trial, mortality in the placebo group was approximately 31%, whereas mortality in RESOLVE was considerably lower at 17%. Because of the low risk of mortality in RESOLVE patients, there was only 31% power in RESOLVE to show a 20% relative risk reduction in mortality for a sample size of 600 patients. Therefore, the results from RESOLVE do not exclude a mortality advantage in children, equivalent to that seen in the PROWESS study.

There may be several reasons for the apparent conflicting effect of DrotAA between children and adults with sepsis:

- There were clear differences between RESOLVE and PROWESS in baseline characteristics, trial design, and statistical power.
- It is likely there are differences in the pathophysiology of paediatric and adult sepsis. Patients in RESOLVE had lower protein C levels, higher D-dimer levels, and higher IL-6 levels than the adult patients in PROWESS. Furthermore, the site of infection and types of bacteria differed substantially between populations.
- It is possible that dosing of DrotAA was insufficient in the children in this study; it might have been more effective if dosed according to protein C levels rather than on a weight basis.

These disparities also emphasize the difficulty in extrapolating results from children to adults, or vice versa. Differences between trials in the natural history of sepsis (e.g. mortality), the comparatively low numbers of patients in RESOLVE, and completely different endpoints, precluded direct extrapolation or comparison of the two trials. Given the inherent limitations of small sample size and the likely imbalances that will inevitably occur, a primary outcome variable with severity adjustment should be considered for future trial designs.

Despite not demonstrating a positive effect, RESOLVE has documented the natural history of severe sepsis and paved the way for future PRCTs in the field of paediatric critical care medicine.

## Conclusions

The challenges for drug development in the PICU are many: the diverse population in terms of age and developmental stages; the multitude of different diseases and injuries; difficulties in study design; the need to conduct multi-center trials; obtaining informed consent from parents; and, selection of clinically durable outcomes that can lead to approval by regulatory authorities. However, the need for new pharmacologic therapies to treat severe and life-threatening diseases is clear. We suggest that the path forward is getting brighter as the PICU medical and research communities along with government and industry collaborators learn from past experiences, develop new methodologies and models of critical illness, join together to form clinical research networks, and work towards successful completion of many promising new therapies.


## References

1　Food and Drug Administration Amendments Act of 2007: United States Congressional Record, 2007.

2　The EU Paediatric Regulation, 2009. (accessed July 11, 2009, at http://www.ema.europa.eu/htms/human/paediatrics/regulation.htm.)

3　Moher D, Schulz KF, Altman DG: The CONSORT statement: revised recommendations for improving the quality of reports of parallel-group randomised trials. Lancet 2001;357:1191–1194.

4　Altman DG, Schulz KF, Moher D, et al: The revised CONSORT statement for reporting randomized trials: explanation and elaboration. Ann Intern Med 2001;134:663–694.

5　ClinicalTrials.gov. 2009. (accessed June 13, 2009, at www.clinicaltrials.gov.)

6　Levin M, Quint PA, Goldstein B, et al: Recombinant bactericidal/permeability-increasing protein (rBPI21) as adjunctive treatment for children with severe meningococcal sepsis: a randomised trial. rBPI21 Meningococcal Sepsis Study Group. Lancet 2000;356:961–967.

7　Giroir BP, Quint PA, Barton P, et al : Preliminary evaluation of recombinant amino-terminal fragment of human bactericidal/permeability-increasing protein in children with severe meningococcal sepsis. Lancet 1997;350:1439–1443.

8　Thomson AP, Sills JA, Hart CA: Validation of the Glasgow Meningococcal Septicemia Prognostic Score: a 10-year retrospective survey. Crit Care Med 1991;19:26–30.

9　Stiehm ER, Damrosch DS: Factors in the prognosis of meningococcal infection. Review of 63 cases with emphasis on recognition and management of the severely ill patient. J Pediatr 1966;68:457–467.

10　Cohen J. Meningococcal disease as a model to evaluate novel anti-sepsis strategies. Crit Care Med 2000;28:S64–S67.

11　Annane D. Improving clinical trials in the critically ill: unique challenge–sepsis. Crit Care Med 2009;37:S117–S128.

12　Gadek JE, DeMichele SJ, Karlstad MD, et al: Effect of enteral feeding with eicosapentaenoic acid, gamma-linolenic acid, and antioxidants in patients with acute respiratory distress syndrome. Enteral Nutrition in ARDS Study Group. Crit Care Med 1999;27:1409–420.

13　Nadkarni V, DeMichele S, Goldstein B, Checchia P, Ayad O, Jacobs BR: Clinical characteristics and outcome in children with ARDS. Crit Care Med 2005;33:A4.

14　Goldstein B, Nadel S, Peters M, et al: ENHANCE: results of a global open-label trial of Drotrecogin alfa (activated) in children with severe sepsis. Pediatr Crit Care Med 2006;7.

15　Bernard GR, Vincent JL, Laterre PF, et al: Efficacy and safety of recombinant human activated protein C for severe sepsis. N Engl J Med 2001;344:699–709.

16　Adelson PD. Hypothermia following paediatric traumatic brain injury. J Neurotrauma 2009;26:429–36.

17　Kochanek PM, Bell MJ, Adelson PD. Hypothermia therapy after traumatic brain injury in children. N Engl J Med 2008;359:1179;author reply 1180.

18　Adelson PD, Ragheb J, Kanev P, et al: Phase II clinical trial of moderate hypothermia after severe traumatic brain injury in children. Neurosurgery 2005;56:740–754; discussion 754.

19　Clifton GL, Miller ER, Choi SC, et al: Lack of effect of induction of hypothermia after acute brain injury. N Engl J Med 2001;344:556–563.

20　An G: In silico experiments of existing and hypothetical cytokine-directed clinical trials using agent-based modeling. Crit Care Med 2004;32:2050–2060.

21　Clermont G, Bartels J, Kumar R, Constantine G, Vodovotz Y, Chow C: In silico design of clinical trials: a method coming of age. Crit Care Med 2004;32:2061–2070.

22　Langley C, Brock C, Brouwer G, et al: Opportunities to replace the use of animals in sepsis research: the report and recommendations of a Focus on Alternatives workshop. Altern Lab Anim 2005;33:641–648.

23　Wakeland W, Agbeko R, Vinecore K, Peters M, Goldstein B: Assessing the prediction potential of an in silico computer model of intracranial pressure dynamics. Crit Care Med 2009;37:1079–1089.

24 Nelson RM: Additional protections for children enrolled in clinical investigations; in Mulberg AE, Silber SA, van den Anker JN (eds): Paediatric Drug Development: Concepts and Applications. Hoboken, Wiley, 2009, pp 81–101.

25 Benjamin DK Jr, Smith PB, Jadhav P, et al: Paediatric antihypertensive trial failures: analysis of end points and dose range. Hypertension 2008;51:834–840.

26 Morris MC, Nelson RM: Randomized, controlled trials as minimal risk: an ethical analysis. Crit Care Med 2007;35: 940–944.

27 Summary of Clinical Review of Paediatric Studies Submitted in Response to a Written Request (Linezolid), 2005. (accessed July 9, 2009, at http://www.fda. gov/downloads/Drugs/DevelopmentApprovalProcess/DevelopmentResources/ UCM164020.pdf.)

28 Food and Drug Administration: International Conference on Harmonisation; Choice of Control Group in Clinical Trials. Fed Register 1999;64:51767–51780.

29 World Medical Association Declaration of Helsinki: Ethical Principles for Medical Research Involving Human Subjects, 2008. (accessed July 9, 2009, at http:// www.wma.net/e/policy/b3.htm.)

30 Holubkov R, Dean JM, Berger J, et al: Is 'rescue' therapy ethical in randomized controlled trials? Pediatr Crit Care Med 2009;10:431–438.

31 Denham EJ, Nelson RM: Self-determination is not an appropriate model for understanding parental permission and child assent. Anesth Analg 2002;94: 1049–1051.

32 Miller VA, Nelson RM: A developmental approach to child assent for nontherapeutic research. J Pediatr 2006;149:S25– S30.

33 Rossi WC, Reynolds W, Nelson RM: Child assent and parental permission in paediatric research. Theor Med Bioeth 2003;24:131–148.

34 Morris MC, Fischbach RL, Nelson RM, Schleien CL: A paradigm for inpatient resuscitation research with an exception from informed consent. Crit Care Med 2006;34:2567–2575.

35 Morris MC, Nadkarni VM, Ward FR, Nelson RM: Exception from informed consent for paediatric resuscitation research: community consultation for a trial of brain cooling after in-hospital cardiac arrest. Paediatrics 2004;114: 776–781.

36 PedsCCM: The Paediatric Critical Care Website: PALISI: Paediatric Acute Lung Injury and Sepsis Investigators. 2009. (accessed July 4, 2009, at http://pedsccm.org/PALISI_network.php.)

37 Lacroix J, Cotting J: Severity of illness and organ dysfunction scoring in children. Pediatr Crit Care Med 2005;6: S126–S134.

38 Randolph AG, Forbes PW, Gedeit RG, et al: Cumulative fluid intake minus output is not associated with ventilator weaning duration or extubation outcomes in children. Pediatr Crit Care Med 2005;6: 642–647.

39 Randolph AG, Wypij D, Venkataraman ST, et al: Effect of mechanical ventilator weaning protocols on respiratory outcomes in infants and children: a randomized controlled trial. JAMA 2002; 288:2561–2568.

40 Tamburro RF, Thomas NJ, Pon S, et al: Post hoc analysis of calfactant use in immunocompromised children with acute lung injury: impact and feasibility of further clinical trials. Pediatr Crit Care Med 2008;9:459–464.

41 The National Collaborative Paediatric Critical Care Research Network, 2009. (accessed July 4, 2009, at http://www. cpccrn.org/.)

42 Willson DF, Dean JM, Newth C, et al: Collaborative Paediatric Critical Care Research Network (CPCCRN). Pediatr Crit Care Med 2006;7:301–307.

43 CureSearch: The Children's Oncology Group and the National Childhood Cancer Foundation, 2005. (accessed July 4, 2009, at http://www.childrensoncologygroup.org/.)

44 Barton P, Kalil AC, Nadel S, et al: Safety, pharmacokinetics, and pharmacodynamics of drotrecogin alfa (activated) in children with severe sepsis. Paediatrics 2004;113:7–17.

45 Nadel S, Goldstein B, Williams MD, et al: Drotrecogin alfa (activated) in children with severe sepsis: a multicentre phase III randomised controlled trial. Lancet 2007;369:836–843.

46 Macias WL, Vallet B, Bernard GR, et al: Sources of variability on the estimate of treatment effect in the PROWESS trial: implications for the design and conduct of future studies in severe sepsis. Crit Care Med 2004;32:2385–2391.

47 Mou SS, Giroir BP, Molitor-Kirsch EA, et al: Fresh whole blood versus reconstituted blood for pump priming in heart surgery in infants. N Engl J Med 2004; 351:1635–1644.

Brahm Goldstein, MD, MCR
Senior Director, Translational Science, Ikaria, Inc.,
Clinton, NJ 08801 (USA)
Tel. +1 908 399 8346, Fax +1 866 219 2448, E-Mail brahm.goldstein@ikaria.com

Rose K, van den Anker JN (eds): Guide to Paediatric Drug Development and Clinical Research.
Basel, Karger, 2010, pp 155–159

# Research and Drug Development in Paediatric Oncology

Giorgio Massimini[a] · Klaus Rose[a] · Gilles Vassal[b] · Kathy Pritchard-Jones[c]

[a]Pharmaceuticals Division, F. Hoffmann-La Roche Ltd., Basel, Switzerland; [b]Institut Gustave Roussy, Villejuif, France and [c]The Institute of Cancer Research and the Royal Marsden Hospital, Sutton, UK

There are few other fields in paediatric medicine that are as challenging as paediatric oncology. Cancer in children is rare in comparison to adults, with approximately 12,000 new cases/year in Europe [1]. As in adult cancer, child cancer is not a uniform disease, but is a group of many different malignant diseases that can develop from almost any tissue in the growing body of the child. The mechanisms that lead to cancer are only partially known, with a mix of genetic predispositions and other influences, probably including environmental factors. The only certainty is that, in contrast to adult cancer, cancer in children is less likely the result of decades of exposure to a noxious environment, although exposure to environment toxics can lead to cancer also in children (e.g. increased cancer frequency in Hiroshima). Present treatment for paediatric cancer is quite effective and more effective than in adults if one considers all types of cancers together; approximately 80% of children with cancer in Europe are now cured with existing treatments while only around 50% of adults enjoy a similar success [2]. As in adults, some cancer types are cured in almost 90% of affected children, while in other cancer types, such as high grade gliomas, the prognosis is still abysmal. The biology of childhood cancer, or better

said the biology of the many different forms of cancer that can affect children, are generally very different from adult cancers. For example, adolescent colorectal cancer (CRC) probably has a much greater genetic component; at present we do not know if it similar biologically to typical adult CRC.

Paediatric oncology has evolved into a well-developed specialty science. It is one area of child medicine where the ongoing need for clinical trials is undisputed and has resulted in very high benefit for patients. Treatment of child cancer represents one of the most prominent success story of modern clinical research (another one is, e.g., development of modern vaccines, see chapter by Ceddia et al. [this vol., pp. 206–211]). Clinical trials in children with cancer started in the 1950s when the first chemotherapy substances became available. An initial nihilistic approach, with concerns about toxicity in the face of poor long-term outcomes, gave way to an increasingly multi-agent treatment approach as some long-term cures came to be seen. Children were better able to tolerate chemotherapeutic agents administered in doses and combinations different from adult cancer, leading to a complex and multi-disciplinary approach to their treatment.

**Table 1.** Relative risks (RRs) of death for children (0–14 years) diagnosed in 2000–2002 compared to those diagnosed in 1995–1999 for each diagnostic group, adjusted by regional grouping, sex and age (from Gatta et al. [2], modified)

| Disease | RR | 95% CI |
|---|---|---|
| Hodgkin lymphomas | 0.62 | 0.35–1.10 |
| Embrional CNS tumours | 0.70 | 0.59–0.84 |
| Lymphoid leukaemias | 0.85 | 0.74–0.97 |
| CNS tumours | 0.85 | 0.77–0.94 |
| Nephroblastoma and other non-epithelial renal tumors | 0.86 | 0.63–1.17 |
| Acute myeloid leukaemias | 0.89 | 0.74–1.06 |
| Non-Hodgkin lymphomas | 0.95 | 0.74–1.22 |
| Astrocytomas | 0.96 | 0.80–1.14 |
| Ependymomas | 0.97 | 0.72–1.30 |
| Neuroblastoma | 0.99 | 0.85–1.17 |
| Osteosarcomas | 0.99 | 0.74–1.32 |
| Rhabdomyosarcomas | 0.99 | 0.78–1.26 |
| Ewing tumour | 1.17 | 0.84–1.62 |

## Present Status and Future Challenges

The mainstay of treatment, as in adults, is a combination of surgery, radiotherapy and chemotherapy, though chemotherapy is used more prominently in these largely chemo-sensitive tumors and radiotherapy tends to be avoided unless essential for local tumor control, due to its long term side effects in the growing child. There are two major differences that distinguish adult from childhood cancer treatment: firstly, cancer in children can often be put into remission and cured in the long term – something unfortunately yet rare in adults, and secondly, participation in a clinical trial has become the standard of care in paediatric oncology. This is largely due to the need for national and international collaboration to make progress in these rare diseases and the consequence of the high success rate observed in clinical trials that encouraged physicians, patients and patients' families to participate. By comparison, while an estimated 90% of children with malignancies have been included in clinical trials, only 5% of the adult patients participate in clinical studies, and the frequency has not changed much over 25 years. The professional organizations of paediatric oncologists and haematologists have played a critical role in systematically testing, applying and developing new therapeutic approaches. Unfortunately, the option of increasing life expectancy and survival by administering higher doses of the same chemotherapeutic agents or by sequencing them in a different way is by and large exhausted, as shown in table 1, where the grey area highlights the diseases where little or no improvement was achieved in reducing the risk of death at the beginning of the present decade versus the previous decade for children aged less than 14 years and similarly for adolescents aged 15–24 years, in many malignant diseases.

The development of modern cancer treatment is more and more focused on therapies directed against specific molecular targets. In general, one can identify three different areas of drug development: treatments directly affecting the tumour, treatment affecting the blood supply to the tumour and treatment affecting the environment from which the tumour depends. An often-quoted example of the first approach is targeting a specific gene-fusion product (bcr-abl) with a tyrosine kinase inhibitor such as imatinib in Philadelphia-positive chronic myeloid leukemia Thereby, these treatments have transformed this leukaemia from a life-threatening disease with a median survival of 3.5 years into a chronic condition with 90% of patients surviving 5 years or more, reducing the need for a bone marrow transplantation to cure the disease [4, 5]; another example is the targeting of specific tumour-overexpressed antigens such as CD20 by monoclonal antibodies such as rituximab, which has significantly improved the outcome of adult and paediatric patients in lymphomas [6, 7]. Another example of the second type of treatment is the targeting of the VEGF receptor pathway by either a tyrosine kinase inhibitor such as sunitinib [6] or by a monoclonal antibody blocking the ligand, VEGF, such as bevacizumab [9]; both approaches result in cutting the blood flow to existing tumours by reducing the sprouting of newly produced vessels induced by tumour-secreted vascular-endothelial growth factor (VEGF) [10]. Modifying the environment in which the tumour grows, such as in hormone-dependent breast cancer by cutting the oestrogen supply through blockage of aromatase, a key enzyme in the estrogen production pathway, has also been successfully tested in adults [11, 12].

Increasingly, targeted therapies are becoming available and improve patients outcome in terms of tumor control, life expectancy and quality of life for patients with breast cancer, colon cancer, chronic leukaemias and many other malignant diseases.

The primary targets of these modern biologics are the rather frequent adult cancer types and their biological features. Where the child cancer biology is comparable to adult cancer biology and/or express the same target, such as CD20 in lymphomas, adult treatment will help to treat affected children as well. Where the childhood cancer biology is different, the therapeutic potential in children of these treatments is an open question.

Another challenge in the development of new treatments in paediatric tumours is the fortunately limited number of patients in need of treatment for cancer. As an example, as shown in table 2, the number of children presenting with lymphoid leukaemia, the most common cancer in Europe is just above 11,000 over 7 years, which means approximately 1,500 new cases per year. With such a limited patient population, the conventional clinical trial approach of phase I followed by phase II and then by confirmatory, randomized phase III is severely challenged insofar even in presence of a very active experimental treatment it will be difficult to enrol sufficient patients to have a definitive answer in a relative short time. This has prompted the use of innovative study designs ('window' studies, etc.) at least for the early-phase clinical trials. The recent introduction of the European Paediatric Regulation has further pushed in this direction. It has to be noted that thousands of new substances are screened in the labs every year and the selection of candidate drugs coupled with a better understanding of the biology of tumours has led to an increase of the success rate in cancer drug development from 5 to 18% [3] which may make paradoxically the development of effective therapies more difficult because of the paucity of cases.

## Conclusions

The goal of paediatric oncology could be described as to save the lives of as many children with cancer as possible and to achieve this with as little long-term side effects and as minimal impairment of their quality of life as possible. The desirable goal of clinical and biological research in paediatric oncology could be described as to have new treatments available to children as soon as possible, improving the excellent cure rate obtained so far, reduce long-term toxicity and improve their quality of life. The rarity of cancer in children limits the new substances that can be tested clinically in patients. There is hope that

**Table 2.** Five-year survival with 95% CIs for Europe as a whole for 15 common cancers diagnosed in children (0–14 years) in 2000–2002 (period analysis) and in 1995–1999 (cohort analysis) (from Gatta et al. [2], modified)

| Disease | 1995–2002 | 2000–2002 | |
| --- | --- | --- | --- |
| | number of cases | population-weighted 5-year survival | 95% CI |
| *Haemopoietic tumours* | | | |
| Lymphoid leukaemia | 11,259 | 85.4 | 83.7–87.1 |
| Acute myeloid leukaemia | 2,037 | 66.8 | 61.8–71.9 |
| Hodgkin lymphoma | 2,169 | 95.2 | 93.0–97.5 |
| Non-Hodgkin lymphoma | 2,066 | 82.3 | 78.2–86.5 |
| Burkitt lymphoma | 719 | 84.4 | 75.2–93.7 |
| *CNS tumours* | | | |
| All CNS tumours | 6,483 | 62.8 | 60.0–65.7 |
| Ependymoma | 840 | 62.0 | 55.7–68.3 |
| Astrocytoma | 2,193 | 62.9 | 57.4–68.5 |
| Astrocytoma (including 9,421/1) | 4,298 | 77.7 | 73.4–82.0 |
| Embryonal CNS tumours | 2,056 | 65.8 | 60.5–71.1 |
| *Other solid tumours* | | | |
| Neuroblastoma | 3,102 | 71.9 | 67.9–75.9 |
| Retinoblastoma (0-4 years old) | 806 | 97.5 | 94.6–100 |
| Nephroblastoma and other non-epithelial renal tumours | 2,382 | 89.1 | 85.8–92.5 |
| Osteosarcoma (10-14 years old) | 710 | 77.3 | 70.8–83.9 |
| Ewing sarcoma | 806 | 66.5 | 58.2–74.7 |
| Rhabdomyosarcoma | 1,480 | 69.1 | 62.9–75.4 |

new technologies will be able to predict the efficacy and possibly the main safety characteristics of new products for specific cancer types, and therefore allow informed decisions on which therapeutic approaches will be potentially more successful and therefore developable. Until now, these technologies are not yet mature enough to allow reliable prediction of efficacy.

## References


1 Steliarova-Foucher E, et al: Geographical patterns and time trends of cancer incidence and survival among children and adolescents in Europe since the 1970s. Lancet 2004;364: 2097–2105.

2 Gatta G, et al: Survival of European children and young adults with cancer diagnosed 1995–2002. Eur J Cancer 2009; 45:992–1005.

3 Walker I, Newell H: Do molecularly targeted agents in oncology have reduced attrition rates? Nat Rev 2009;1:1–2.

4 O'Brian S, et al: Imatinib compared with interferon and low-dose cytarabine for newly diagnosed chronic-phase chronic myeloid leukaemia. N Engl J Med 2003;348:994–1004.

5 Hochaus A, et al: Six-year follow-up of patients receiving imatinib for the first-line treatment of chronic myeloid leukemia. Leukemia 2009;23:1054–1061.

6 Reiter A: Diagnosis and treatment of childhood non-Hodgkin's lymphoma. Hematology 2007;285–296.

7 Link M, Weinstein H: Malignant non-Hodgkin lymphomas in children; in: Principles and Practice of Pediatric Oncology, ed 5. Philadelphia, Lippincott Williams & Wilkins, 2006, pp 722–747.

8 Favre S, et al: Safety, pharmacokinetic, and antitumor activity of SU11248, a novel oral multitarget tyrosine kinase inhibitor, in patients with cancer J Clin Oncol 2009;24:25–35.

9 Ferrara N: VEGF as a therapeutic target in cancer. Oncology 2005; 69(suppl 3):11–16.

10 Ferrara N, Gerber HP, LeCouter J: The biology of VEGF and its receptors. Nature Med 2003;9:669–676.

11 Hamilton A, Piccart M: The third-generation non-steroidal aromatase inhibitors: a review of their clinical benefits in the second-line hormonal treatment of advanced breast cancer. Ann Oncol 1999;10:377–384.

12 Geisler J, King N, Anker G, et al: In vivo inhibition of aromatization by exemestane, a novel irreversible aromatase inhibitor, in postmenopausal breast cancer patients. Clin Cancer Res 1998;4:2089–2093.

Giorgio Massimini, MD
F. Hoffmann-La Roche Ltd., Pharmaceuticals Division
CH–4070 Basel (Switzerland)
Tel. +41 61 687 1249, Fax +41 61 688 7085
E-Mail giorgio.massimini@roche.com

Rose K, van den Anker JN (eds): Guide to Paediatric Drug Development and Clinical Research.
Basel, Karger, 2010, pp 160–163

# Paediatric Cancer Treatment in Africa

Lorna A. Renner

Korle-Bu Teaching Hospital, Accra, Ghana

Childhood cancers lack priority when it comes to considering conditions causing death among African children, but 80% of children with cancer live in developing countries including much of Africa. Inadequate epidemiological data from most parts of Africa makes assessing accurately the incidence and significance of this condition to morbidity and mortality virtually impossible. There is a general lack of awareness about childhood cancer in Africa but despite this, one has to bear in mind the fact that the United Nations Convention on the Rights of the Child makes it our moral duty to ensure children affected worldwide by all disease conditions, including cancer, have access to acceptable standards of care. This is also in line with the mission statement of WHO/AFRO non-communicable disease unit to contribute to the reduction of the burden of non-communicable diseases in the countries of the region, as well as improving the quality of life and the life expectancy of the populations [1].

Childhood cancer in Africa is now emerging as a potentially important disease condition.

With most health system resources being directed to combating infectious diseases including HIV/AIDS, TB, malaria and other conditions such as malnutrition, it is expected that these conditions will be brought under control. Childhood cancer, which has been relatively neglected, will be on the ascendancy as an important cause of morbidity and mortality.

## Challenges

Childhood cancer care in Africa is beset by many challenges. The level of care varies from no paediatric cancer units in several countries to high level care in a few others such as South Africa and some North African countries. The general lack of awareness about childhood cancer is compounded by adverse socio-cultural practices and limited access to services, with few health workers trained in paediatric cancer management. Other limitations include inadequate diagnostic services, unavailability of chemotherapeutic agents, limited access to suitable protocols, inadequate supportive care, and unaffordable costs of treatment. Improving care for childhood cancers would entail stiff competition for scarce resources.

### Epidemiology

Lack of cancer registries in many countries has led to the seeming insignificance of childhood cancers in Africa. It is known that some cancers have a higher incidence, e.g. Burkitt's lymphoma being endemic in some parts of Sub-Saharan Africa and Kaposi's sarcoma linked with HIV. The incidence of leukaemia is not as high as in developed countries according to data from some countries [2], but to diagnose these, one needs a good haematology service including the capacity to perform bone marrow aspirates. Symptoms of leukaemia in childhood may be attributed to infections and is often inadequately investigated resulting in death before ascertainment of the diagnosis hence the likelihood of under diagnosing and under reporting. On the other hand, the solid tumors are more readily recognized as such by the lay public and health workers and are referred on to treatment facilities. It is most likely that brain tumours are also under diagnosed as access to diagnostic scans is limited. Many steps are required for a child with cancer to be diagnosed and registered and barriers occur at all stages in low income countries [3], a group to which most African countries belong.

*Diagnosis*

Diagnosing childhood cancers is fraught with difficulties in most places. Health facilities that have the expertise to diagnose and manage cancers are few and far between in most African countries. The use of radiological imaging is not optimal as apart from xray facilities and ultrasound scans that are widespread and readily available in most major health facilities, other more sophisticated but essential diagnostic equipment are not. Resources are invested in the barest minimum of laboratory equipment and laboratories rely on the use of light microscopy with limited access to other diagnostic techniques.

*Management*

Costs involved and distances families have to travel lead to delays in seeking treatment. Traditional healers play an important role in delivering healthcare to the majority of people in rural Africa and they can be the rate-limiting factor before a child is brought to see orthodox medical practitioners. Access to chemotherapy is limited even in some places that have paediatric cancer units. Families oftentimes cannot afford the cost of treatment. To reduce this, generic drugs are sometimes utilized and the efficacy of some of these drugs is uncertain. The potency of generic drugs needs to be assessed by the various country licensing agencies as substandard drugs are common on the market. There is also the real problem of storage of drugs in some parts of Africa where there are frequent power outages.

Some of the protocols used in developed countries are intensive and are associated with side effects and toxicities that may be difficult to manage as there are limitations to supportive care in most parts of Africa. This can result in treatment related deaths [4]. Suitable protocols tailored to the prevailing conditions found in most parts of sub-Saharan Africa are not widely available and need to be developed. There are few paediatric cancer clinical trials ongoing in Africa. Unlike the Western world where national protocols are in place and collaborative trials are undertaken, clinicians managing childhood cancer cases often make do with whatever protocols are available and there are few countries where treatment is standardized. Currently, the International Society for Paediatric Oncology (SIOP) and the Franco-African Childhood Cancer group are some of the few international groups that are actively involved in collaborative studies in Africa.

Other modalities of treatment include surgery and radiotherapy. Radiotherapy requires skilled expertise and there are few radiotherapy centres in Africa.

Supportive care, including the use of blood and blood products, antibiotics and good nutrition, is an essential component of care. Lack of adequate supportive care is a factor for the inability to use some protocols without modifications to the dose intensity. Children also often present with co-morbidities such as malnutrition, severe anaemia, HIV and other infections leading to increased risk of death before, during and soon after chemotherapy.

Palliative care is of huge importance as children who need it should be able to have a reasonably pain free, acceptable quality of life, causing less distress to their families. Opioids and other required drugs are not always readily obtainable. There is the strong perception by health workers about the negative addictive effects of opioids even in terminal cases leading to these drugs being withheld unnecessarily even when available.

*Treatment Outcome*

The multiple factors stated above including, lack of knowledge, loss of family income, duration of treatment and the demands of other family members leads often times to abandonment of treatment. The Franco-African Childhood Cancer group and also studies involving Malawi, Cameroun and Ghana have shown it is possible to achieve very good results using protocol modifications [4, 5]. Results of outreach programmes between St. Jude's Children's Hospital and centres in South America have shown likewise [6]. However, for the majority of children in Africa the prognosis is bleak. Follow-up of survivors is a challenge that needs to be tackled in order to determine any long-term effects of treatment.

## Way Forward

National cancer control plans should be developed in-country and these will inform and guide governments, stakeholders including health providers, international organizations, industry, NGOs and the lay public.

Strong advocacy for resources for cancer control programmes that include prevention, early detection and care is required.

Training health professionals so that there are functioning teams for paediatric cancer units is a necessity.

Suitable protocols must be developed and made available for trained health professionals.

Drug pricing agreements for concessions for developing countries would help improve affordability.

Cancer registries, hospital based and population based, should be established and this must go along with building diagnostic and treatment capacity in countries in Africa.

Twinning programmes between centres in more advanced countries and centres in Africa can play a major role in capacity building and also facilitate research.

## Research

There is a huge gap in the area of research between the developed world and African countries. Appropriate research would be very helpful and should be used to strengthen health systems on the continent.

Research in the African continent can be quite challenging. There is the probability of parents being coerced into participating because that might be the only way their child would receive treatment. Consent and assent in some countries would require several different languages as it is not uncommon to have over 20 different languages being spoken in one country. Reducing the numbers lost to follow-up would also require active measures to ensure results of studies are valid.

Pharmaceutical industry involvement could be in drug development research and drug pharmacokinetics in African children.

Clinical trials of modified treatment protocols that will achieve good cure rates with minimal toxicity need to be undertaken.

Vaccine research, for example malaria vaccine, EBV vaccine, HIV vaccine and any others found to be associated with the development of some cancers, could be beneficial.

Socio-cultural factors that impact negatively on management of cancers require investigating and strategies to address these should be adopted.

Studies to determine risks for and causative factors of childhood cancer for example genetics and environmental factors in the African continent would be helpful. This would not only benefit children of African descent but also throw more light on these aspects of cancer control for global benefit.

## Conclusion

In conclusion, childhood cancer in Africa is a very neglected area which has to compete with other pressing health care needs for limited resources. Support is required in several areas including capacity building, research, establishment of cancer registries, treatment protocol development, and drug supply management. Multi-stakeholder collaboration between academia, pharmaceutical industry, teaching hospitals, international agencies and National governments represents a useful way forward.


## References

1   WHO/AFRO: Chronic diseases accessed at www.afro.who.int/cdp/index.html

2   Parkin DM, Kramarova E, Draper GJ, et al: International Incidence of Childhood Cancer. Lyon, International Agency for Cancer Research, 1998, vol II, pp 1–391.

3   Howard SC, Metzger ML, Williams JA, et al: Childhood cancer epidemiology in low-income countries. Cancer 2008; 112:461–472.

4   Harif M, Barsaoui S, Benchekroun S, et al: Treatment of B-cell lymphoma with LMB modified protocols in Africa – report of the French-African Pediatric Oncology Group (GFAOP). Paediatr Blood Cancer 2008;50:1138–1142.

5   Hesseling P.B, Molyneux E, Tchintseme F, et al: Treating Burkitt's lymphoma in Malawi, Cameroon and Ghana. Lancet Oncol 2008;9:512–513.

6   Howard SC, Ortiz R, Baez LF, et al: Protocol based treatment for children with cancer in low income countries in Latin America: a report on the recent meetings of the Monza International School of Pediatric Hematology/oncology. Pediatr Blood Cancer 2007;48:486–490.



Prof. Lorna A. Renner, MD
Consultant Paediatric Oncologist
University of Ghana Medical School, Korle Bu Teaching Hospital
P.O. Box 4236, Accra (Ghana)
Tel. +233 21 665405, Fax +233 21 681080, E-Mail lornarenner@gmail.com

Rose K, van den Anker JN (eds): Guide to Paediatric Drug Development and Clinical Research.
Basel, Karger, 2010, pp 164–169

# Paediatric Clinical Research in Immunology and Inflammation

C. Bolte[a] · L. Senolt[c] · S. Gay[b]

[a]F. Hoffmann-La Roche Ltd., Pharmaceuticals Division, Basel, and [b]Department of Rheumatology, University Hospital Zürich, Zurich, Switzerland; [c]Department of Experimental Rheumatology, Institute of Rheumatology, Prague, Czech Republic

Autoimmune-mediated inflammatory diseases comprise a wide range of medical conditions across different therapeutic areas. Depending on disease activity and duration many of these conditions are associated with increased morbidity and even mortality not only because of specific end-organ damage but also systemic damage mediated by common inflammatory pathways. Table 1 provides a non-exhaustive overview of autoimmune inflammatory conditions structured by organ systems involved.

Some of the better-defined conditions serve as target indications for the development of new medicines, including biologic agents, which provide novel treatment options also for paediatric patients [1].

## Unmet Needs in Children

Paediatric legislation exists now in Europe and the US with the objective to foster the development of safe and efficacious medicines for children. In order to comply with EMA regulations, a paediatric investigation plan (PIP) has to be submitted at an early stage in clinical drug development (typically around phase 2) [2]. Data from paediatric studies are required for each indication, dosage form, dosage regimen and route of administration per relevant age groups, unless a waiver or deferral has been granted.

The EMA paediatric working party (predecessor to the paediatric committee) has assessed paediatric needs under 'Immunology' and 'Rheumatology' [2]. These needs apply to already approved medicines, where a formal indication is lacking for certain or sometimes all paediatric age groups according to ICH. It is implied that for molecules still in development a PIP is submitted as outlined above.

## Developmental Challenges

Regulations and unmet paediatric needs aside there are three key challenges to the development of novel medicines with respect to autoimmune-mediated conditions in children:
1 Translational
2 Clinical
3 Operational (logistical)

**Table 1.** A selection of autoimmune-mediated inflammatory conditions

| |
|---|
| **CNS:** multiple sclerosis |
| **Cardio-vascular:** vasculitides; secondary pulmonary arterial hypertension |
| **Haematopoetic:** autoimmune cytopaenias (ITP, PRCA, AIHE, etc.); Castleman's disease |
| **Endocrine:** Grave's disease/morbus Basedow, type 1 diabetes |
| **Gastrointestinal:** Crohn's disease, ulcerative colitis, various hepatides, primary biliary cirrhosis |
| **Renal:** various nephropathies (membranous, proliferative glomerulonephritis), lupus nephritis, nephrotic syndrome |
| **Musculo-skletal:** rheumatoid arthritis – JIA in children; connective tissue diseases |
| **Dermatological:** pemphigus vulgaris, psoriasis, dermatomyositis, scleroderma |

*Translational*

A true conundrum unfolds: to develop a compound for paediatric use at such an early stage, with only scarce adult data available, sometimes no validated animal model and limited utility of pharmacokinetic-pharmacodynamic (PK-PD) simulation, especially if the dose-response relationship is not linear – the extra- or interpolation from adult to paediatric cohorts simply based on weight or body surface area as is not feasible in most cases.

In addition to identifying an appropriate dosage regimen for each relevant age group (based on adult or animal data, where such a paediatric animal model exists), one also needs to consider special aspects for biologic compounds like immunogenicity (human anti-chimeric or anti-human antibodies, in some cases neutralising), altered immune response to typical childhood vaccinations, and in general longer-term effects on the maturing immune system.

Genetic predisposition and general health aside children are in a constant process of actively developing and adapting an immunological memory state as a result of frequent exposure to all sorts of pathogens and vaccinations. Hence, it is believed that the immune system of an immunological immature or even naïve individual is likely to be lymphatically more active than a juvenile or adolescent with a more 'adapted' immune system.

With future advances in gene expression profiling, it is to be expected that paediatric cohorts can also be stratified according to their predicted likelihood of responding to certain treatments. Recent investigations have linked the activation of disease-specific genes to clinical disease phenotypes. Functional variants provide strong evidence for a primary effect of the targeted gene, but a whole genome analysis is necessary for a comprehensive susceptibility genes search, as well as for drug response. For personalised healthcare (PHC) to become reality in this setting both phenotype and genotype matching will be necessary.

PHC also stands for identifying and validating surrogate genomic or proteomic 'biomarkers' that allow selecting the optimal therapeutic regimen for each particular patient to predict a clinical response and/or potential adverse events. Additionally, PHC will help to prevent losing time and cost for ineffective therapies, and reduce the number of patients exposed to unnecessary health risks [3].

For instance, some auto-immune-mediated diseases bear the hallmark of a 'B cell signature', hence B cell-depleting treatment with chimeric, humanised or fully human anti-CD20 monoclonal antibodies (rituximab, ocrelizumab, ofatumumab) would be justified for selected autoimmune and oncologic conditions, at least in clinical trials, provided the benefit-risk ratio is favourable in general for such a cohort and no other effective treatment options are available.

Many cytokines and immune cells are suggested to be involved in the pathology of autoimmune process in chronic arthritis [4]. The challenge here is to develop efficacious medicines without long-term safety data for children, since the starting point, at least in the past, have been adult studies with scarce or limited long-term safety data.

Another translational aspect is immunogenicity: minimum immunogenicity for paediatric patients would be appreciated, hence humanised or fully human antibodies represent important agents to be used. Progress in manufacturing technology led recently to the development of humanised (ocrelizumab) and fully human (ofatumumab) B-cell depleting agents, which are currently in phase 3 clinical trials in adult RA patients and may represent a beneficial treatment option with a favourable benefit-risk ratio also for children.

Additionally, the parenteral (intravenous, subcutaneous) administration of these large molecules is associated with an increased risk of several adverse events, which led to the search for agents suitable for oral administration. Orally administered drugs particularly target complex intracellular signalling pathways that have been tested with a variable clinical response in adult RA patients [5].


*Clinical*

The next challenge for autoimmune mediated inflammatory diseases is to agree on corresponding paediatric indications, which goes beyond just simply transferring the same disease entity from an adult population to a younger age group. In fact, sometimes the paediatric manifestation doesn't even bear similar clinical features. A good example is rheumatoid arthritis (RA).

While the manifestation of adult RA is confined mainly (not exclusively) to synovial tissues, childhood RA is a more systemic inflammatory disease with high mortality and a sometimes devastating impact on the overall development of the child. The nomenclature has evolved from juvenile RA (jRA) to systemic juvenile idiopathic arthritis (sJIA) with a well-defined polyarticular as well as oligoarticular subset of JIA (pJIA/oJIA), depending on the pattern of joint involvement (table 2 – ILAR).

JIA represents a heterogeneous group of arthritides of unknown cause beginning before the age of 16 years. According to the latest classification, it consists of several subtypes including systemic arthritis, oligoarthritis, polyarthritis (RF-negative, RF-positive), psoriatic arthritis, enthesis-related arthritis, and undifferentiated arthritis [7]. Compared to adult rheumatoid arthritis, JIA is a distinct disease with several clinical features. Thereby, the targeted therapy may also be not unique and may differ according the classification.

There is a trend towards early aggressive treatment in adult RA patients with the aim of improving long-term outcomes. Similar treatment strategy may be applied also to paediatric patients with chronic inflammatory diseases inadequately responding to conventional therapy in order to decrease specific end-organ as well as systemic damage.

Cytokines IL-1 and IL-6 appear to be the primary molecules involved in the pathogenesis of systemic arthritis. Hence, the IL-6 inhibiting humanised antibody tocilizumab is also being developed for juvenile RA indications [8], both sJIA and pJIA, and has already obtained regulatory approval for these indications in Japan (marketed as Actemra™).

TNF-α represents another major pro-inflammatory cytokine in the pathogenesis of oligoarticular and polyarticular JIA. Based on positive

| Subset | % frequency | Age at onset | Gender ratio |
|---|---|---|---|
| Systemic JIA | 4–17 | throughout childhood | F = M |
| Oligoarthritis | 27–56 | early childhood; peak at 2–4 years | F >>> M |
| RF-positive polyarthritis | 2–7 | late childhood or adolescence-peak at 10–14 years | F >> M |
| RF negative polyarthritis | 11–28 | biphasic distribution; early peak at 2–4 years and later peak at 6–12 years | F >> M |
| Enthesis | 3–11 | late childhood or adolescence | M >> F |
| Psoriatic arthritis | 2–11 | biphasic distribution; early peak at 2–4 years and later peak at 9–11 years | F >> M |

Source: Ravelli et al. [6].

results of randomised controlled clinical trials showing sustained efficacy and acceptable safety profile, etanercept (a soluble fully human TNF-receptor) and recently also adalimumab (a human anti-TNF-α monoclonal antibody) have been approved for moderate-to-severe active polyarticular-course JIA [9, 10].

T cell-targeted drugs have already demonstrated clinical benefits in the therapy of adult RA and also polyarticular JIA patients. A key role of a subset of memory T cells (Th17 subtype) has been recently described in the pathogenesis of autoimmune inflammation. Cell differentiation into Th17 cells is predominantly supported by cytokine IL-23 that has become a promising target of therapy for several autoimmune diseases [11]. Ustekinumab, a specific monoclonal antibody against the p40 subunit of cytokines IL-12 and IL-23, has very recently generated promising results in psoriasis and one proof-of-concept study demonstrated that besides associated psoriatic skin lesions, ustekinumab can also reduce the signs and symptoms of arthritis in patients with psoriatic arthritis [12].

Excipients, inactive ingredients, which serve to stabilise a specific formulation and also alter absorption, metabolism, distribution and excretion have to be taken into account as well. This been raised by a UK-based research team, which has described the excipient exposure in vulnerable preterm babies in a single centre. They found that 38 premature infants born over a 14-month period were exposed to more than 20 different excipients, including ethanol and propylene glycol, both of which are associated with significant neurotoxicity. The group also found that infants were exposed to high levels of sorbitol, with some of them exposed to higher than recommended adult levels [13].

Finally, in order to reduce potential child-specific and systemic toxicity, intra-articular therapy with both old traditional and new biological agents targeting cytokines, proliferation and/or apoptosis of synovial cells could represent a prospective therapeutic option particularly for paediatric patients with mono- to oligoarticular manifestation.

*Operational (Logistic)*

According to current nomenclature and terminology, this is a challenge of numbers – in the form of low incidences and prevalences. Not many reliable sources and publications exist that provide accurate epidemiological figures for paediatric autoimmune-mediated inflammatory diseases.

In order to investigate novel medicines for paediatric use one needs to find children and parents willing to participate in especially designed clinical trials that lead to the withdrawal of the young patient in case the subject is not responding to the investigational drug. Typically, the comparator arm consists of standard-of-care regimens with steroids, sometimes in combination with more established, non-biologic disease-modifying anti-rheumatic drugs. Children participating in clinical trials should at least receive standard-of-care therapy, regardless whether the trial bears a withdrawal or parallel-group design with rescue therapy.

National and International clinical research networks of referral centres with GCP-trained investigators and dedicated research personnel are available for the evaluation of new treatment strategies, including the validation of child-specific response criteria and outcome measures. Such child-specific outcome measures have been developed for a number of different rheumatologic diseases for monitoring disease progression as well as evaluating new treatment modalities in clinical trials.

Examples for disease-specific research networks:
- CARRA (Childhood Arthritis and Rheumatology Research Alliance) http://www.arthritis.org/carra.php)
- PRCSG (Paediatric Rheumatology Collaborative Study Group) http://www.cincinnatichildrens.org/research/div/rheumatology/resources/prcsg.htm
- PRINTO (Paediatric Rheumatology International Trials Organisation) http://www.printo.it/
- SCTC (Scleroderma Clinical Trials Consortium) http://www.sctc-online.org/index.htm

## Outlook

This guide is designed to give the non-specialist clinical researcher some insight into the novel strategies to treat children, one has to discuss first the lessons and limitations learnt in adults with all the novel 'biologic agents'. So far, despite tremendous progress made in the treatment of various forms of arthritis no therapy for RA has been able to reach an ACR 70 in over 60% of the treated patients. Interesting is also the fact that the same results and limitations have been observed in targeting T cells, B cells and monocytes. So, one has to ask the following questions:
- Why can't we do better and cure the disease?
- Why do most biologic agents benefiting RA patients do not work at all in patients with SLE?
- Why haven't we made more progress with PHC – personalised health care – in clinical practice?

All these questions need to be addressed with novel future research strategies. Since the successful sequencing of the human genome has so far provided only very limited new insights into health and disease and not resulted in the discovery of novel loci related to immunology and inflammation, it is currently emphasised to search for the regulation of the expression of the known genes in development and disease. In this regard, *epigenetics* is moving rapidly into the limelight of molecular research, in particular here rheumatic diseases [14].

Based on the fact that the regulation of gene expression is tightly controlled by specific epigenetic modifications, including acetylation, methylation, phosphorylation, ubiquitination and micro-RNAs, present research in the leading laboratories is focussed on the role of histone acetyltransferases (HATs), specific histone deacetylases (HDACs), DNA methyltransferases (DNAMTs) and over 1,000 micro-RNAs to be targetted already therapeutically with very selective antagomirs. In this regard it is more than obvious that drugs designed to correct aberrant epigenetic processes are on the cutting edge of science in future drug development to target, for example the synovial fibroblast [15].

Also novel approaches have to be found to predict responding patients for personalised healthcare in the future and detecting early potential 'off target c' effects by using detailed FACS analysis of mononuclear cells in the blood and gene expression as well as micro-RNA profiling [16] especially for small molecular drugs [5].

Finally, it is conceivable that a number of medical conditions together with their terminology and classification, which were based on early 20th century histo-morphological findings will be redefined and re-classified according to emerging immunological evidence and more insight into disease-specific inflammatory pathways. Hence, new medicines with novel mechanisms of action can be developed in a much more targeted fashion, in particular for paediatric cohorts.

## References


1 Gartlehner G, Hansen RA, Jonas BL, Thieda P, Lohr KN: Biologics for the treatment of juvenile idiopathic arthritis: a systematic review and critical analysis of the evidence. Clin Rheumatol 2008;27:67–76.

2 EMA Paediatric Working Party recommendations. http://www.ema.europa.eu/pdfs/human/paediatrics/38192206.pdf

3 Smolen JS, Aletaha D, Grisar J, Redlich K, Steiner G, Wagner O: The need for prognosticators in rheumatoid arthritis. Biological and clinical markers: where are we now? Arthritis Res Ther 2008; 10:208.

4 Gay S, Gay RE, Koopman WJ: Molecular and cellular mechanisms of joint destruction in rheumatoid arthritis: two cellular mechanisms explain joint destruction? Ann Rheum Dis 1993; 52(suppl 1):S39–S47.

5 Stanczyk J, Ospelt C, Gay S: Is there a future for small molecule drugs in the treatment of rheumatic diseases? Curr Opin Rheumatol 2008;20:257–262.

6 Ravelli A, Martini A: Juvenile idiopathic arthritis. Lancet 2007;369:767–778

7 Petty RE, Southwood TR, Manners P, et al: International League of Associations for Rheumatology. International League of Associations for Rheumatology classification of juvenile idiopathic arthritis, revision 2. Edmonton, 2001. J Rheumatol 2004;31:390–392.

8 Woo P: Systemic juvenile idiopathic arthritis – diagnosis, management and outcome. Nat Clin Pract Rheumatol 2006;2:28–34.

9 Lovell DJ, Giannini EH, Reiff A, et al: Etanercept in children with polyarticular juvenile rheumatoid arthritis. Paediatric Rheumatology Collaborative Study Group. N Engl J Med 2000;342:763–769.

10 Lovell DJ, Ruperto N, Goodman S, et al: Paediatric Rheumatology Collaborative Study Group; Paediatric Rheumatology International Trials Organisation. Adalimumab with or without methotrexate in juvenile rheumatoid arthritis. N Engl J Med 2008;359:810–820.

11 Tan ZY, Bealgey KW, Fang Y, Gong YM, Bao S: Interleukin-23: Immunological roles and clinical implications. Int J Biochem Cell Biol 2009;4:733–735.

12 Gottlieb AB, Mendelsohn A, Shen YK, Menter A: Randomized, placebo-controlled phase 2 study of ustekinumab, a human interleukin-12/23 monoclonal antibody, in psoriatic arthritis. Ann Rheum Dis 2008;67(suppl II):99.

13 Whittaker A, Mulla H, Turner MA, et al: Toxic Additives in Medications to Preterm Infants. Arch Dis Child Fetal Neonatal Ed, published online Jan 21 2009 doi: 10.1136/adc.2008.146035.

14 Huber LC, Stanczyk J, Jungel A, Gay S: Epigenetics in inflammatory diseases, Arthritis Rheum 2007;56:3523–3531.

15 Karouzakis E, Gay RE, Gay S, Neidhart M: Epigenetic control in rheumatoid synovial fibroblasts. Nat Rev Rheumatol 2009;5:266–272.

16 Ospelt C, Gay S: Antirheumatic drugs and gene signatures. Curr Opin Investig Drugs 2007;8:385–389.

17 Yokota S, Imagawa T, Mori M, et al: Efficacy and safety of tocilizumab in patients with systemic-onset juvenile idiopathic arthritis: a randomised, double-blind, placebo-controlled, withdrawal phase III trial. Lancet 2008; 371:998–1006.



Claus Bolte, MD, MBA
Pharmaceuticals Division: Global Medical Director (Immunology)
F. Hoffmann-La Roche Ltd., Pharmaceuticals Division
Grenzacherstrasse 74, bldg 74/4 Ost/106
CH–4070 Basel (Switzerland)
Tel. +41 414101426, E-Mail clausmannyc@netscape.net

Rose K, van den Anker JN (eds): Guide to Paediatric Drug Development and Clinical Research.
Basel, Karger, 2010, pp 170–177

# Clinical Trials of Anti-Infective Agents in Paediatrics

Irja Lutsar[a] · Ian Friedland[b]

[a]University of Tartu, Tartu, Estonia; [b]Cubist Pharmaceuticals, Lexington, Mass., USA

Antimicrobial agents are unique in that they continually lose efficacy over time because of the emergence of antimicrobial resistance, which can spread rapidly and widely. Unlike other classes of drugs, there is a perpetual need to develop new antimicrobial agents to counter the continual development of resistance [1]. Differences in the epidemiology of resistance in adults compared with paediatric populations necessitate specific considerations in the design of clinical studies in the different populations. In this chapter, issues specifically affecting the design of paediatric trials with antibacterial and antifungal agents will be discussed. The development of antiretroviral agents has several unique issues and will not be covered.

## General Principles

The efficacy of an anti-infective agent largely depends on the susceptibility (as measured with in vitro laboratory tests) of a micro-organism in relation to the concentration of a particular antibiotic at the site of infection. The antibacterial effect is likely to be similar in different age groups, provided that similar drug exposure is achieved. Thus, the results from adequate clinical studies in adults can often be extrapolated to the paediatric population.

Still, several differences between children and adults exist which could confound the extrapolation of results from adult studies. First, the pharmacokinetic (PK) properties of any medicine, including anti-infective agents, depend on the maturation of the body systems involved in absorption, distribution and elimination [2]. Second, there are situations (e.g. acute otitis media, pharyngotonsillitis, exacerbation of *Pseudomonas aeruginosa* infection in cystic fibrosis (CF), congenital immunodeficiencies) where the disease process or incidence differs between children and adults. Third, in neonates and infants below 3 months of age infections are often not limited to one organ system and tend to present as a systemic disease with sepsis-like symptoms prevailing over local signs, regardless of the site of infection. In all these situations, the data obtained in adults cannot reliably be extrapolated. Drugs may have unknown short-term toxicities peculiar to children or unknown long-term effects that could affect growth and development. Thus, safety trials should almost always be conducted in children.

## Issues to Consider when Conducting Paediatric Studies

### Timing of Paediatric Studies

In line with the EU paediatric regulation, a paediatric investigation plan (PIP) should be submitted early in the development of new drugs to ensure that appropriate development in children is incorporated. The timing of paediatric studies depends on whether the new agent is indicated for a disease where several marketed alternatives are available (e.g. a new antibiotic for otitis media) or whether the new agent could fulfil a significant unmet medical need (e.g. new inhaled antibiotic with activity against multi-resistant *Pseudomonas* spp. with potential use in CF). In the first scenario, paediatric studies could be delayed until safety and efficacy in adults has been proven. In the second scenario, however, paediatric studies could justifiably start immediately after the phase 1 programme in adults.

*Placebo-Controlled Trials*

Determining the treatment effect of an antibacterial agent compared with the course of a disease treated only with supportive care is an important goal. A placebo-controlled, randomised, double-blind trial is the most likely way to achieve this and is most applicable to diseases with causes in addition to bacteria or those with a self-limited course (e.g. otitis media, sinusitis). Although placebo-controlled studies in these situations are scientifically justifiable, paediatric placebo-controlled trials are likely to be challenged by the medical community, regulatory agencies or parents, especially in indications where there is evidence of the superiority of antibacterial agents over placebo, e.g. moderate to severe CAP or skin and soft tissue infections (SSTI) [3]. Even in indications as otitis media, in which the benefit of antibacterial therapy is questionable [4], placebo-controlled studies are problematic. Parents' expectations that their child should receive antibiotics will make obtaining consent challenging.

*Uncontrolled versus Comparative Trials*

Patients with immunocompromising underlying conditions (e.g. cancer, immunodeficiency syndromes) have the greatest need for new antibiotics with a wide spectrum. They are also prone to many adverse events, either from their underlying illness or from the multiple medicines they receive. Because of the complex nature of assessing the safety profile of a new drug in such circumstances, comparative trials are preferred over uncontrolled studies as they can better distinguish drug-associated reactions from those caused by other factors. To best evaluate a new drug, the use of a single (or at most two) comparator agent simplifies the safety analysis. Where possible, comparator agents should be chosen from those approved by regulatory agencies for the indication under study. However, where approved agents are limited or the optimal dose is not known, consideration of authoritative guidelines or expert advice could be appropriate.

Usually, clinical development of new agents requires multinational studies; this can be impeded if the potential comparator agents are approved only in selected countries. For example, linezolid is indicated for treatment of paediatric SSTI in the US but not in the EU. In such circumstances, two different comparator agents may be needed in each region. In some countries, regulatory agencies and ethics committees do allow trials to be conducted with 'unapproved' comparator agents provided there are sufficient safety and efficacy data in the paediatric population. In multi-centre trials, it is often challenging to find one or two comparator agents acceptable to all study sites. However, the choice of comparator agents should be limited because studies that allow the investigators to select comparator agents (i.e. 'standard of care' studies) are generally too confounded to be acceptable for unambiguous safety analysis.

*Studies in Immunocompromised Patients*

New anti-infective agents are especially needed for immunocompromised patients who are often infected with micro-organisms resistant to available agents. Unfortunately, clinical trials tend to exclude a large proportion of immunocompromised children, leaving critical knowledge gaps in the treatment of the immunocompromised host. It would be desirable not to exclude paediatric subjects from clinical trials solely because of immunocompromised states (whether congenital or acquired). However, it is appreciated that immunocompromising conditions are heterogeneous, many specific conditions are rare, and the susceptibility of patients to specific infections varies with different illnesses, e.g. patients with chronic granulomatous disease are prone to aspergillosis and staphylococcal infection whereas those with advanced stage HIV infection often suffer from viral infection (e.g. herpesviruses) or non-tuberculous mycobacteria. Thus, the inclusion of immunosuppressed patients in general, and which specific disorders to include, should be considered carefully, depending on the target pathogens of the new agent.

*Effect of Antibiotics on Normal Microflora and Emergence of Resistance*

The effect of antibiotics on normal microflora has been reviewed in detail elsewhere [5]. Antibacterial agents affect indigenous microbiota in several ways of which the emergence of antimicrobial resistance and development of antibiotic-associated diarrhoea (AAD) caused by *Clostridium difficile* are best documented. Recovery of normal microflora to pre-treatment levels can be prolonged.

The number of appropriate studies in this field is fairly limited. To evaluate the composition of human microbiota is time- and labour-consuming and has mostly been undertaken in small groups of subjects and in specialised laboratories. For reliable results several specimens per timepoint at various times should be collected. New DNA based methodologies are preferred.

Also in antibiotic clinical trials in children it is important to monitor the emergence of bacteria resistant to the study agents. The frequency of AAD should also be followed and reported.

## Type of Studies

*Pharmacokinetic Studies and Dose Selection*

Some aspects of the PK of anti-infective agents (e.g. absorption, elimination half-life) differ in adult and paediatric populations. Other aspects, such as dose linearity and protein binding, tend to be similar. In addition, PK values are likely to be more widely distributed in children if the entire paediatric population is considered. Differences are more pronounced in the most immature patients, such that dosing regimens for extremely premature babies are usually very different from those in adults and older children [6]. A detailed description of the PK characteristics in children is considered elsewhere [2, 7, 8].

In order to identify appropriate doses of a new anti-infective agent, PK studies in all age categories should be conducted before safety/efficacy trials. Age categories are defined in the ICH-11 guideline. Historically, a staggered approach, starting with older age cohorts and conducting an interim analysis before moving to the next cohort, has usually been followed. However, the scientific rationale and benefit of such an approach with anti-infective agents is questionable and some recent paediatric PK studies have enrolled age cohorts (except neonates) concurrently. A staggered approach may unnecessarily delay the start of subsequent safety/efficacy studies.

In general, paediatric PK studies aim to determine doses that approximate the exposure with standard dosing in adults, enabling the extrapolation of efficacy data from the adult studies [9]. More specifically than comparing the drug exposure in paediatric and adult patients, paediatric PK studies should target appropriate PK/PD parameters [e.g. peak/MIC, AUC/MIC ratio or time above MIC (T > MIC)], which have been shown to be major determinants of in vivo efficacy [10–12], e.g. the antibacterial effect of beta-lactam antibiotics is known to be time-dependent. T > MIC values of 30–40% of the dosing interval are often accepted in adults and the same target is assumed in children. However, higher targets, based on expert opinion rather than scientific evidence, e.g. 40–50% for penicillins and of 50–60% for cephalosporins, are assumed to be needed in neonates because of their immature immune system [13].

The Helsinki Declaration precludes the use of healthy volunteers in paediatric studies. Thus, PK studies of new antibiotics are conducted in patients with proven or suspected infections. Nevertheless, at the time of PK studies the effective dosing regimen of a new agent in children awaits confirmation and, thus it is acceptable to give the agent as an add-on to standard-of-care antibiotic treatment. In this situation, care is needed to avoid potential drug-drug interactions or cumulative toxicity. As highlighted elsewhere, the need to conduct single- or multiple-dose studies mainly depends on the PK characteristics of the drug (http://www.ema.europa.eu/pdfs/human/ich/271199en.pdf). If a new agent has linear PK properties in adults (and thus presumed likely in children) the conduct of single dose studies might be sufficient. If, however, the PK pattern is non-linear, multiple dose studies, with sample collection at steady state, are recommended.

An important consideration for a new agent, especially one with a very wide spectrum of antibacterial activity, is that it will be used in patients with complex disease, impaired immunity and will often be used in combination with several other agents. In such situations, the likelihood of drug-drug interactions and inter-patient variability in PK parameters is high. Thus, the within patient dose-escalation/reduction methodology as described in the recent voriconazole paediatric PK studies could be used to avoid potential biases introduced by drug-drug interactions [9,

14]. Of note, formal drug interaction studies are generally not conducted in the paediatric population and can be extrapolated from adult studies. However, additional or confirmatory information may become apparent from analyses of concomitant medication use in paediatric studies.

Clinical susceptibility breakpoints of a microorganism are determined by different agencies in Europe and the US (European Committee on Antimicrobial Susceptibility Testing [EUCAST] and the Clinical Laboratory Standards Institute [CLSI], respectively) resulting in many differences in recommendations in the two regions [15]. This can add additional complexity to international studies and should be borne in mind when considering appropriate PK/PD targets. This potential complexity is not specific for paediatrics. Different dosing recommendations may be reached in different regions.

The invasiveness related to pain/anxiety and blood loss precludes collection of a large number of blood samples in many instances, particularly in neonates and infants. Population approaches, which rely on PK-PD modelling, are particularly appealing in such situations because these models can utilize sparse data and thus avoid distress and pain [16]. In a recent study, gatifloxacin exposure in children with recurrent otitis media was estimated using just one blood sample per patient [17]. In the voriconazole clinical programme, the recommended dose for children from 2 to 12 years was defined using population-PK modelling from several PK studies [9].

*Evaluating Efficacy in Paediatric Population*

Once PK studies have identified an appropriate dose, adequately powered efficacy trials should be considered. Adequate and well-controlled efficacy studies have not always been needed to support approval in children, partially because of the difficulties in achieving a microbiological diagnosis and partially because often the number of paediatric subjects is too limited to perform statistically powered studies [3]. In addition, in most cases the disease process in children is similar to that in adults and efficacy can be extrapolated from the adult, provided that similar drug exposure is achieved in both populations (http://www.ema.europa.eu/pdfs/human/ich/271199en.pdf). However, efficacy trials in the paediatric population can be required for approval. First, some infections, such as otitis media, are very common in the paediatric population but occur rarely in adults. Thus, for new agents potentially active against bacteria causing otitis, especially those targeting resistant micro-organisms, adequate and well-controlled studies in this indication might be required. This becomes more critical if bacterial resistance appears to be emerging more rapidly in paediatric infections, as occurred recently with emergence of pneumococcal resistance and community-acquired MRSA. Second, there are debilitating conditions, e.g. CF or congenital immunodeficiencies that are more common in children than in adults, although most CF patients now survive into adulthood [18]. New antibacterial agents targeted for use in CF and active against *Pseudomonas* spp. and/or *S. aureus,* including coverage of multi-resistant strains, could appropriately be studied in children alone or concurrently with adults. Third, paediatric efficacy trials might be needed in situations where the disease process in children differs from that in adults. For example, the eradication rate of group A-beta-haemolytic streptococci (GABHS) in paediatric patients with pharyngotonsillitis and treated with penicillin is lower than that in adults [19]. In addition, GABHS pharyngotonsillitis is a paediatric disease that mostly occurs between 5 and 15 years. For the indication of GABHS pharyngotonsillitis paediatric efficacy trials should be conducted.

Fourth, there is an urgent need for efficacy studies in neonates, an understudied patient population. Neonates are unique because of their immature immune and other organ systems [20].

Because of their poor systemic and local immunity, infection often spreads from the original focus leading to systemic infection. Systemic infection in neonates mimics many other conditions making establishment of a diagnosis difficult and resulting in frequent use of empiric broad-spectrum antibiotic therapy. In addition, the precarious fluid balance and immature kidney function in neonates result in PK characteristics very different from older age groups necessitating very careful attention to dosing regimens [21]. These factors necessitate caution in extrapolating data from studies conducted in older age groups. Concerns in neonates are compounded in the most vulnerable population of extremely premature babies in whom almost no adequately designed studies with anti-infective agents have been conducted. Published studies have either been retrospective or underpowered [22, 23]. Despite this antibiotics are very widely used in this population; 94–100% of extremely premature neonates receive antibiotics for prophylaxis or treatment of suspected bacterial infections [24]. Therefore, neonates, including those with extreme prematurity, should be included in clinical studies of antimicrobial agents unless exclusion is justified on grounds of safety or predicted lack of therapeutic benefit. While it may not be possible to conduct adequately powered efficacy studies in a number of different indications in neonates, neonatal sepsis is an important target for study with new antimicrobial medicinal products. With the implementation of new paediatric legislation and introduction of an EU and NIH funding schemes for off-patent medicines, new data are expected in the near future.

Guidelines for the conduct of efficacy trials with antiinfective agents, including those in paediatric populations, are provided by the EMA and the US FDA. In general, selection of patients (inclusion and exclusion criteria, with appropriate age adjustments), statistical considerations, and validation of primary and secondary endpoints are similar in paediatric and adult studies. In both populations, the ideal endpoint would be the bacterial eradication rate. However, in many indications (e.g. pneumonia, SSTI, and neonatal sepsis) this may not be possible as patients are generally diagnosed on clinical signs and symptoms and quantitative microbiological evaluations are not generally feasible. Even obtaining adequate qualitative microbiological specimens (e.g. sputum) is more problematic in children. Even if microbiological evaluations are obtained at baseline, follow-up cultures may not be feasible. For example, the ethics review committees in most industrialised countries are unlikely to accept repeated tympanic taps in patients with clinically improving otitis media or repeat lumbar punctures in patients with bacterial meningitis. Indications such as pneumonia or SSTI infection suffer from lack of availability of suitable specimens for follow-up cultures once patients are clinically improved. Invasive techniques, such as bronchoalveolar lavage, to diagnose CAP are unlikely to be acceptable to families, physicians or ethics committees [3]. Therefore, the generally accepted primary endpoint in most indications (except urinary tract infections) is the clinical cure rate at a follow-up visit as determined by the investigator. Still, as in adult studies, repeat microbiological cultures should be collected and reported wherever feasible. In addition, other outcome measures such as mortality, reinfection and relapse rates should be collected.

*Evaluating Safety in the Paediatric Population*

In contrast to efficacy data, safety should always be evaluated in children as it might be very different. Although the safety profile of most antimicrobial agents is similar in adults and children (especially those of school age), in the past, several antibacterial agents have had harmful effects specific to children, including chloramphenicol (shock in neonates), sulphonamides (kernicterus), tetracyclines (discoloured or damaged bones and teeth) and quinolones (potential cartilage damage) [25]. The mechanisms responsible for the different safety profile of such drugs in children are varied and often related to the immaturity of drug metabolising enzymes [7] or to effects on developing organs. The likelihood of specific paediatric safety issues cannot easily be predicted, hence the need for dedicated paediatric safety studies.

Similar to efficacy studies, safety studies should only commence once PK studies have identified the appropriate dosing regimen(s) for all age categories. As a rule, safety trials should be conducted in populations in which a new agent is potentially indicated.

Many new antimicrobial agents have the potential to be used against antibiotic-resistant micro-organisms and, as much as possible, the study population should include patients with resistant bacterial infections; this often necessitates inclusion of patients with complex underlying conditions or impaired immunity. For example, MRSA often infects patients with impaired immunity (although it is also common in those with normal immunity) such as those with CF and extremely premature babies.

Agents belonging to a class with a well-described safety profile could be studied in several paediatric age cohorts simultaneously whereas a cautious approach may be more appropriate with agents with a benefit to risk profile that is not clearly defined or is less favourable. In the latter case, a staggered approach would be preferred, starting with studies in adolescents and moving sequentially into younger age groups. Although this approach is frequently recommended, there is little published evidence of the benefit of such an approach.

There is little regulatory guidance concerning sample size estimations for safety trials. The frequency of adverse events observed in adult studies or known to occur with similar agents could serve as the basis for sample size calculations. A safety database of 300–400 patients across all paediatric age categories is usually sufficient to identify safety issues occurring with a frequency of 1% or greater. As in adults, rare events may not be uncovered in initial paediatric studies and thus postmarketing surveillance or sometimes even active registries may be necessary.

When assessing safety of anti-infective agents, it is imperative to consider the growth and development characteristics of children (including neonates) as well as the impact that organ maturation has throughout the different stages of childhood. Therefore, long-term follow-up is sometimes appropriate, especially when the new agent belongs to a new class or has shown effects that affect growth and development in juvenile animals. The exact duration of follow-up should be decided on a case by case basis depending on PK properties, duration of therapy and specific safety concerns.

Safety studies should also evaluate relationships between adverse events and drug exposure. Thus, sparse blood (and, if appropriate, urine) samples should be collected; through population PK analysis and modelling, relationships between drug exposure and side effects should be described, as appropriate [16].

## Future Directions

Our knowledge of how best to design paediatric studies of antimicrobial agents has much room for improvement. First, better diagnostic techniques for bacterial and fungal infections are essential for enrolment of children into clinical trials who are most likely to benefit from the therapy under study. Although new nucleic acid based methods have been developed recently they are not validated and thus cannot be recommended presently for patient enrolment. Another factor critical in every clinical trial is the inclusion of appropriate diagnostic criteria for the indication under study. These are better defined in some indications and age groups than in others. Diagnostic criteria are most poorly defined in the neonatal age group.

Future research should focus on developing new design methodologies for paediatric studies that would allow enrolment of fewer subjects and the extrapolation of results across different populations. This would enable new medicines to be approved faster for use in paediatric subjects and could avoid unnecessary studies with potential reduction in the cost and timelines of paediatric studies.

## References


1 Spellberg B, Guidos R, Gilbert D, Bradley J, Boucher HW, Scheld WM, Bartlett JG, Edwards J Jr: The epidemic of antibiotic-resistant infections: a call to action for the medical community from the Infectious Diseases Society of America. Clin Infect Dis 2008;46:155–164.
2 Kearns GL, Abdel-Rahman SM, Alander SW, Blowey DL, Leeder JS, Kauffman RE: Developmental pharmacology–drug disposition, action, and therapy in infants and children. N Engl J Med 2003;349:1157–1167.
3 Bradley JS, McCracken GH: Unique considerations in the evaluation of antibacterials in clinical trials for pediatric community-acquired pneumonia. Clin Infect Dis 2008;47(suppl 3):S241–S248.
4 Glasziou PP, Del Mar CB, Sanders SL, Hayem M: Antibiotics for acute otitis media in children. Cochrane Database Syst Rev 2004;CD000219.
5 Sullivan A, Edlund C, Nord CE: Effect of antimicrobial agents on the ecological balance of human microflora. Lancet Infect Dis 2001;1:101–114.
6 Metsvaht T, Oselin K, Ilmoja ML, Anier K, Lutsar I: Pharmacokinetics of penicillin g in very-low-birth-weight neonates. Antimicrob Agents Chemother 2007;51:1995–2000.
7 Hines RN: The ontogeny of drug metabolism enzymes and implications for adverse drug events. Pharmacol Ther 2008;118:250–267.
8 Alcorn J, McNamara PJ: Pharmacokinetics in the newborn. Adv Drug Deliv Rev 2003;55:667–686.
9 Karlsson MO, Lutsar I, Milligan PA: Population pharmacokinetic analysis of voriconazole plasma concentration data from pediatric studies. Antimicrob Agents Chemother 2009;53:935–944.
10 Craig WA: The hidden impact of antibacterial resistance in respiratory tract infection. Re-evaluating current antibiotic therapy. Respir Med 2001;95(suppl A): S12–S19; discussion S26–S27.
11 Drusano GL: Antimicrobial pharmacodynamics: critical interactions of 'bug and drug'. Nat Rev Microbiol 2004;2: 289–300.

12  van den Anker JN, Pokorna P, Kinzig-Schippers M, Martinkova J, de Groot R, Drusano GL, Sorgel F: Meropenem pharmacokinetics in the newborn. Antimicrob Agents Chemother 2009;53:3871–3879.

13  de Hoog M, Mouton JW, van den Anker JN: New dosing strategies for antibacterial agents in the neonate. Semin Fetal Neonatal Med 2005;10:185–194.

14  Walsh TJ, Karlsson MO, Driscoll T, Arguedas AG, Adamson P, Saez-Llorens X, Vora AJ, Arrieta AC, Blumer J, Lutsar I, Milligan P, Wood N: 'Pharmacokinetics and safety of intravenous voriconazole in children after single- or multiple-dose administration.' Antimicrob Agents Chemother 2004;48:2166–2172.

15  Kahlmeter G: Breakpoints for intravenously used cephalosporins in Enterobacteriaceae–EUCAST and CLSI breakpoints. Clin Microbiol Infect 2008; 14(suppl 1):169–174.

16  Tod M, Jullien V, Pons G: Facilitation of drug evaluation in children by population methods and modelling. Clin Pharmacokinet 2008;47:231–243.

17  Rubino CM, Ambrose P, Cirincione B, Arguedas A, Sher L, Lopez E, Saez-Llorens X, Grasela DM: Pharmacokinetics and pharmacodynamics of gatifloxacin in children with recurrent otitis media: application of sparse sampling in clinical development. Diagn Microbiol Infect Dis 2007;59:67–74.

18  Doring G, Elborn JS, Johannesson M, de Jonge H, Griese M, Smyth A, Heijerman H: Clinical trials in cystic fibrosis. J Cyst Fibros 2007;6:85–99.

19  Brook I: A pooled comparison of cefdinir and penicillin in the treatment of group a beta-hemolytic streptococcal pharyngotonsillitis. Clin Ther 2005;27: 1266–1273.

20  Wynn JL, Neu J, Moldawer LL, Levy O: Potential of immunomodulatory agents for prevention and treatment of neonatal sepsis. J Perinatol 2009;29:79–88.

21  Drukker A, Guignard JP: Renal aspects of the term and preterm infant: a selective update. Curr Opin Pediatr 2002;14: 175–182.

22  Mtitimila EI, Cooke RW: Antibiotic regimens for suspected early neonatal sepsis. Cochrane Database Syst Rev 2004; CD004495.

23  Stoll BJ, Hansen NI, Higgins RD, Fanaroff AA, Duara S, Goldberg R, Laptook A, Walsh M, Oh W, Hale E: Very low birth weight preterm infants with early onset neonatal sepsis: the predominance of gram-negative infections continues in the National Institute of Child Health and Human Development Neonatal Research Network, 2002–2003. Pediatr Infect Dis J 2005;24:635–639.

24  Shani L, Weitzman D, Melamed R, Zmora E, Marks K: Risk factors for early sepsis in very low birth weight neonates with respiratory distress syndrome. Acta Paediatr 2008;97:12–15.

25  Ramachandrappa A, Jain L: Iatrogenic disorders in modern neonatology: a focus on safety and quality of care. Clin Perinatol 2008;35:1–34, vii.

Prof. Irja Lutsar, MD
University of Tartu
Ravila 19
Tartu 50411 (Estonia)
Tel. +372 737 4171, Fax +372 737 4172, E-Mail irja.lutsar@ut.ee

Rose K, van den Anker JN (eds): Guide to Paediatric Drug Development and Clinical Research.
Basel, Karger, 2010, pp 178–186

# Obesity in Children

Johannes Hebebrand

Department of Child and Adolescent Psychiatry, LVR-Klinikum Essen, University of Duisburg-Essen, Essen, Germany

## Definition and Epidemiology

Overweight is present if body weight adjusted for height exceeds a specified cut-off; obesity implies an excessive fraction of total body weight comprised of fat mass. In clinical practice, the body mass index (BMI) defined as weight in kilograms divided by squared height in meters has become widely accepted as the optimal weight-height index throughout childhood and adolescence and as a surrogate measure of adiposity. The correlations between BMI and percent body fat are high. In adults obesity is conventionally defined via a BMI ≥30; for children and adolescents different definitions exist: The Centers for Disease Control and Prevention (CDC) discriminate 'at risk of overweight' children between ages 2 and 19 years with a BMI between the 85th and 95th percentile from 'overweight' children who have a BMI ≥95th percentile (fig. 1). According to German recommendations, overweight and obese children have a BMI between the 90th and 97th and ≥97th centiles, respectively, of the reference sample (http://www.mybmi.de). The International Obesity Task Force advocates using those BMI centiles that pass through the adult cut-off points for overweight and obesity of 25 and 30 kg/m$^2$ at age 18 years. If a child is obese, the risk of persistence into adulthood increases

with the degree of adiposity, age of the child and parental obesity [1].

Worldwide mean BMI and as a consequence prevalence rates for overweight and obesity in children, adolescents and adults have been on the rise in both industrialized and developing countries [2]. Children and adolescents have been affected strongly by this secular trend. In the USA, the National Health Examination Surveys have revealed a fourfold increase in the prevalence of overweight among children aged 6–11 and a threefold increase for adolescents aged 12–19 between the 1960s and the most recent survey conducted between 1999 and 2002 [3]; in the 1999–2002 survey 16% of the children aged 6 through 19 years were overweight as defined via a BMI ≥95th centile of the surveys in the 1960s. An additional 16% of children were classified as at risk of overweight. Most recently, the obesity rates in the USA have seemingly levelled off: The prevalence of high BMI for age among children and adolescents showed no significant changes between 2003–2004 and 2005–2006 and no significant trends between 1999 and 2006 [4]. Single European studies have also provided evidence that obesity rates have not increased any further during the last few years in the respective countries. However, it is too early to tell whether these findings indeed represent a true levelling off.

## Medical and Psychological Sequelae

Cardiovascular disorders including hypertension, impaired glucose tolerance, type 2 diabetes mellitus, dyslipidaemia and metabolic syndrome have become more prevalent during adolescence as a consequence of the obesity epidemic [1]. The associations of higher BMI with coronary heart disease are stronger in boys than in girls and increase with the age of the child in both sexes [5]. Sleep apnoea, pseudotumour cerebri, and Blount's disease represent further sources of morbidity [1]. Childhood and adolescent obesity has been associated with an increased mortality even upon adjustment for adult BMI. Assessment of body fat distribution is important for the estimation of future risks; both a high waist circumference and a high waist-hip ratio entail elevated risks for medical consequences. The economic implications of childhood obesity are dire: Elevated BMI in childhood has been estimated to entail USD 14.1 billion in additional prescription drug, emergency room, and outpatient visit costs annually [6].

Obesity entails considerable stigmatisation; nevertheless, rates of psychiatric disorders are not elevated in population-based obese adolescents. However, in children and adolescents who enlist in weight reduction programs, rates of mood, anxiety and eating disorders are increased. Quality of life is reduced in obese children and adolescents; the reduction is, however, more pronounced if the young individual feels overweight, irrespective of whether or not overweight defined in medical terms is actually present or not [7].

## Risk Factors

Parental obesity is the strongest risk factor for childhood and adolescent obesity. The risk is influenced by the degree of parental obesity and is further elevated if both parents are obese [8] (table 1). Twin, family and adoption studies have led to the conclusion that the strong predictive value of parental BMI mainly stems from genetic rather than environmental factors. Twin studies have produced the most consistent and highest heritability estimates in the range of 0.6–0.9 for BMI, estimates based on family and adoption studies have typically been lower [9].

Monogenic forms of childhood obesity are based on functionally relevant mutations in genes involved in body weight regulation including those coding for leptin, leptin receptor, pro-opiomelanocortin, and melanocortin-4 receptor *(MC4R)*. Whereas most of such monogenic forms of obesity are exceedingly rare, *MC4R* mutations leading to autosomal-dominant inheritance of obesity can be detected in 2–4% of extremely overweight children and adolescents [9, 10]. More recently, genome-wide association studies have led to the identification of a number of polygenes including the 'fat mass and obesity associated gene' *(FTO)* and the *MC4R*. The respective variants act in an additive manner; the effect sizes of predisposing alleles range from below 200 g to a maximum of 1.5 kg [10].

Secular changes in energy intake and expenditure in interaction with a common genetic predisposition to overweight are assumed to underlie the recent obesity epidemic. Attempts to unequivocally pinpoint relevant environmental mechanisms even within a single country or society have proven difficult. For example, the relationship between TV consumption and obesity has been studied repeatedly in cross-sectional studies. Most studies have shown a clear cut association; however, only single longitudinal studies have been performed which allow a causal inference [1]. A longitudinal study of 980 children followed-up biannually from age 3–15 and at ages 21 and 26 revealed that the population-attributable fraction for overweight at age 26 due to viewing between ages 5 and 15 was 17% after adjustment for potential confounders [11].

Children spend only 2% of their time pursuing moderate to vigorous activity. Overweight and obesity are associated with a poorer body gross

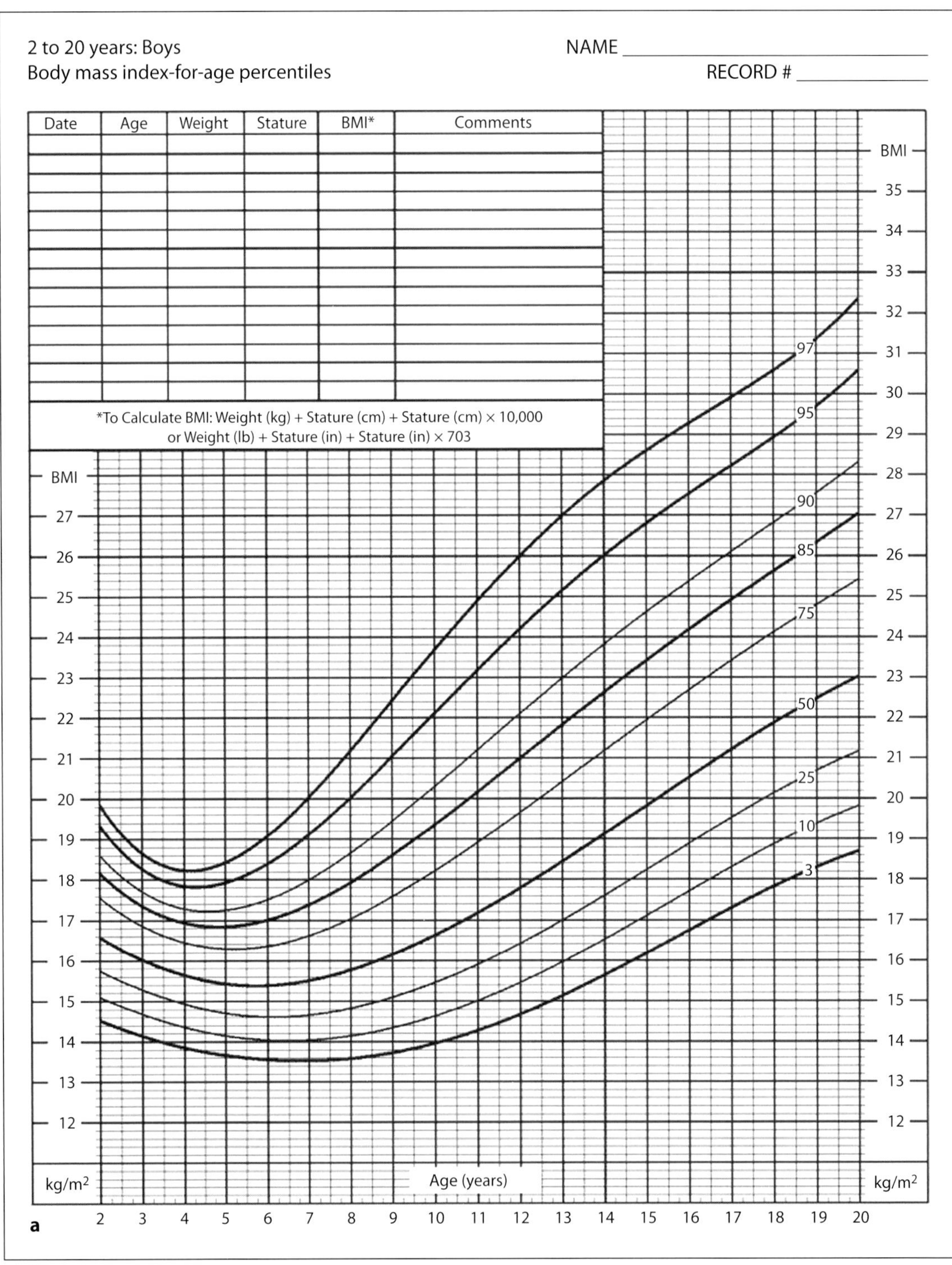


**Fig. 1. a**, **b** BMI-for-age percentiles for boys (**a**) and girls (**b**) for the US population (http://www.cdc.gov/growthcharts).

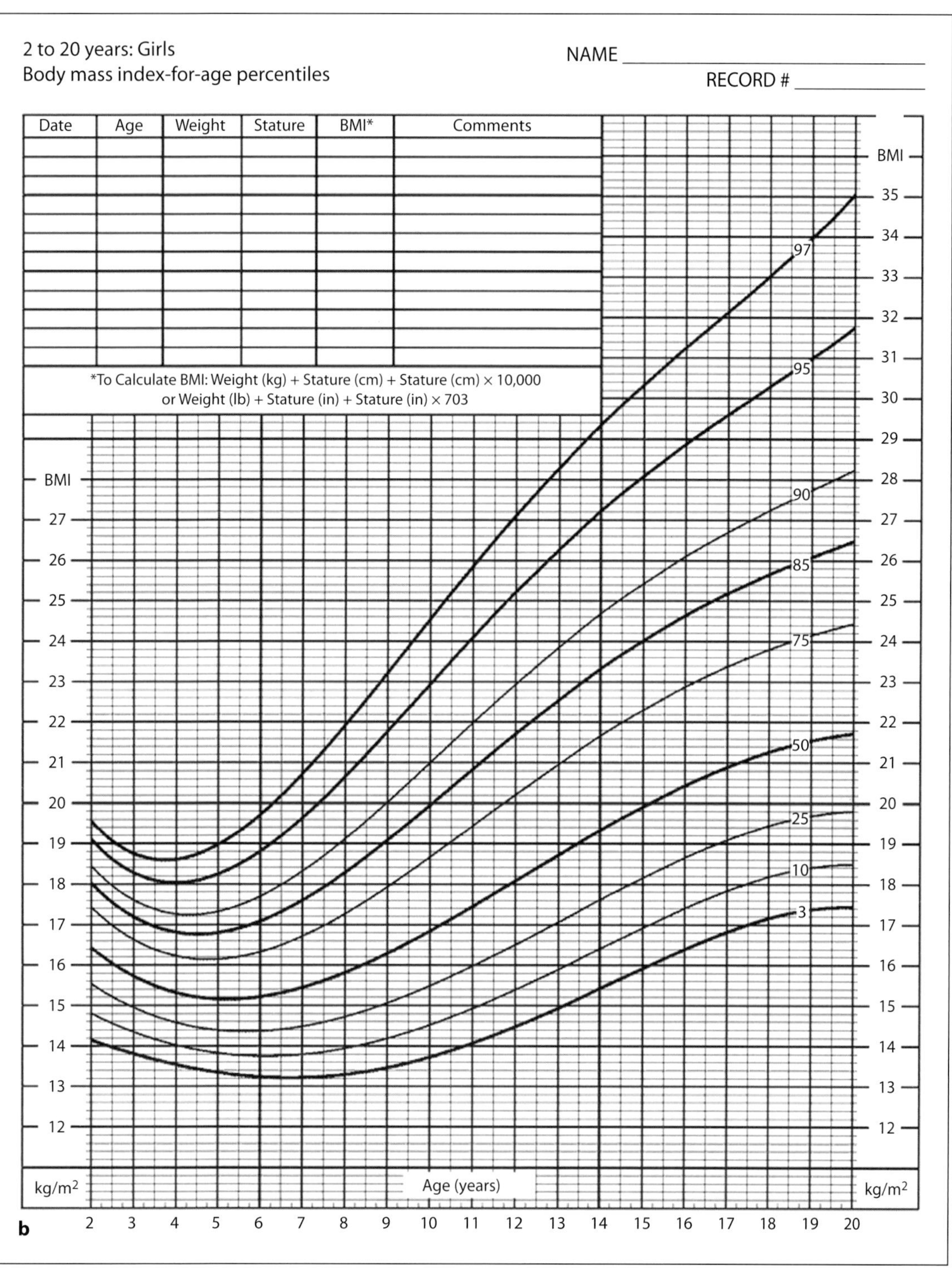

2 to 20 years: Girls
Body mass index-for-age percentiles
NAME
RECORD #
Date
Age
Weight
Stature
BMI*
Comments
*To Calculate BMI: Weight (kg) + Stature (cm) + Stature (cm) × 10,000
or Weight (lb) + Stature (in) + Stature (in) × 703
BMI
BMI
35
34
33
32
31
30
29
28
27
27
26
26
25
25
24
24
23
23
22
22
21
21
20
20
19
19
18
18
17
17
16
16
15
15
14
14
13
13
12
12
97
95
90
85
75
50
25
10
3
kg/m²
kg/m²
Age (years)
b
2
3
4
5
6
7
8
9
10
11
12
13
14
15
16
17
18
19
20

**Table 1.** Association of risk factors and obesity at age 7 years in the Avon longitudinal study of parents and children using multivariable binary logistic regression models [8]

| Risk factor | Prevalence of childhood obesity[1] in % (n = 7,758) | Final model adjusted odds ratio (95% CI; n = 5,493)[2] |
|---|---|---|
| Birth weight, continuous (100 g units) | 8.4 | 1.05 (1.03–1.07) |
| Maternal smoking during pregnancy | | |
| None | 7.5 | 1.00 |
| 1–9 | 11.5 | 1.76 (1.21–2.52) |
| 10–19 | 11.3 | 1.59 (1.08–2.34) |
| >= 20 | 13.8 | 1.80 (1.01–3.39) |
| Parental obesity | | |
| Both parents BMI <30 | 6.2 | 1.00 |
| Father BMI >30 | 16.2 | 2.54 (1.72–3.75) |
| Mother BMI >30 | 23.6 | 4.25 (2.86–6.32) |
| Both parents BMI >30 | 43.8 | 10.44 (5.11–21.32) |
| Time spent watching TV | | |
| <= 4 h/week | 5.2 | 1.00 |
| 4.1–8 h/week | 8.3 | 1.37 (1.02–1.83) |
| >8 h/week | 10.3 | 1.55 (1.13–2.12) |
| Duration of night-time sleep, h | | |
| First quartile | 10.3 | 1.45 (1.10–1.89) |
| Second quartile | 8.8 | 1.35 (1.02–1.79) |
| Third quartile | 6.4 | 1.04 (0.76–1.42) |
| Fourth quartile | 6.8 | 1.00 |

Non-significant variables: infant feeding (breast-feeding, age at introduction of solids), dietary patterns (junk food, healthy food, traditional, fussy).
Variables that did not enter the model: parity, season of birth, gestational age, number of foetuses, number of siblings, ethnicity of child, age of mother at delivery, time in car per day.
[1] BMI ≥95th centile relative to the 1990 British reference population.
[2] Odds ratio is adjusted for maternal education, energy intake at 3 years and sex; all listed variables significant at the p < 0.01 level.

motor development and endurance performance. Dietary changes including increased energy intake and portion sizes, elevations in fat and/or carbohydrate intake, reduced intake of fruits and vegetables and increased consumption of soft drinks have all been implicated in the obesity epidemic. Consumer trends and food marketing strategies including advertisement have also been deemed important. Most of these factors are viewed controversially and unequivocal data casually linking the obesity epidemic to any one of these factors are virtually absent. Maternal smoking during pregnancy has been associated with an increased risk of childhood obesity. A minor protective effect of breast feeding has been observed repeatedly, which according to some studies is still detectable in adolescence. Cross-sectional studies have revealed that a shorter duration of sleep is associated with obesity. Longitudinal studies have revealed a predictive value of depressive symptoms in childhood and adolescence for obesity in later childhood, adolescence and adulthood [1].

Many of the (assumed) risk factors are more prevalent in families with a low socio-economic background; accordingly, a low socio-economic status is associated with higher rates of obesity in both children and adults. It appears that parental education is particularly important within this context [1].

*Treatment:* High attrition rates of approximately 25–35% apply to both conventional and drug treatment studies of paediatric obesity; high dropout rates warrant attention because individual drop-outs may be due to failure to lose weight [12]. Most treatment studies were of short duration only; long-term data are scanty. The efficacies of both conventional and pharmacological treatments of obesity have been re-analysed recently based on 61 [13] and 64 [14] randomized controlled trails. Non-pharmacological treatments are typically based on dietary, physical activity and/or behavioural interventions; currently, the evidence is insufficient to favour one treatment program over another. Both reviews pointed to methodological limitations inherent to many non-pharmacological childhood obesity intervention studies. The conclusions differed somewhat: McGovern et al. [13] found no effect of physical activity on BMI and a moderate effect on adiposity; combined lifestyle interventions led to only small changes in BMI. These authors stress that limited evidence supports the short-term efficacy of lifestyle interventions; the long-term efficacy and safety of paediatric obesity treatments were judged as unclear; side effects were not analyzed in most studies. According to Oude-Luttikhuis et al. [14] combined behavioural lifestyle interventions compared to standard care or self-help can produce a significant and clinically meaningful reduction in overweight in both children and adolescents. The limited efficacy of interventions can be viewed as evidence for the complex regulation of body weight and its resistance to change.

In adults with extreme obesity bariatric surgery has proven to be the most effective mode of treatment; however, considerable caution is warranted upon use of surgery in adolescents. No surgical intervention was eligible for inclusion in the recent Cochrane Database Systematic Review of paediatric treatment interventions [14].

According to expert recommendations [15] use of medications can be considered in severely obese youths (tertiary care intervention); their effect was judged as modest. Currently, two obesity drugs – orlistat (Xenical®) and sibutramine (Meridia®) – have been approved by the Food and Drug Agency (FDA) for use in adolescents ≥16 years [12]. Only orlistat has been approved for use in paediatric subjects in the age range ≥12 years.

The two largest randomized, double-blind, controlled trails (RCT) to assess the efficacy of obesity drugs for the treatment of paediatric obesity each included over 500 participants:

1  Orlistat reversibly inhibits gastric and pancreatic lipase, which catalyzes the conversion of triglycerides into absorbable free fatty acids. Safety and efficacy of orlistat were evaluated in a 54-week long-large RCT of 539 obese adolescents [16]. For inclusion adolescents were required to have a BMI 2 units or higher than the US weighted mean for the 95th percentile based on age and sex (adolescents with BMI ≥44 were excluded); the minimum BMI ranged from 28.5 in boys and 29.5 in girls at 12 years to 31.8 and 31.9, respectively, at 16 years. The study was funded by F. Hoffmann-La Roche Ltd. Participants were maintained on a nutritionally balanced, hypocaloric diet designed to produce an initial weight loss of 0.5–1.0 kg per week; the 32 participating study centres had behavioural modification programs in place using a study-specific manual as a guideline. Patients treated with orlistat had a mean reduction in BMI of 0.55 compared with an average increase of 0.31 in placebo-treated patients. Compared

with 15.7% of the placebo group, 26.5% of orlistat-treated participants had a 5% or higher decrease in BMI and 4.5% of the placebo group and 13.3% of the orlistat group had a 10% or higher decrease in BMI. 3% of adolescents in each treatment group had a serious adverse effect (SAE); a symptomatic cholelithiasis that led to cholecystectomy in a 15-year-old girl treated with orlistat was considered the only SAE possibly related to study medication by the investigators. In general, the side effects were similar to those described in adults and included fatty/oily stool, oily spotting, and oily evacuation. Because orlistat can interfere with the absorption of fat-soluble vitamins, patients are recommended to take a daily multivitamin that contains vitamins A, D, E, K, and beta-carotene at least 2 h prior to orlisat.

2   The second FDA-approved drug sibutramine acts centrally as a serotonin and norepinephrine transporter blocker. The largest paediatric RCT to assess efficacy and side effects of this drug included 498 adolescents aged 12–16 years with BMIs of 28.1 to 46.3; the study was sponsored by Abbott Laboratories and conducted over a 12-month period in 33 US clinics [17]; BMI inclusion criteria were similar to those of the aforementioned orlistat study. Candidates with systolic and diastolic blood pressure >130 and >85 mm Hg, respectively, or a pulse rate >95 beats per minute were excluded, but hypertensive subjects stable on therapy were permitted. Eligible subjects were randomly assigned in a 3:1 ratio to receive either single daily doses of sibutramine 10 mg or placebo; all participants received site-specific instruction in lifestyle behaviour modification. At month 6, subjects who had not lost >10% of their initial BMI were up-titrated in a blinded fashion to 15 mg of sibutramine or

placebo. Significantly more subjects (76 vs. 62%) in the sibutramine group completed the study. Withdrawal rates of 6% and 5% were similar in both groups. Treatment with sibutramine plus behavioural therapy resulted in a statistically significant reduction in mean (SE) BMI from baseline to the end point in the intention-to-treat population of –2.9 (0.15) compared with –0.3 (0.24) for placebo plus behavioural therapy with a mean treatment difference of 2.6 (SE: 0.27; 95% CI: 2.0–3.1), in favour of sibutramine. A BMI reduction of 5 and 10% occurred in 62.3 and 38.8% of subjects treated with sibutramine compared with 18.1 and 5.5% of subjects treated with placebo, respectively. There were no statistically significant differences in blood pressure between obese adolescents treated with sibutramine and those given placebo. Both treatment groups showed small mean decreases in blood pressure and pulse rate; the decrease in mean blood pressure in sibutramine treated subjects was less than that in placebo treated subjects who achieved an equivalent change in BMI.

In their Cochrane Database Systematic Review, Oude-Luttikhuis et al. [14] included a total of 10 drug-intervention (orlistat, sibutramine and met-formin) RCTs in their analysis with a follow-up duration of at least 3 months. They concluded that consideration should be given to the use of either orlistat or sibutramine in obese adolescents, as an adjunct to lifestyle interventions, although this approach needs to be carefully weighed up against the potential for adverse effects.

It is currently largely unknown which obese adolescents benefit from pharmacotherapy. It appears that Caucasian adolescents respond better to both orlistat and sibutramine than African-Americans. In patients with additional insulin resistance, the oral anti-diabetic metformin that decreases hepatic glucose production (approved by the FDA for treatment of type 2 diabetes mellitus in patients ≥ 10 years) can lead to weight loss. According to a RCT based on 28 patients aged 9–18 years, metformin led to significantly greater weight loss. Topiramate and other drugs have been used off-label for the treatment of adolescent obesity; however, due to the potential for serious side effects including psychiatric ones substantial care must be taken upon prescription of such drugs [12].

Delineation of autosomal-recessively inherited leptin deficiency has led to the successful treatment of such rare patients with recombinant leptin [18].

Prior to the initiation of conventional or pharmacological treatment, adolescents need to be informed that normalization of body weight appears highly unlikely; their high expectations need to be reflected upon critically to avoid disappointment and frustration. Patients should be medically monitored throughout the treatment period. The adolescent should also be informed that weight regain usually occurs once the intake of the drug is discontinued. Because the long-term side-effects of drug interventions are unknown, the physician must carefully weigh the options of drug treatment versus other modes of treatment.

## Prevention

Of the 22 studies included in the 2005 Cochrane analysis by Summerbell et al. [19] less than half lasted for at least 1 year. 19 were school/pre-school-based interventions, one was a community-based intervention targeting low-income families, and two were family-based interventions targeting non-obese children of obese or overweight parents. Six of the 10 long-term studies combined dietary education and physical activity interventions; five resulted in no difference in overweight status between groups and one resulted in improvements for girls receiving the intervention, but not boys. Of the two studies focussing on physical activity alone, a multimedia approach appeared to be effective in preventing obesity. The two studies that focused on provision of nutrition education were ineffective. Of the 12 short-term studies 10 did not have a significant impact on obesity prevention. Two of the four studies that focused on interventions to increase physical activity levels resulted in minor reductions in overweight status in favour of the intervention. Nearly all of the 22 studies resulted in some improvement in diet or physical activity. More recently, Kamath et al. [20] analyzed paediatric obesity prevention programs encompassing a total of 9981 participants. The interventions caused only small changes in target behaviours and no significant effect on BMI compared with controls.

## Outlook

Particularly children are affected by the obesity epidemic; as a result their health is compromised early on in life. In many aspects, the environment for children has become unfavourable. Recent research indicates that within the context of our current obesogenic environment an obesity prone individual stands only a limited chance of avoiding an elevated body weight. Even if obesity prevalence rates might be levelling off, the high personal toll and the magnitude of socioeconomic costs of obesity have become evident. Even small reductions in mean BMI of a population would translate into large effects in terms of obesity prevalence rates. On the other hand, we are seemingly largely resistant to minor lifestyle changes; it seems that many changes are required if they are to have a significant effect on BMI. Instead of focussing on individuals or families, a more promising approach may be to promote structural changes via political actions. For extremely obese children and adolescents, research into novel pharmacological interventions is required.

## Note Added in Proof

In an early communication dated 11/20/2009, the FDA reported on an ongoing review of preliminary data indicative of a higher rate of cardiovascular events in sibutramine versus placebo-treated adult patients; regulatory action has not been taken. However, the European Medicines Agency has recently (1/21/2010) recommended the suspension of marketing authorisations for sibutramine by concluding that the risks outweigh the benefits. It has been suspended from use in the UK and the EU.


## References

1 Hebebrand J: Obesity; in Martin A, Volkmar FR, Lewis M (eds): Lewis's Child and Adolescent Psychiatry: A Comprehensive Textbook. Philadelphia, Lippincott Williams & Wilkins, a Wolters Kluwer business, 2007, pp 602–614.

2 Ebbeling CB, Pawlak DB, Ludwig DS: Childhood obesity: public health crisis, common sense cure. Lancet 2002;360: 473–482.

3 Hedley AA, Ogden CL, Johnson CL, Caroll MD, Curtin LR, Flegal KM: Prevalence of overweight and obesity among US children, adolescents, and adults, 1999–2002. JAMA 2004;291:2847–2850.

4 Ogden CL, Carroll MD, Flegal KM: High body mass index for age among US children and adolescents, 2003–2006. JAMA 2008;299:2401–2405.

5 Baker JL, Olsen LW, Sørensen TIA: Childhood body-mass index and the risk of coronary heart disease in adulthood. N Engl J Med 2007;357:2329–2337

6 Trasande I, Chatterjee S: The impact of obesity on health service utilization and costs in childhood. Obesity (Silver Spring) 2009;17:1749.

7 Hebebrand J, Herpertz-Dahlmann B: Psychological aspects of childhood obesity. Child Adolesc Psychiatr Clin N Am 2009;18:49–46.

8 Reilly JJ, Armstrong J, Dorosty AR, Emmett PM, Ness A, Rogers I, Steer C, Sherriff A: Avon Longitudinal Study of Parents and Children Study Team: early life risk factors for obesity in childhood: cohort study. BMJ 2005;330:1357.

9 Hinney A, Hebebrand J: Polygenic obesity in humans. Obesity Facts 2008;1: 35–42.

10 Hinney A, Hebebrand J: Three at one swoop! Obesity Facts 2009;2:3–8.

11 Hancox RJ, Milne BJ, Poulton R: Association between child and adolescent television viewing and adult health: a longitudinal birth cohort study. Lancet 2004; 364:257–262.

12 Powers PS, Bruty H: Pharmacotherapy for eating disorders and obesity. Child Adolesc Psychiatr Clin N Am 2009;18: 175–187.

13 McGovern L, Johnson JN, Paulo R, Hettinger A, Singhal V, Kamath C, Erwin PJ, Montori VM: Clinical review: treatment of pediatric obesity: a systematic review and meta-analysis of randomized trials. J Clin Endocrinol Metab 2008;93:4600–4605.

14 Oude-Luttikhuis H, Baur L, Jansen H, Shrewsbury VA, O'Malley C, Stolk RP, Summerbell CD: Interventions for treating obesity in children. Cochrane Database Syst Rev 2009;1:CD001872.

15 Barlow SE and the Expert Committee: Expert committee recommendations regarding the prevention, assessment, and treatment of child and adolescent overweight and obesity: summary report. Pediatrics 2007;120:S164–S192.

16 Chanoine JP, Hampl S, Jensen C, Boldrin M, Hauptman J: Effect of orlistat on weight and body composition in obese adolescents: a randomized controlled trial. JAMA 2005;293:2873–2883.

17 Daniels SR, Long B, Crow S, Styne D, Sothern M, Vargas-Rodriguez I, Harris L, Walch J, Jasinsky O, Cwik K, Hewkin A, Blakesley V; Sibutramine Adolescent Study Group: Cardiovascular effects of sibutramine in the treatment of adolescents: results of a randomized, double-blind, placebo-controlled study. Pediatrics 2007;120;e147–e157.

18 Farooqi IS, Jebb SA, Langmack G, Lawrence E, Cheetham CH, Prentice AM, Hughes IA, McCamish MA, O'Rahilly S: Effects of recombinant leptin therapy in a child with congenital leptin deficiency. N Engl J Med 1999;341:879–884.

19 Summerbell CD, Waters E, Edmunds LD, Kelly S, Brown T, Campbell KJ: Interventions for preventing obesity in children. Cochrane Database Syst Rev 2005;3: CD001871.

20 Kamath CC, Vickers KS, Ehrlich A, McGovern L, Johnson J, Singhal V, Paulo R, Hettinger A, Erwin PJ, Montori VM: Clinical review: behavioral interventions to prevent childhood obesity – a systematic review and metaanalyses of randomized trials. J Clin Endocrinol Metab 2008;93:4606–4615.



Professor Johannes Hebebrand, MD
Department of Child and Adolescent Psychiatry, LVR-Klinikum
University of Duisburg-Essen, Virchowstrasse 174
DE–45147 Essen (Germany)
Tel. +49 201 7227465, Fax +49 201 7227302, E-Mail Johannes.Hebebrand@uni-duisburg-essen.de

Rose K, van den Anker JN (eds): Guide to Paediatric Drug Development and Clinical Research.
Basel, Karger, 2010, pp 187–195

# Familial Dyslipidaemia in Children

D.M. Kusters[a,b] · Hans J. Avis[a,b] · Maud N. Vissers[a] ·
Barbara A. Hutten[c] · John J.P. Kastelein[a] · Albert Wiegman[b]

Departments of [a]Vascular Medicine, [b]Pediatrics, and [c]Clinical Epidemiology, Biostatistics and Bioinformatics, Academic Medical
Centre, Amsterdam, The Netherlands

Unlike in adults, dyslipidaemia is a relatively rare condition in children, although its prevalence is on the rise in conjunction with the obesity epidemic [1]. Particularly, if dyslipidaemia is present in a non-obese child, the underlying cause is likely to be familial [2]. In such cases, it concerns a chronic condition that requires early intervention and careful surveillance to maximize long-term symptom-free survival.

Classically, familial dyslipidaemia is incorporated in the Fredrickson classification, which is based on the concentrations of various lipoproteins in the circulation. Importantly, this classification was designed before the significance of high-density lipoprotein cholesterol (HDL-C) was recognised as a prognostic indicator. In Fredrickson type I, chylomicrons are increased; type IIa implies elevation of low-density lipoprotein cholesterol (LDL-C) and type IIb elevation of both LDL and very-low-density lipoprotein cholesterol (VLDL-C). Type III implies elevation of chylomicron and VLDL remnants, type IV elevation of VLDL-C and type V elevation of VLDL-C as well as chylomicrons [3]. Since nowadays the molecular background of many familial dyslipidaemias has been elucidated, a classification based on genotype is currently preferred (table 1).

Of the familial dyslipidaemias that affect children, familial hypercholesterolaemia (FH) is the best studied, due to its high prevalence and well-understood biochemical and molecular background. Another relatively prevalent condition is familial combined hyperlipidaemia (FCH). As opposed to FH, the pathophysiology of this polygenic complex disease is yet to be clarified. Other familial dyslipidaemias, including autosomal-recessive hypercholesterolemia (ARH), familial hyperchylomicronaemia, sitosterolaemia and hypo-alpha-lipoproteinaemia are rare and will be discussed briefly below.

## Familial Hypercholesterolaemia

FH is the most common autosomal-dominant monogenic disorder with a prevalence of 1 per 500 in the general population. It results from a mutation in the gene encoding for a liver cell-surface receptor that removes LDL-C particles from the circulation. In approximately 5% of cases, the disorder is caused by familial defective apolipoprotein B (FDB), which results from mutations in the gene encoding for the LDL receptor-binding domain of apolipoprotein B (ApoB). Also, gain-of-function

| Dislipidaemia | Frederickson classification | Mutated gene | Biochemical features | Clinical features | Cardiovascular risks | Treatment |
|---|---|---|---|---|---|---|
| Familial hypercholesterolaemia | type IIa | LDLR/ PSCK9/ APOB | HeFH: LDL-C ↑ <br> HoFH: LDL-C ↑↑ | HeFH: sometimes: arcus corneae, xanthelasmas, tendon xanthomas <br> HoFH: arcus corneae, tendon xanthomas | HeFH: premature atherosclerosis, CVD during adulthood <br> HoFH: premature atherosclerosis, CVD before age 30 | HeFH: diet, life-style modifications; lipid-lowering medication, usually statins <br> HoFH: lipid-lowering medication, usually statins, LDL apheresis |
| Familial combined hyperlipidaemia | type IIb (type IV) | not known yet | TC ↑ / TG ↑ / TC ↑ + TG ↑ | obesity | premature atherosclerosis and CVD in adulthood | diet, life-style modifications; consider lipid-lowering medication |
| Autosomal-recessive hypercholesterolaemia | type IIa | ARH | LDL ↑↑ | arcus corneae, tendon xanthomas | premature atherosclerosis and CVD | lipid-lowering medication, usually statins |
| Sitosterolaemia | not in classification | ABCG5/ ABCG8 | plasma sitosterol and campestrol ↑↑ | xanthomas, haemolytic anaemia and thrombocytopenia, abnormal liver function tests | premature atherosclerosis and CVD | diet colestyramine, ezetimibe |
| Hyperchylomicronaemia | type I | LPL or Apo C-II | TG ↑↑ | colicky abdominal pain, acute pancreatitis, failure to thrive, hepatosplenomegaly, xanthomas | no increased risk | diet |
| Tangier disease | not in classification | ABCA1 | HDL ↓↓ | enlarged tonsils, hepatosplenomegaly, corneal clouding, peripheral neuropathy | premature atherosclerosis and CVD in adulthood | no consensus |
| LCAT deficiency | not in classification | LCAT | HDL ↓↓ | FLD: corneal opacity, anaemia, proteinuria FED: corneal opacity | unclear | FLD: diet FED: no treatment |
| Apo A-I deficiency | not in classification | Apo A-I | HDL ↓↓ | corneal opacity | unclear | no consensus |

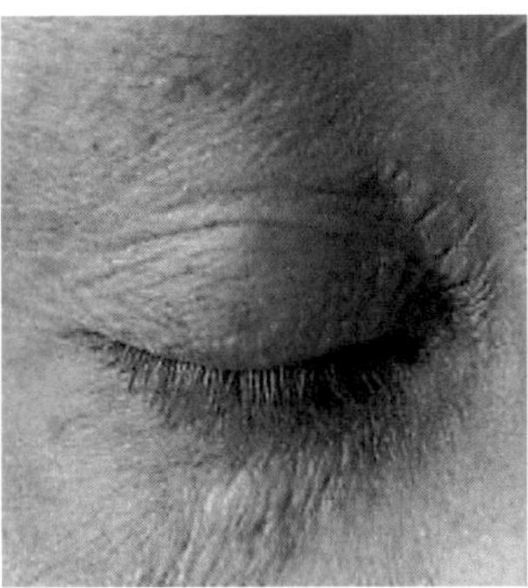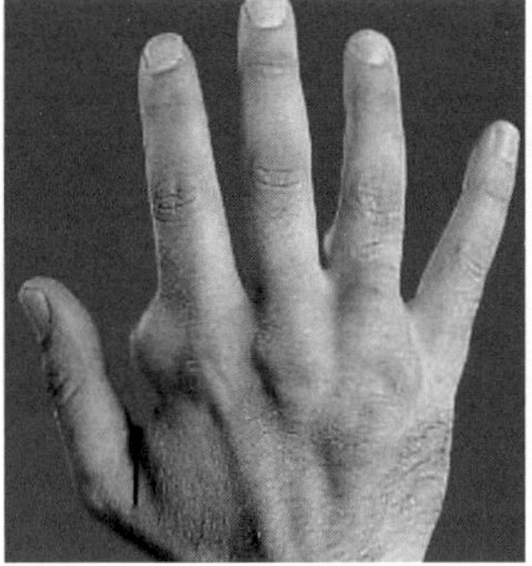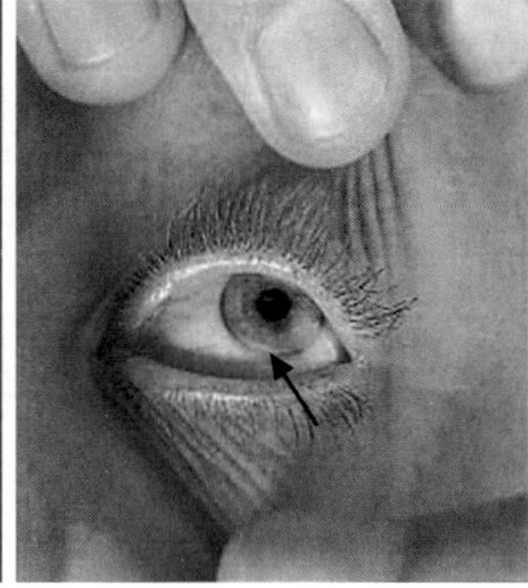

**Fig. 1.** Xanthelasmas, tendon xanthoma, arcus corneae.

mutations in the gene encoding for proprotein convertase subtillisin-kexin type 9 (PCSK9) may underlie the FH phenotype, by promoting degradation of the LDL receptor in the liver and thus increasing LDL-C particles in plasma. Both FDB and PCSK9 have the same biochemical and clinical features, the same age of presentation and long-term cardiovascular risk as FH [4]. More than a 1,000 different mutations, mostly in the LDL receptor gene, are currently listed on the internet at http://www.umd.necker.fr. FH is characterized by severely elevated levels of LDL-C from birth onwards, clinically leading to premature atherosclerosis and cardiovascular disease (CVD). Physical examination may reveal cholesterol deposits in the skin, eyes or tendons known as xanthelasmas, arcus corneae and tendon xanthomas, respectively (fig. 1). Homozygous patients are uncommon (1:1,000,000) and exhibit a far more severe phenotype with extremely elevated LDL-C levels of at least >10 mmol/l (385 mg/dl). If left untreated, most of these patients will develop symptomatic coronary atherosclerosis before the age of 30 [5].

## Clinical Characteristics and Diagnosis

The primary manifestation in children with FH is the marked elevation of LDL-C, usually two or three times above the upper limit of normal. Children generally present without any complaints or symptoms; a family history positive for premature CVD often raises an initial suspicion for FH. In a cohort of over a 1,000 children with heterozygous FH, 31% had a first-degree relative with a history of premature CVD, and 57% a second- and/or third-degree relative [6]. Albeit in a minority of cases, physical examination may reveal tendon xanthomas (mainly on the Achilles tendons and the extensor tendons of the hand), subcutaneous tuberous xanthomas (mainly over the elbows), arcus corneae, or palpebral xanthomas (xanthelasmas). Yet, xanthelasmas are not pathognomonic for FH. In a cohort of 539 children with FH, approximately 30% (161) reported a painful Achilles tendon even though without xanthomas [unpubl. data].

The above-mentioned findings are the main criteria for a clinical diagnosis of FH. A child with an LDL-C ≥3.5 mmol/l (135 mg/dl) and one parent with definite FH has a 0.98 (95% CI: 0.96–0.99) probability of a LDL receptor mutation. According to the Dutch Lipid Clinic criteria, adjusted for children [7], the lipid profile suggests the presence of FH if the LDL-C level is raised above the 95th percentile for age and gender, or above 3.5 mmol/l (135 mg/dl) when FH is confirmed in a first-degree family member. Family history for CVD is judged positive if CVD is present before the age of 55 in men and before the age of 60 in women. When the LDL-C criterion is present in combination with a positive family history for CVD or physical symptoms like tendon xanthomas, a diagnosis of FH is considered highly likely. The Dutch criteria resemble the Simon Broome diagnostic criteria for FH, which specify that patients under 16 should have total cholesterol above 6.7 mmol/l (260 mg/dl) or LDL-C above 4.0 mmol/l (155 mg/dl) to suspect FH [8]. If possible, a clinical diagnosis of FH should preferably be confirmed by molecular genetic testing.

Despite the absence of complaints, several abnormalities suggesting the first steps on the road to atherosclerosis are already present in children with FH. Increased inflammatory activity, the key pathologic process underlying atherosclerosis, is reflected by elevated levels of high-sensitivity C-reactive protein (hsCRP) in children with heterozygous FH, when compared to their unaffected siblings [9]. Furthermore, functional and morphological changes of the arterial wall can be observed in children with FH. This is illustrated by an impaired flow-mediated dilatation (FMD) of the brachial artery [10] and an increased intima-media thickness (IMT) of the carotid artery [11]. Whereas decreased FMD has only be suggested as an indicator of the atherosclerotic process, IMT is well established as a surrogate marker that predicts CVD risk in adults [12]. These findings thus indicate that enhanced atherogenesis is already present in young children with FH.

*Molecular Diagnosis and Screening*

Due to the long preclinical phase of atherosclerosis and because early diagnosis and treatment reduces the risk of premature CVD, screening for FH is advocated. In several countries, nationwide screening programmes are currently being set up or running. For example, in the Netherlands, a screening programme is currently ongoing in which all first-degree family members of an index patient are identified and genetically tested for FH. Cascade screening is then performed to screen more distant relatives using the inheritance pattern across the pedigree. Over the last 14 years, more than 16,000 relatives with an FH mutation have been identified which is almost half of the total number of FH carriers in The Netherlands.

One could argue vis-à-vis the need for genetic screening in children. Nevertheless, we recommend screening of all first-degree relatives of a confirmed FH patient already from the age of 6. The reason for this is twofold. First, albeit in simple terms, children of that age are able to understand the background and consequences of their (probable) condition as well as why screening is necessary. We feel that (parents of) children with FH should be thoroughly aware of their condition, preferably some time before pharmacological therapy is initiated. Second, these children could be well made aware of what is 'good' and 'bad' with respect to lifestyle and earlier implementation of a healthy lifestyle may lead to better adherence to this lifestyle in later life.

*Treatment*

The functional and morphological changes of the arterial wall already present in children with FH have led to the hypothesis that treatment initiated early in life could reduce the incidence of CVD later in life. Life-style modifications focussing on LDL-C lowering and reduction of other risk factors for CVD are a first step. All children with FH should be advised to adhere to a low saturated fat and low cholesterol diet, physical activity should be promoted, and smoking strongly discouraged. However, lifestyle modifications alone do not sufficiently reduce LDL-C levels and drug therapy should be considered [13].

Various lipid-lowering drugs have been shown to effectively lower LDL-C levels and reverse abnormal FMD or IMT in children with FH [14].

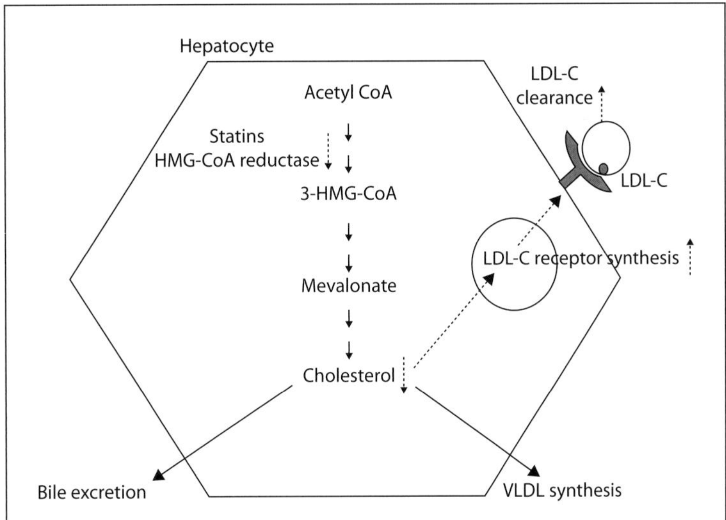



**Fig. 2.** Mechanism of action by statins.

Statins are the mainstay of lipid-lowering treatment in both adults and children with FH. They lower HMG-CoA reductase, thereby reducing intracellular cholesterol production in hepatocytes. This leads to increased LDL-receptor synthesis and increased LDL-C clearance (fig. 2). A meta-analysis of randomized placebo-controlled trials in children with FH showed that statin therapy significantly reduces TC, LDL-C and ApoB [15]. With respect to vascular function, statin therapy reversed impaired FMD in children with FH [10]. Furthermore, a randomized placebo-controlled trial demonstrated that 2 years of pravastatin therapy induced regression of carotid IMT in 8- to 18-year-old children with FH, whereas a trend towards progression of IMT was observed in the placebo group [11]. These children continued with or, in case they received placebo, switched to statin therapy and were treated for on average 4.5 years, which showed that age at statin initiation was positively associated with carotid IMT after follow-up, indicating that early statin initiation retards IMT progression. This longest follow-up study of statin therapy in childhood so far showed no adverse effects on growth, sexual maturation, or liver or muscle tissue [13]. In the meta-analysis, which included studies with a duration of 3–24 months, safety outcomes were favourable as well [15]. However, further studies are required to assess lifelong safety.

The above-mentioned findings led to the development of several guidelines advocating early initiation of lipid-lowering treatment. According to a recent policy statement from the American Academy of Paediatrics on cholesterol in childhood [16], statin treatment should be considered for children aged 8–18 years with FH and LDL-C levels above 4.1 mmol/l (160 mg/dl). Target LDL-C levels as low as 3.35 mmol/l (130 mg/dl) or even 2.8 mmol/l (110 mg/dl) may be warranted, especially when there is a strong family history for premature CVD. If with statin therapy alone the recommended LDL-C goals cannot be reached, co-administration of ezetimibe may be considered. In a multicenter study with 10- to 17-year-old children, co-administered ezetimibe and simvastatin resulted in a significantly greater reduction of LDL-C compared with simvastatin monotherapy, and was well tolerated [17].

Pravastatin is registered for children >8 years (20 mg is advised when <14 years of age and 40 mg when aged ≥14) and ezetimibe 10 mg is registered for children >10 years of age by the American Food and Drug Administration (FDA) and the European Medicines Agency. Simvastatin 10–40 mg, lovastatin 10–40 mg and atorvastatin 10–20 mg are registered by the FDA for children >10 years of age.

Considering the extreme phenotype in children with homozygous FH (HoFH), a more aggressive treatment regimen is needed. It is now common practice to start lipid-lowering medication already during the first year of life, or immediately after the patient is diagnosed. Efficacy of statin therapy is often poor in these patients because statins act through LDL-C receptor up-regulation (fig. 2). LDL apheresis is currently the only effective treatment available, but this procedure is costly and invasive. However, for children this has proven to be safe and children who have been treated now for many years have shown normal growth and development. The procedure is usually initiated at the age of 6–7 years, or even earlier [18].

**Other Familial Dyslipidaemias**

*Familial Combined Hyperlipidaemia*

Familial combined hyperlipidaemia (FCH) occurs in about 1–3% of the adult population. It is defined as a metabolic disorder characterized by increased total cholesterol and/or triglycerides in at least two members of the same family, intra-individual and interfamilial variability of the lipid phenotype, and increased risk of premature coronary heart disease. Typically, the phenotype is variable regarding dyslipidaemia: about one third of patients exhibit hypercholesterolaemia, one third hypertriglyceridaemia, and one third exhibits both. Most of the affected individuals also have low HDL levels [19]. However, even for adults the cut-off points for cholesterol and triglyceride levels are not well defined. It has been considered that the clinical expression of FCH is delayed until early adulthood, but some studies showed that this may not be true. In a Japanese screening programme in 1,190 children aged 9–13 years, a prevalence of FCH of 0.4% was found. Based on these findings, the authors suggest that at least half of all patients with FCH already demonstrate hyperlipidaemia in childhood [20]. Another study concluded that FCH is expressed three times more frequently in children visiting a lipid clinic than FH [21]. However, both these studies are not very recent and no molecular genetic testing was performed, so it might be possible that some of these children were in fact FH patients. Hence, the degree of FCH expression in childhood remains controversial.

There is a strong association between obesity and the FCH phenotype in children. Also, there is a greater correlation between relative weight and plasma lipoproteins in children with FCH compared to their unaffected siblings [22]. Whether (the tendency toward) obesity is part of the genetic background needed for early presentation of FCH is unknown. Not surprisingly, many studies have shown an association with the metabolic syndrome, which makes the definition of FCH even more complicated. FCH is associated with premature CVD: approximately 20% of patients with a premature myocardial infarction have FCH [23].

Treatment of patients with FCH starts with dietary and life-style modifications. In case of severe hypercholesterolaemia lipid-lowering drugs can be considered. However, paediatric studies in this specific population are scarce and most FCH children treated in a research setting participated in studies that included both subjects suffering from FCH and FH. Recommended levels for hypertrigyceridaemia or low HDL-C for the initiation of drug therapy have not been established for children, and there is very little experience in children with compounds such as fibrates and nicotinic acid for these types of lipid abnormalities.

*Autosomal-Recessive Hypercholesterolaemia*

Autosomal-recessive hypercholesterolaemia (ARH) is a rare monogenic lipid disorder mostly found in people of Italian, especially Sardinian origin. Mutations in ARH prevent normal internalization of the LDL receptor, and therefore LDL receptor protein accumulates at the cell surface. The clinical phenotype and cardiovascular risk is somehow similar to that of HoFH, but is more variable and less severe [24]. Patients with ARH generally respond better to lipid-lowering medication (statins) than patients with HoFH.

*Familial Hyperchylomicronaemia*

Hyperchylomicronaemia is a rare disorder mostly caused by a deficiency in lipoprotein lipase (LPL) or one of its co-factors, mostly apolipoprotein C-II (Apo C-II), and very rarely by a recently identified mutation in glycosylphosphatidylinositol-anchored high-density lipoprotein-binding protein 1 (GPIHBP1), which blocks the ability of GPIHBP1 to bind LPL and chylomicrons [25]. LPL deficiency concerns an autosomal-recessive disorder of triglyceride metabolism that affects an estimated 1 per 1,000,000 individuals, and Apo C-II deficiency is even less common. These dyslipidaemias are characterized by impaired peripheral lipolysis of triglycerides by LPL, leading to extremely elevated plasma triglyceride levels, often above 10 mmol/l (885 mg/dl). Clinically, it presents in early childhood with indistinctive symptoms including repetitive colicky abdominal pain and failure to thrive. Acute pancreatitis, of which the underlying pathology is unknown, is the most severe complication of the disease. Hepatosplenomegaly and eruptive xanthomas may occur as a result of triglyceride uptake by macrophages in the liver, spleen and skin [26]. Blood plasma is typically lactescent, which is often a first clue of the disease.

In the management of LPL deficiency and Apo C-II deficiency, dietary modification plays a key role since triglyceride-lowering agents all act through LPL up-regulation and are therefore ineffective in this condition. Dietary fat should be restricted as much as possible, and agents that are known to increase plasma triglyceride such as alcohol, estrogens and steroids should be avoided. A recent study showed promising results for gene therapy by intramuscular administration of adeno-associated virus subtype 1 (AAV1) lipoprotein lipase [27].

The main complication is (recurrent) pancreatitis. Though the common, milder forms of hypertriglyceridaemia are associated with an increased risk of developing atherosclerotic cardiovascular disease, this does not seem to occur in LPL-deficient patients, despite high triglyceride concentrations [28].

*Sitosterolaemia*

Sitosterolaemia, also known as phytosterolaemia, is a very rare disorder. It is characterized by increased plasma levels of plant sterols, such as sitosterol and campesterol, of which the chemical structure is almost similar to that of cholesterol. As plant sterols are derived from plants only, as suggested by the name, diet is the only source. Normally, they are taken up by the enterocytes and directly excreted again by ATP-binding cassette, sub-family G member 5 (ABCG5) and ABCG8 proteins. As a consequence, their net absorption and plasma levels are usually low. Mutations in either ABCG5 or ABCG8 genes lead to the inability of the G5G8 transporter to pump these plant sterols from the enterocytes back into the intestinal lumen and from the liver into bile, which results in the accumulation of plant sterols in blood, plasma, erythrocytes, and different tissues, most commonly in xanthomas and the arterial wall. Clinical characteristics include premature atherosclerosis, tendon xanthomas, chronic haemolytic anaemia and thrombocytopenia, and abnormal liver function tests. Patients are advised to keep a diet low in plant and shellfish sterols. Both colestyramine and ezetimibe lower cholesterol and plant sterols levels [29].

*Hypo Alpha Lipoproteinaemia*

A number of rare genetic lipid disorders can lead to reduced plasma HDL levels. The one with the most pronounced phenotype, Tangier disease, is characterized by a near absence of HDL in plasma and by the accumulation of cholesteryl esters in tissues like tonsils, liver, spleen, lymph nodes, thymus, intestinal mucosa, peripheral nerves and the cornea. It is caused by mutations in the gene that codes for the ATP-binding cassette transporter 1 (ABC1). Even though children with Tangier disease have low LDL levels, they appear to have an increased risk of CVD during adulthood. There is no consensus regarding treatment since there is no experience with HDL modifying agents in children. Lipid-lowering medication in order to decrease the LDL-C/HDL-C ratio is usually initiated later in life [30].

Lecithin cholesteryl acyltransferase (LCAT) deficiency and Apo A-I deficiency are other causes of extremely low plasma HDL. LCAT deficiency can lead to the development of two distinct syndromes: familial LCAT deficiency (FLD) and fish eye disease (FED). The clinical presentation can be variable and signs seen in Tangier disease such as corneal clouding, commonly appear during adulthood. For FED, treatment is mostly not needed. Patients with FLD should keep a fat-restricted diet and further treatment is symptomatic [29]. It is not clear yet whether these patients have an increased cardiovascular risk.

## Conclusions

Among the known familial dyslipidaemias presenting in childhood, FH and FCH are relatively prevalent disorders that may require early diagnosis and treatment. For children with FH, guidelines have been published recently advocating initiation of dietary and statin therapy before puberty. In FCH, dietary therapy seems even more important and effective. Future research should further assess CVD risk and necessity of childhood initiated drug treatment in this condition. Other familial dyslipidaemias are rare and require follow-up by specialized paediatricians and/or lipidologists. In all familial dyslipidaemias, the ultimate question of whether childhood initiated therapy results in a lower CVD incidence in adulthood remains to be answered. Studies answering this question should be set out in the future.


## References

1 Reilly JJ, Methven E, McDowell ZC, Hacking B, Alexander D, Stewart L, Kelnar CJ: Health consequences of obesity. Arch Dis Child 2003;88:748–752.

2 Graaf van der A, Avis HJ, Vissers MN, Hutten B, Defesche JC, Wiegman A, Fouchier S, Kastelein JJ: Phenotype and genotype of familial hypercholesterolemia in over 2000 children. Symp Int Atherosclerosis Soc, Boston, 2009.

3 Fredrickson DS, Lees RS: A system for phenotyping hyperlipoproteinemia. Circulation 1965;31:321–327.

4 Soutar AK, Naoumova RP: Mechanisms of disease: genetic causes of familial hypercholesterolemia. Nat Clin Pract Cardiovasc Med 2007;4:214–225.

5 Goldstein JL, Hobbs HH, Brown MS: Familial hypercholesterolemia; in Scriver CR, Beaudet AL, Valle D, Sly WS (eds): The Metabolic and Molecular Bases of Inherited Disease, ed 8. New York, McGraw Hill, 2001, pp 2863–2913.

6 Wiegman A, Rodenburg J, de Jongh S, Defesche JC, Bakker HD, Kastelein JJ, Sijbrands EJ: Family history and cardiovascular risk in familial hypercholesterolemia: data in more than 1000 children. Circulation 2003;107:1473–1478.

7 Defesche JC: Familial hypercholesterolaemia; in Betteridge DJ (ed): Lipids and Vascular Disease. London, Martin Dunitz, 2000, pp 65–76.

8 Scientific Steering Committee on behalf of the Simon Broome Register Group: Risk of fatal coronary heart disease in familial hypercholesterolaemia. BMJ 1991;303:893–896.

9 Ueland T, Vissers MN, Wiegman A, Rodenburg J, Hutten B, Gullestad L, Ose L, Rifai N, Ridker PM, Kastelein JJ, Aukrust P, Semb AG: Increased inflammatory markers in children with familial hypercholesterolaemia. Eur J Clin Invest 2006;36:147–152.

10 de Jongh S, Lilien MR, op't Roodt J, Stroes ES, Bakker HD, Kastelein JJ: Early statin therapy restores endothelial function in children with familial hypercholesterolemia. J Am Coll Cardiol 2002; 40:2117–2121.

11 Wiegman A, de Groot E, Hutten BA, Rodenburg J, Gort J, Bakker HD, Sijbrands EJ, Kastelein JJ: Arterial intima-media thickness in children heterozygous for familial hypercholesterolaemia. Lancet 2004;363:369–370.

12 Sankatsing RR, de Groot E, Jukema JW, de Feyter PJ, Pennell DJ, Schoenhagen P, Nissen SE, Stroes ES, Kastelein JJ: Surrogate markers for atherosclerotic disease. Curr Opin Lipidol 2005;16:434–441.

13 Rodenburg J, Vissers MN, Wiegman A, van Trotsenburg AS, van der Graaf A, de Groot E, Wijburg FA, Kastelein JJ, Hutten BA: Statin treatment in children with familial hypercholesterolemia: the younger, the better. Circulation 2007; 116:664–668.

14 Avis HJ, Vissers MN, Wijburg FA, Kastelein JJ, Hutten BA: The use of lipid-lowering drug therapy in children and adolescents. Curr Opin Investig Drugs 2009;10:224–231.

15 Avis HJ, Vissers MN, Stein EA, Wijburg FA, Trip MD, Kastelein JJ, Hutten BA: A systematic review and meta-analysis of statin therapy in children with familial hypercholesterolemia. Arterioscler Thromb Vasc Biol 2007;27:1803–1810.

16 Daniels SR, Greer FR: Lipid screening and cardiovascular health in childhood. Pediatrics 2008;122:198–208.

17 van der Graaf A, Cuffie-Jackson C, Vissers MN, Trip MD, Gagne C, Shi G, Veltri E, Avis HJ, Kastelein JJ: Efficacy and safety of coadministration of ezetimibe and simvastatin in adolescents with heterozygous familial hypercholesterolemia. J Am Coll Cardiol 2008;52:1421–1429.

18 Naoumova RP, Thompson GR, Soutar AK: Current management of severe homozygous hypercholesterolaemias. Curr Opin Lipidol 2004;15:413–422.

19 Goldstein JL, Hazzard WR, Schrott HG, Bierman EL, Motulsky AG: Hyperlipidemia in coronary heart disease. I. Lipid levels in 500 survivors of myocardial infarction. J Clin Invest 1973;52:1533–1543.

20 Iwata F, Okada T, Kuromori Y, Hara M, Harada K: Screening for familial combined hyperlipidemia in children using lipid phenotypes. J Atheroscler Thromb 2003;10:299–303.

21 Cortner JA, Coates PM, Gallagher PR: Prevalence and expression of familial combined hyperlipidemia in childhood. J Pediatr 1990;116:514–519.

22 Shamir R, Tershakovec AM, Gallagher PR, Liacouras CA, Hayman LL, Cortner JA: The influence of age and relative weight on the presentation of familial combined hyperlipidemia in childhood. Atherosclerosis 1996;121:85–91.

23 de Graaf J, van der Vleuten GM, Stalenhoef AF: Diagnostic criteria in relation to the pathogenesis of familial combined hyperlipidemia. Semin Vasc Med 2004;4:229–240.

24 Soutar AK, Naoumova RP, Traub LM: Genetics, clinical phenotype, and molecular cell biology of autosomal recessive hypercholesterolemia. Arterioscler Thromb Vasc Biol 2003;23:1963–1970.

25 Beigneux AP, Franssen R, Bensadoun A, Gin P, Melford K, Peter J, Walzem RL, Weinstein MM, Davies BS, Kuivenhoven JA, Kastelein JJ, Fong LG, linga-Thie GM, Young SG: Chylomicronemia with a mutant GPIHBP1 (Q115P) that cannot bind lipoprotein lipase. Arterioscler Thromb Vasc Biol 2009;29:956–962.

26 Feoli-Fonseca JC, Levy E, Godard M, Lambert M: Familial lipoprotein lipase deficiency in infancy: clinical, biochemical, and molecular study. J Pediatr 1998;133:417–423.

27 Stroes ES, Nierman MC, Meulenberg JJ, Franssen R, Twisk J, Henny CP, Maas MM, Zwinderman AH, Ross C, Aronica E, High KA, Levi MM, Hayden MR, Kastelein JJ, Kuivenhoven JA: Intramuscular administration of AAV1-lipoprotein lipase S447X lowers triglycerides in lipoprotein lipase-deficient patients. Arterioscler Thromb Vasc Biol 2008; 28:2303–2304.

28 Brunzell JD, Deeb SS: Deficiencies of lipoprotein lipase, apo C-II, and hepatic lipase; in Scriver CR, Beaudet AL, Valle D, Sly WS (eds): The Metabolic and Molecular Bases of Inherited Disease, ed 8. New York, McGraw Hill, 2001, pp 2789–2816.

29 Salen G, von Bergmann K, Lutjohann D, Kwiterovich P, Kane J, Patel SB, Musliner T, Stein P, Musser B: Ezetimibe effectively reduces plasma plant sterols in patients with sitosterolemia. Circulation 2004;109:966–971.

30 Assmann G, von Eckardstein A, Brewer HB Jr: Familial analphalipoproteinemia: Tangier disease; in Scriver CR, Beaudet AL, Valle D, Sly WS (eds): The Metabolic and Molecular Bases of Inherited Disease, ed 8. New York, McGraw Hill, 2001, pp 2937–2960.

Albert Wiegman, MD, PhD
Academic Medical Centre, Department of Pediatrics
Meibergdreef 9
NL–1105 AZ Amsterdam (The Netherlands)
Tel. +31 20 566 3468, Fax +31 20 691 9854, E-Mail a.wiegman@amc.uva.nl

Rose K, van den Anker JN (eds): Guide to Paediatric Drug Development and Clinical Research.
Basel, Karger, 2010, pp 196–205

# Paediatric Anti-Hypertensive Clinical Trials and Various Factors Influencing Trial Success or Failure

Jennifer S. Li[a] · Daniel K. Benjamin, Jr.[a] · Thomas Severin[c] · Ronald J. Portman[b]

[a]Department of Paediatrics and Duke Clinical Research Institute, Durham, N.C., and [b]Bristol Myers Squibb, Princeton, N.J., USA; [c]Novartis Pharma AG, Basel, Switzerland

Systemic hypertension occurs in 1–4% of children [1–5], and the prevalence is increasing because of the epidemic of childhood obesity and insulin resistance [6, 7]. The prevalence of paediatric hypertension is not only increasing, but is frequently under-diagnosed [8, 9]. In younger children, hypertension is often secondary to an underlying disorder (e.g. renal disease, renal artery stenosis, Cushing's syndrome, coarctation of the aorta, pheochromocytoma, systemic lupus erythematosus, hyperaldosteronism, or hyperthyroidism) [10]. Primary (or essential) hypertension, however, accounts for up to 95% of the cases in adolescents [11]. Hypertension in this age group is linked to obesity and risk factors associated with metabolic syndrome that can lead to cardiovascular disease in later life, including lipid abnormalities and insulin resistance. This is a significant public health concern because over the past 3 decades, childhood obesity has increased dramatically and has been deemed an epidemic by the Centres for Disease Control and Prevention [12]. The 2002 National Health and Nutrition Examination Survey reported that the prevalence of overweight and obese children aged 6–19 years was 31%, a 45% increase from the previous survey

[13]. Obesity has been linked to co-morbid conditions in children, including type 2 diabetes mellitus, hypertension, and hyperlipidemia [14, 15].

There is widespread concern that the increasing prevalence of these cardiovascular risk factors in children will lead to a dramatic rise in adult cardiovascular disease and neurologic events. The presence of obesity, diabetes, hyperlipidaemia, and hypertension in childhood has been linked to elevated left ventricular mass and carotid intima-media thickness, as well as peripheral endothelial dysfunction [15–18]. The presence and severity of coronary atherosclerotic plaque in asymptomatic young adults is related to the number of risk factors present, including higher body mass index, hypertension, and hyperlipidaemia [19]. A Danish study of 275,835 adults found that childhood body mass index was significantly associated with coronary artery events and death in adulthood [20].

Given these trends, the number of children prescribed antihypertensive medications is likely to increase in coming years. Therapy for this condition is hampered, however, by uncertainty over the efficacy and safety of antihypertensive medicines in children. Agents that have been extensively tested and that have a long history of use in adults are often not supported by adequate data obtained in children; drug treatment of hypertension therefore presents a challenge for the paediatrician.

In response to a paucity of clinical trials in children, Congress passed the Food and Drug Administration Modernization Act (FDAMA) in 1997 providing for an additional 6-month period of marketing exclusivity to a drug company that responds to a Food and Drug Administration (FDA)-issued written request for studies of their drug in paediatric patients [21, 22]. The program was extended in January 2002 when Congress passed the Best Pharmaceuticals for Children Act and was renewed in September 2007. This program has been very successful in stimulating drug studies in children, and, as a result of the program, >200 drug labelling changes have been enacted for children [22–24]. The European Medicines Agency has recently started to require drug studies in children [25] and has begun to receive paediatric investigation plans (PIPS) for new molecular entities, including antihypertensive products. Also, under the EU Paediatric Regulation, for already authorized and patented medicinal products a PIP is required if a sponsor applies for a variation of an existing marketing authorization (e.g. to add a new indication (including paediatric), a new pharmaceutical form, or a new route of administration). Further, for off-patent medicines developed specifically for paediatric use and with an appropriate formulation, a new marketing authorization – the paediatric-use marketing authorization (PUMA) – can be obtained [25].

Since the program's inception in the USA, approximately half of the products studied have been found to have substantive differences in dosing, safety, or efficacy in children when compared with adult populations [26]. Twenty-nine of 131 drugs examined were found to be ineffective when studied in children. Several products that did not demonstrate efficacy (or for which a statistically significant dose-response was not observed) were

oral antihypertensive agents known to be effective in adults.

This chapter will present an overview of the paediatric anti-hypertensive studies done to date and will focus on the clinical trial design and factors associated with success or failure of the clinical trials.

## Paediatric Anti-Hypertensive Clinical Trial Design

The FDA allows for several types of trial designs in the written request for an antihypertensive agent. The written request, generally issued by FDA before initiation of paediatric exclusivity studies, contains the required elements of the requested studies, including indication, number of studies, sample sizes, trial design, age ranges, and need for a paediatric formulation [22]. In the written requests for antihypertensive drugs, the FDA allows for 4 efficacy trial designs (fig. 1) [27]. Of note, it is not necessary for the dose-ranging trial to show that a certain drug is effective in treating paediatric hypertension in order for its manufacturer to be eligible for exclusivity. However, trial data must be 'interpretable,' in accordance with the guidelines in order for the drug manufacturer to be eligible for patent extension. In other words, the study should show that the drug is either effective or ineffective. Thus, a failed trial is one that does not show a clear result; not one that shows a medication to be ineffective. Conducting these trials is further complicated by ethical and methodological issues unique to paediatric research, in addition to compliance with the formal guidelines.

### Trial Design A

In trial design A, patients are randomized to placebo or 1 of a few different dosages of the test medication (fig. 1). It is recommended that the dosages be chosen to provide exposure in a range from slightly

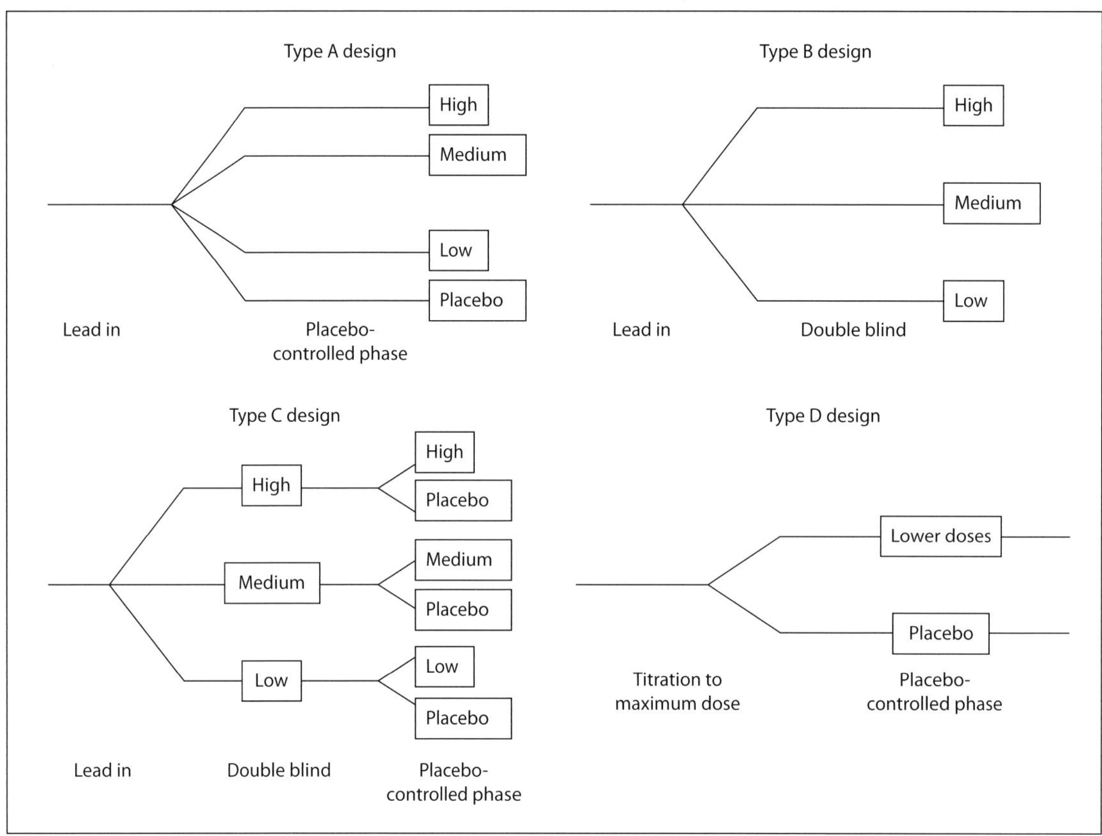



**Fig. 1.** Paediatric trial design options for antihypertensive agents.

less than those achieved by the lowest approved adult dosage to slightly more than those achieved by the highest approved adult dosage. After 2 weeks of treatment, the trial is analyzed by examining the slope of the placebo corrected change in blood pressure from baseline as a function of dosage. A negative slope (i.e., the reduction in blood pressure increases as treatment dosage increases) indicates that the trial was successful, or that the test drug was effective. If the slope was not different from zero, the drug is considered ineffective. The major advantage of this trial type is its straightforward design and analysis. Both successful and unsuccessful trials are considered to be interpretable, and therefore responsive to the written request.

However, the placebo-controlled design can lead to slow recruitment because parents are often uncomfortable with the possibility that their child may be placed on placebo. These trials can employ a 3:1 randomization scheme (thereby 3 times as many children receive active product) some parents still have significant concerns about their child's participation, especially if the trial drug is available off-label. The knowledge that one could use a 3:1 randomization scheme was not evident in the early days of paediatric antihypertensive trials and thus this option was not frequently chosen by companies. Some question the ethics of conducting placebo-controlled trials in children in general, in part due to the potential risk of adverse events while not on active therapy [28]. We have recently evaluated adverse events in subjects while on placebo in 10 antihypertensive trials and observed no differences in the rates of adverse events reported between the patients who received placebo and those who received active drug. Short-term exposure to placebo in paediatric trials of antihypertensive medications thus appears to be safe [29].

*Trial Design B*

To avoid the issues associated with a placebo-controlled trial, trial design B involves randomization to 1 of 3 dosages of the test medication as in trial A, but without a placebo arm (fig. 1). If analysis of trial design B reveals a negative slope of the dose-response curve, the trial is considered successful and responsive to the written request. However, if the slope were zero, it would not be possible to determine whether this was due to the absence of an effect, or if all doses were too low or too high. Therefore, the trial would be considered a failure, and uninterpretable. Thus, a negative trial would be unresponsive to the written request. This trial has the simplest design of the 4 and avoids ethical and patient recruitment issues associated with placebo-controlled trials in children. However, it involves significant risk for manufacturers compared with the other trials, in that only a positive outcome is considered responsive to the written request. More importantly, the ethics of enrolling paediatric patients in a trial in which the outcome may not be interpretable are questionable. Finally, the lack of controls does not allow adequate assessment of safety.

*Trial Design C*

Trial design C employs a more complicated design in order to avoid use of a true placebo arm as in trial design B, while adding the power to obtain interpretable results regardless of the outcome of the trial, as in trial A (fig. 1). Trial design C begins like trial design B with randomization to 1 of 3 dosages of the test product. In addition, it includes a randomized withdrawal phase. At the end of the treatment period, patients are re-randomized to continue on their assigned treatments or to be withdrawn to placebo, with close follow-up and withdrawal to open-label treatment. The analysis of the treatment phase is similar to that of trial design B. If the slope of the dose-response curve is negative, the trial is considered successful and responsive to the written request. However, if the slope is zero during the treatment phase, the addition of the withdrawal phase allows further analysis and interpretation of the trial. For example, if the treatment phase dose-response curve slope was zero, but the withdrawal phase demonstrated a rise in blood pressure with withdrawal to placebo, this indicates that the dosages used during the treatment phase were too high. If blood pressure did not change significantly with withdrawal to placebo, this suggests that all dosages were too low, or that the drug was ineffective. Thus, as in trial design A, the trial would be considered interpretable regardless of the outcome, and therefore, responsive to the written request. Having two chances to meet eligibility for exclusivity is a major advantage of this trial design. In addition, minimizing the use of an explicit placebo arm likely makes this type of trial more appealing when presented to parents.

*Trial Design D*

In trial design D, the entire trial is built around randomized drug withdrawal (fig. 1). In this trial, patients are force-titrated to maximal tolerated dosages of the drug, and then randomly withdrawn to lower dosages, including placebo, with close follow up, and discretionary withdrawal to open-label therapy. The analysis of this type of trial is similar to that of trial design C. Much like

**Table 1.** Overview of completed paediatric anti-hypertensive efficacy trials

| Drug | Trial design | Sample size | Dose response | Label change |
|---|---|---|---|---|
| Amlodipine | C | 268 | no | yes |
| Benazepril | D | 107 | no | yes |
| Bisoprolol | A | 94 | yes | no |
| Candesartan | A | 240 | no | no |
| Enalapril | C | 110 | yes | yes |
| Eplerenone | C | 304 | no | yes (negative) |
| Felodipine | D | 133 | no | no |
| Fosinopril | C | 253 | no | yes |
| Irbesartan | C | 318 | no | yes (negative) |
| Lisinopril | C | 115 | yes | yes |
| Losartan | C | 175 | yes | yes |
| Metoprolol | A | 140 | no | yes |
| Quinapril | A | 112 | no | no |
| Ramipril | D | 219 | no | no |
| Valsartan | C | 351 | no age 1–5/yes age 6–16 | yes |

trial design C, trial design D minimizes the use of a placebo arm. However, the close follow-up and risk of adverse events that come with titration to maximal dosages are considerable disadvantages, and can result in recruitment problems. Further, since all patients begin the placebo withdrawal period at the highest dose of study drug, a very effective or long acting drug may still be effective even after the short 2- to 3-week withdrawal period and be interpreted as a negative study as the placebo dose would not rise (ramipril study).

## Clinical Efficacy Studies

The passage of the Food and Drug Administration Modernization Act in 1997 has been the single greatest stimulus for the recent proliferation of industry-sponsored trials of anti-hypertensive agents in children [30].

Table 1 lists the various studies completed to date. The results of many, but not all, of the clinical trials of anti-hypertensive agents in children have resulted in publications in scientific journals [31–43]. Furthermore, the Best Pharmaceuticals for Children Act now requires the FDA to publish the results of its internal analyses of the trial results submitted by sponsors on the Internet [24]. A recent review summarizes the advances in our knowledge about the use of anti-hypertensive agents in children and provides updated recommendations on the optimal use of anti-hypertensive agents in children and adolescents who require pharmacologic treatment [30]. Of note, however, most of these studies failed to show a dose response. As a pattern of failed paediatric antihypertensive trials emerged, we sought to determine why these trials failed to show dose response in children and hypothesized that difficulties in dosing might be the cause of trial failure [44]. Using meta-analytic techniques, we determined that several factors are important which were predictive of trial success. These factors are discussed below.

*Dose Range*

The dose-range received by children randomly assigned to low- and high-dosage groups is extremely variable between trials. For example, in the amlodipine trial which did not show a clear dose response, there was only a 2-fold difference between the high-dosage and low-dosage groups with children in the high dosage group received 5 mg and children in the low dosage group received 2.5 mg. In the fosinopril and irbesartan trials a similar pattern of lack of dose response was also seen with small, dosing ranges at 6- and 9-fold, respectively. The enalapril, lisinopril, and losartan trials (which were successful in demonstrating a dose response) had considerably higher dosing ranges, at 32-, 32- and 20-fold, respectively. The successful trials thus incorporated a wide range of doses. The lowest clinical trial dose should be lower than the lowest approved dose in adults, and the highest clinical trial dose should at least be 2-fold higher than the highest approved dose in adults, unless contraindicated for safety concerns. In some of these situations, there had been a conflict between FDA, investigators and IRB's in this regard. The FDA has requested higher doses than approved in adults leaving investigators and IRBs in a difficult situation of using a dose higher than its approval in adults. With the knowledge from these early trials, this issue should not arise in future trials.

None of the failed trials investigated dose ranges higher than the corresponding adult doses. For example, the highest irbesartan dosage was 4.5 mg/kg, whereas adult data indicate that most adults need dosages up to 150–300 mg (~2–4 mg/kg for a 75-kg child) for better blood pressure control. Data obtained from irbesartan use in adults showed that effects on blood pressure increase at dosages ≥600 mg (~8 mg/kg for a 75-kg child), and the maximum irbesartan dosage studied in adults was 900 mg. These doses, however, were not included in the drug's label making IRB approvals of this high dose problematic at the time.

In contrast, successful trials provided large differences across low-, medium-, and high-dosage strata. Successful trials used dosages much lower (nearly placebo) than the dosages approved in adults. For example, the recommended initial lisinopril dose in adults is 10 mg, and the usual dose range is 20–40 mg. The lowest dosage used in the paediatric clinical trial was 0.625 mg, thus providing a wider range for exploring the dose response.

The selection of wide dosage ranges has important pharmacokinetic/pharmacodynamic implications because closely spaced dosages will likely yield overlapping exposures among dose groups. If overlap is substantial, the dose response could appear flat and, thus, fail to demonstrate a significant dose response relationship.

Another important aspect of early antihypertensive trials in children was that pharmacokinetic studies were often performed simultaneously with safety and efficacy trials and thus the information was not available for use in determining dosing. Under current paediatric drug development programs, PK/PD studies are performed before embarking on subsequent phase 3 trials in children.

*Dose by Weight*

Weight-based dosing strategies were inconsistent in the trials. The amlodipine trial did not incorporate individual subject weight in dosing but rather gave all children in the low-dosage arm 2.5 mg of product and all children in the high-dosage arm 5 mg of product. This dosing strategy resulted in the following paradox: a 100-kg subject randomly assigned to 'high' dosage received 0.05 mg/kg, and a 20-kg subject randomly assigned to 'low' dosage received 0.125 mg/kg. In the low-dosage group, one fourth of subjects received >0.06 mg/kg, and one fourth of the high-dosage group received <0.06 mg/kg. Although blood pressure did not show a dose response to amlodipine as randomized, increased dosage on a milligram per kilogram basis was associated with a decrease in blood pressure.

The fosinopril trial also failed to demonstrate a dose-response, although it incorporated individual subject weight into the dosing. However, the weight-based strategy of dosing in this trial was limited in that no child received a dosage >40 mg. Thus, children randomly assigned to medium dosage who weighed <30 kg received more fosinopril (in mg/kg) than the heaviest subjects randomly assigned to high dosage. Similar to the amlodipine trial, blood pressure dose response was not associated with product as randomized, but increased dosing on a milligrams per kilogram basis was associated with blood pressure reduction.

*Development and Use of a Liquid Formulation*

Several of the trials of orally administered antihypertensive agents (particularly those used in the failed trials) did not develop a paediatric (e.g. liquid) formulation and, thus, exhibited a wide range in exposure within each weight stratum. This is because precise dosing is not feasible using a limited number of tablets; liquid formulations allow for more precise dosing per kilogram. Development of a liquid formulation is often challenging because bioavailability can be unreliable, and dissolving the agent in liquid can require high concentrations of alcohol. In addition, stability and bioequivalence testing of liquid formulations also require additional time and expense. Moreover, it is important that the liquid formulation be palatable and often crushed tablets suspended in an aqueous medium are bitter which ultimately will affect drug compliance. Despite these issues, paediatric formulations should be requested in the Paediatric Drug Development Programs whenever possible. Development of these formulations is now more economically feasible because of benefits provided to companies for successfully completing trials requested by FDA as part of this program.

*Primary Endpoint*

Many successful trials used change in diastolic blood pressure (DBP) as the primary endpoint. Several unsuccessful studies (e.g. trials of amlodipine, fosinopril, and irbesartan) used change in sitting systolic blood pressure (SBP) as the primary outcome. We evaluated the reduction in SBP and DBP related to several agents and found that a reduction in DBP was more closely related to the dosage of agent administered. For example, in the enalapril trial where DBP elevation was the entry criteria, the dosage was more closely related to a reduction in DBP than SBP (coefficient 0.19 [p = 0.001] versus coefficient 0.12; p = 0.08). We also observed a closer relationship between DBP reduction and dosage in the lisinopril trial (coefficient 0.12 [p = 0.001] vs. coefficient 0.08; p = 0.09).

The reason for this closer relationship between DBP reduction and dosage may relate to the fact that there is less variability associated with measurement of DBP compared to SBP. DBP may have less physiological variability but also the change in DBP may be more difficult to detect by BP measurement. This reduction in variability may contribute to the success of DBP as the primary endpoint. Perhaps more likely is the fact that inclusion of DBP as a primary entry criteria tends to select children with secondary forms of hypertension. These patients are more likely to respond to drugs affecting the renin-angiotensin-aldosterone system as seen with enalapril, lisinopril and losartan studies.

Systolic hypertension is, however, 3-fold more common than diastolic hypertension, and the motivation to use SBP as the primary endpoint may derive from feasibility, a common problem in conducting paediatric drug trials. However, another important consideration is that SBP is a surrogate measurement that has been long accepted in adult patients because of its close relationship with hard endpoints of stroke, congestive heart failure and myocardial infarction. These events are rare in children but the best BP correlate to any form of end organ damage in children, i.e.

left-ventricular hypertrophy, is SBP. Thus, it seems that there would be definite benefit to the patient to test an antihypertensive medication for reduction in SBP. A primary study endpoint of mean arterial blood pressure that incorporates both SBP and DBP values might prove advantageous, and this possibility should be explored in future trials. Perhaps, even more beneficial would be the use of ambulatory BP monitoring in paediatric clinical trials for antihypertensive medications.

## Conclusion

As a result of legislative initiatives for paediatric drug development, much has been learned about the treatment of hypertension in children and adolescents in the last decade. This expansion of our knowledge base allows for improved understanding of efficacy and safety of these agents. Understanding clinical trial design in paediatric studies is paramount:

- poor dose selection,
- failure to fully incorporate weight and paediatric pharmacology into trial design, and
- lack of liquid formulation development,

likely led to the difficulties observed in several antihypertensive paediatric exclusivity trials. Which parameter of BP measurement to use as the primary endpoint of these trials remains controversial.

These data may be applicable to efforts to improve paediatric clinical trial design by government agencies, clinicians, and pharmaceutical sponsors in both North America and Europe. In the future, we recommend that paediatric antihypertensive trials do the following:

- (1) develop an exposure-response model using adult data and published paediatric data and use this model to perform clinical trial simulations of paediatric studies and to explore competing trial designs and analysis options;
- (2) work with FDA/EU PDCO to design global paediatric trials by leveraging previous quantitative knowledge;
- (3) routinely collect blood samples at informative time points to assess the pharmacokinetics in each subject to ascertain exposure response analysis; perform these PK/PD trials before the initiation of safety and efficacy trials.
- (4) Consider the use of ambulatory blood pressure monitoring as part of the clinical trial.

In addition, studies of the comparative effectiveness, long-term safety, and effects on growth, development and neurocognitive development are needed. Additional studies might also explore the effects on vascular reactivity and the impact of pharmacologic treatment on outcomes such as development of cardiovascular morbidity and mortality.


## References

1 Rames LK, Clarke WR, Connor WE, Reiter MA, Lauer RM: Normal blood pressure and the evaluation of sustained blood pressure elevation in childhood: the Muscatine study. Paediatrics 1978;61:2245–2251.

2 Reichman LN, Cooper BM, Blumenthal S, Block G, O'Hare D, Chaves AD, Alderman MH, Deming QB, Farber SJ, Thomson GE: Hypertension testing among high school students. I. Surveillance procedures and results. J Chronic Dis 1975;28:161–171.

3 Kilcoyne MM, Richter RW, Alsup PA: Adolescent hypertension. I. Detection and prevalence. Circulation 1974;50:758–764.

4 Fixler DE, Laird WP: Validity of mass blood pressure screening in children. Paediatrics 1983;72:459–463.

5 Sinaiko AR, Gomex-Marin O, Prineas RJ: 'Significant' diastolic hypertension in pre-high school black and white children: the Children and Adolescent Blood Pressure Program. Am J Hypertens 1988;1:178–180.

6  Sorof J, Daniels S: Obesity hypertension in children: a problem of epidemic proportions. Hypertension 2002;40:441–447.

7  Ogden CL, Flegal KM, Carroll MC, John CL: Prevalence and trends in overweight among US children and adolescents, 1999–2000. JAMA 2002;288:1728–1732.

8  Sorof JM, Lai D, Turner J, Poffenbarger T, Portman RJ: Overweight, ethnicity, and the prevalence of hypertension in school-aged children. Paediatrics 2004;113:475–482.

9  Hansen ML, Gunn PW, Kaelber DC: Underdiagnosis of hypertension in children and adolescents. JAMA 2007;298:874–879.

10  Luma GB, Spiotta RT: Hypertension in children and adolescents. Am Fam Physician 2006;73:1558–1568.

11  Flynn JT: Evaluation and management of hypertension in childhood. Prog Pediatr Cardiol 2001;12:177–188.

12  Strauss RS, Pollack HA. Epidemic increase in childhood overweight, 1986–1998. JAMA. 2001;286:2845–2848.

13  Hedley AA, Ogden CL, Johnson CL, Carroll MD, Curtin LR, Flegal KM: Prevalence of overweight and obesity among US children, adolescents, and adults, 1999–2002. JAMA 2004;291:2847–2850.

14  Berenson GS, Pickoff AS: Preventive cardiology and its potential influence on the early natural history of adult heart diseases: the Bogalusa Heart Study and the Heart Smart Program. Am J Med Sci 1995;310(suppl 1):S133–S138.

15  Chinali M, de Simone G, Roman MJ, Lee ET, Best LG, Howard BV, Devereux RB: Impact of obesity on cardiac geometry and function in a population of adolescents: the Strong Heart Study. J Am Coll Cardiol 2006;47:2267–2273.

16  Woo KS, Chook P, Yu CW, Sung RY, Qiao M, Leung SS, Lam CW, Metreweli C, Celermajer DS: Overweight in children is associated with arterial endothelial dysfunction and intima-media thickening. Int J Obes Relat Metab Disord 2004;28:852–857.

17  Davis PH, Dawson JD, Riley WA, Lauer RM: Carotid intimal-medial thickness is related to cardiovascular risk factors measured from childhood through middle age: the Muscatine Study. Circulation 2001;104:2815–2819.

18  Raitakari OT, Juonala M, Kahonen M, Taittonen L, Laitinen T, Maki-Torkko N, Jarvisalo MJ, Uhari M, Rokinen E, Ronnemaa T, Akerblom HK, Viikari JS: Cardiovascular risk factors in childhood and carotid intima-media thickness in adulthood: the Cardiovascular Risk in Young Finns Study. JAMA 2003;290:2277–2283.

19  Berenson GS, Srinivasan SR, Bao W, Newman WP III, Tracy RE, Wattigney WA: Association between multiple cardiovascular risk factors and atherosclerosis in children and young adults. N Engl J Med 1998;338:1650–1656.

20  Baker JL, Olsen LW, Sorensen TIA: Childhood body-mass index and the risk of coronary heart disease in adulthood. N Engl J Med 2007;357:2329–2337.

21  Food and Drug Administration Modernization Act of 1997. 111 Stat 2296, Vol 105, 105th Congress ed, 1997, pp 107–109.

22  Benjamin DK Jr, Smith PB, Murphy MD, Roberts R, Mathis L, Avant D, Califf RM, Li JS: Peer-reviewed publication of clinical trials completed for paediatric exclusivity. JAMA 2006;296:1266–1273.

23  Li JS, Eisenstein EL, Grabowski HG, Reid ED, Mangum B, Schulman KA, Goldsmith JV, Murphy MD, Califf RM, Benjamin DK Jr: Economic return of clinical trials performed under the paediatric exclusivity program. JAMA 2007;297:480–488.

24  Food and Drug Administration Website: Paediatric exclusivity labeling changes. http://www.fda.gov/Drugs/DevelopmentApprovalProcess/DevelopmentResources/UCM076610

25  Regulation (EC) No 1901/2006 of the European Parliament and of the Council of 12 December 2006 on medicinal products for paediatric use. http://ec.europa.eu/enterprise/pharmaceuticals/eudralex/vol-1/reg_2006_1901/reg_2006_1901_en.pdf

26  Rodriguez W, Selen A, Avant D, Chaurasia C, Crescenzi T, Gieser G, Di Giacinto J, Huang SM, Lee P, Mathis L, Murphy D, Murphy S, Roberts R, Sachs HS, Suarez S, Tandon V, Uppoor RS: Improving paediatric dosing through paediatric initiatives: What we have learned. Paediatrics 2009, in press.

27  Pasquali SK, Sanders SP, Li JS: Oral antihypertensive trial design and analysis under the paediatric exclusivity provision. Am Heart J 2002;144:608–614.

28  American Academy of Paediatrics: Guidelines for the ethical conduct of studies to evaluate drugs in paediatric populations. Paediatrics 1995;95:286–294.

29  Smith PB, Li JS, Murphy MD, Califf RM, Benjamin DK Jr: Safety of placebo controls in paediatric hypertension trials. Hypertension 2008;51:1–5.

30  Flynn JT, Daniels SR: Pharmacologic treatment of hypertension in children and adolescents. J Pediatr 2006;149:746–754.

31  Flynn JT, Newburger JW, Daniels SR, Sanders SP, Portman RJ, Hogg RJ: A randomized, placebo-controlled trial of amlodipine in children with hypertension. J Pediatr 2004;145:353–359.

32  Sorof JM, Cargo P, Graepel J, et al: Beta-blocker/thiazide combination for treatment of hypertensive children: a randomized double-blind, placebo-controlled trial. Pediatr Nephrol 2002;17:345–350.

33  Trachtman H, Hainer JW, Sugg J, Teng R, Sorof JM, Radcliffe J, Candesartan in Children with Hypertension (CINCH) Investigators: Efficacy, safety, and pharmacokinetics of candesartan cilexetil in hypertensive children aged 6 to 17 years. J Clin Hypertens (Greenwich) 2008;10:743–750.

34  Wells T, Frame V, Soffer B, et al: A double-blind, placebo-controlled, dose-response study of the effectiveness and safety of enalapril for children with hypertension. J Clin Pharmacol 2002;42:870–880.

35  Flynn J, Li JS, Davis I, Portman R, Ogawa M, Pressler M: Randomized, Double-Blind Trial of the Aldosterone Receptor Antagonist (ARA) Eplerenone in Hypertensive Children. Washington, Paediatric Academic Society, 2008.

36  Trachtman H, Frank R, Mahan JD, et al: Clinical trial of extended-release felodipine in paediatric essential hypertension. Pediatr Nephrol 2003;18:548–553.

37  Li JS, Berezny K, Kilaru R, et al: Is the extrapolated adult dose of fosinopril safe and effective in treating hypertensive children? Hypertension 2004;44:289–293.

38  Sakarcan A, Tenney F, Wilson JT, et al: The pharmacokinetics of irbesartan in hypertensive children and adolescents. J Clin Pharmacol 2001;41:742–749.

39  Soffer B, Zhang Z, Miller K, Vogt BA, Shahinfar S. A double-blind, placebo-controlled, dose-response study of the effectiveness and safety of lisinopril for children with hypertension. Am J Hypertens 2003;16:795–800

40  Shahinfar S, Cano F, Soffer BA, et al: A double-blind, dose–response study of losartan in hypertensive children. Am J Hypertens 2005;18:183–190.

41  Batisky DL, Sorof JM, Sugg J, Llewellyn M, Klibaner M, Hainer JW, Portman RJ, Falkner B, Toprol-XL Paediatric Hypertension Investigators: Efficacy and safety of extended release metoprolol succinate in hypertensive children 6 to 16 years of age: a clinical trial experience. J Pediatr 2007;150:134–139, 139.e1.

42  Blumer JL, Daniels SR, Dreyer WJ, et al: Pharmacokinetics of quinapril in children: assessment during substitution for chronic angiotensin-converting enzyme inhibitor treatment. J Clin Pharmacol 2003;43:128–132.

43  Flynn JT, Meyers KEC, Neto JP, Meneses R, Zurowska A, Bagga A, Mattheyse L, Shi V, Gupte J, Solar-Yohay S, Han G, Paediatric Valsartan Study Group: Efficacy and safety of the angiotensin receptor blocker valsartan in children with hypertension aged 1 to 5 years. Hypertension 2008;52:222–228.

44  Benjamin DK Jr, Smith PB, Jadhav P, Gobburu JV, Murphy MD, Hasselblad V, Baker-Smith C, Califf RM, Li JS: Paediatric antihypertensive trial failures: analysis of endpoints and dose range. Hypertension 2008;51:834–840.

Thomas Severin, MD
Novartis Pharma AG
Novartis Campus
CH–4002 Basel (Switzerland)
Tel. +41 61 324 5424, Fax +41 61 324 2130, E-Mail thomas.severin@novartis.com

Rose K, van den Anker JN (eds): Guide to Paediatric Drug Development and Clinical Research.
Basel, Karger, 2010, pp 206–211

# Paediatric Vaccination Trials

Francesca Ceddia[a] · Audino Podda[b] · Timo Vesikari[c]

[a]GlaxoSmithKline Biologicals, Wavre, Belgium, [b]Novartis Vaccines Institute for Global Health, Siena, Italy, and [c]Vaccine Research Center, University of Tampere, Tampere, Finland

Eradication of smallpox is considered as perhaps the most important public health achievement of the 20th century. As a result, smallpox vaccinations could be stopped globally in 1979. Eradication of poliomyelitis is targeted next in the early 21st century. Other viral infections, such as measles and rubella, which are limited to humans with no animal reservoir, might eventually be eradicated by extensive immunization of young children, freeing mankind from these diseases that cause high mortality or permanent disability.

In other cases, immunization of children will prevent most of the serious diseases while elimination of the infectious disease agent is not possible at present. Such diseases include diphtheria, tetanus, pertussis, *Haemophilus influenzae b* (Hib) infections, meningococcal and pneumococcal disease and more. In such cases it will be necessary to maintain immunization programmes for the foreseeable future. However, even though these vaccines already exist, there is need for constant improvement for better efficacy or greater safety or both.

Although most of the vaccines currently available target young children, adolescents may also be targeted by certain vaccination programmes, particularly such as the one against human papilloma virus for the prevention of cervical cancer. In each case, it is necessary to evaluate the vaccines, whether new or improvements of existing ones, in the particular age group the vaccines are intended to be used for. Therefore, most of the clinical studies needed for vaccine development need to be performed in paediatric populations.

## Characteristics of Vaccine Development

A number of substantial differences exist between vaccine and drug development.

Firstly, the majority of vaccines to date have been developed for prevention of infectious diseases, and therefore their target population is most often represented by healthy individuals, especially children. For this reason, and, in consideration of the large number of subjects the vaccines may be potentially administered to, it is of utmost importance that vaccination benefits greatly outweigh risks. Therefore, the clinical databases requested for registration of vaccines for human use include tens of thousands subjects, or significantly more than what is normally required for the registration of a drug. Sometimes, to obtain an even more precise assessment of safety and to rule out rare vaccine associated adverse effects, post marketing commitments for additional, even larger, post-registration trials are required by the regulators.

Childhood vaccines may be combined to include multiple antigens: for example against diphtheria, tetanus, pertussis, *Haemophilus influenzae* type B, hepatitis B and poliovirus. All new combinations will require testing for safety and immunogenicity even though the components may be well known and already licensed vaccines.

Unlike drugs, which are mostly chemical agents, vaccines are biological products and therefore it is essential to evaluate the consistency of their manufacturing process both in pre-clinical and clinical development.

Additionally, unlike drugs, often developed for adults and subsequently 'adapted to children', many vaccines have primarily a paediatric target population and therefore the definition of their clinical profile should primarily occur in children.

Finally, also from a clinical operations perspective, the infrastructure utilized for vaccine trials is also unique; in fact children are usually referred to special health care units, like vaccination clinics or well baby clinics, rather than to hospitals and in most of the cases trials involve healthy children only.

In this chapter, we will review the most important elements to be considered for the clinical development of paediatric vaccines.

## Regulations for Paediatric Vaccine Clinical Development

Despite the differences highlighted above, both vaccines and drugs are covered by the same regulations.

According to ICH E11, children are considered a vulnerable population and as such, regulations have also become more stringent over time, even for vaccines where paediatric development has always been the rule rather than the exception.

In USA, vaccines and drugs are covered by the Pediatric Research Equity Act (PREA), which came into force in 2003 and requirements for safety and efficacy are similar (http://www.fda.gov/opacom/laws/prea.html.).

In the EU, a new Paediatric Regulation entered into force in 2007 for both drugs and vaccines. The Paediatric Regulation requires early submission of a Paediatric Investigational Plan, aimed at ensuring that the necessary data are obtained through studies in children aged 0–17 years, when it is safe to do so, to support the authorisation of the medicine for children (www.ema.europa.eu/htms/human/pediatrics/classwaivers).

### Stages of Clinical Development of Paediatric Vaccines

The main goal for clinical development of a vaccine is to demonstrate efficacy and safety of the candidate vaccine. Efficacy is normally demonstrated through field trials based on clinical endpoints.

Similar to drugs, clinical development of vaccines includes different stages, and paediatric clinical development holds a number of peculiarities within these stages.

### Phase I

Before testing a new vaccine in children, a phase I study is usually conducted in healthy adults, even if the ultimate target of the test vaccine is the paediatric population. Although phase I studies are primarily aimed to look at the tolerability profile of the new vaccine, they are also used to get an initial information on its immunogenicity, both at the serological and at the cellular level. Additionally, these studies may look at different doses and regimens of administration including or not a control licensed vaccine if that is available.

### Phase II

Normally with an age de-escalation approach (i.e. progressive testing in adults, adolescents, older children and infants) during phase II the new paediatric vaccine is tested in the target population.

Several issues should be addressed in phase II in the context of randomized and controlled studies. Among them, the most relevant are the following:

(a) Definition of the most appropriate vaccine formulation; this includes the selection of the antigen(s) concentration and the assessment of the potential need for an adjuvant to induce a sufficient immune response. Typically, these studies are conducted in the specific target population or in the age closest to the target population (e.g. either infants or toddlers, if the target population is infants). Ideally, the selected vaccine formulation should be the same for all age groups. However, in some cases the same vaccine may require different formulations for adults and children. In the case of influenza and hepatitis, the dose in children is lower than in adults, whereas in the case of diphtheria and pertussis, the (booster) dose in adults is lower than that for children.

(b) Characterization of the tolerability (local and systemic post-immunization reactions) and safety (vaccine related serious and non-serious adverse events) profile of the new vaccine in the target age group. Post-immunization reactions vary according to the age group. In infants, the most commonly reported reactions for an injectable vaccine include: tenderness, erythema and induration at the injection site, fever, changes in eating habits, sleepiness, irritability, persistent crying, diarrhea and rash.

(c) Assessment of the ability of the vaccine to induce an immune response both from a qualitative and a quantitative point of view. As part of the immunogenicity assessment, it is important to also look at the ability of the vaccine to prime the individuals and, on a booster vaccination, induce an anamnestic or memory response so that a subsequent exposure to that same antigen results in a faster, greater and longer antibody response and ultimately a more effective protection from the disease. Assessment of memory response can be investigated in different ways including the use of a polysaccharide vaccine after priming with conjugates, or by investigating the cell-mediated immune response.

(d) Assessment of the kinetics of the immune response. Although duration of protection is normally assessed with follow-up surveillance studies after registration, the pre-licensure immunological characterization of the vaccine should include evaluation of the persistence of antibody titers and the need for a booster dose in order to maintain an adequate level of circulating antibodies.

(e) Definition of the most appropriate schedule of immunization to be used later in phase III clinical trials pivotal for registration. Children of different ages may need a different number of doses to induce an optimal immunological response. Infants, due to a less mature immune system, may need multiple doses (e.g. between 2 and 4 doses within the first 2 years of life) while older children may require fewer doses (e.g. 1–2 doses in toddlers up to a single dose in pre-school children or adolescents). Looking at this objective, it is important on one side to identify the most appropriate spacing among doses to get an optimal immunological response, but on the other side to keep in mind all different vaccination regimens already existing worldwide. Ideally, in order to achieve a high coverage and to reduce additional costs of vaccine delivery, the new vaccine should be administrable according to the established multiple schedules of immunization for paediatric vaccines in Europe (2, 3, 4 months; 2, 4, 6 months and 3, 5, 12 months), USA (2, 4, 6 months) and developing countries (6, 10 and 14 weeks of age, as recommended by the EPI Programme of the WHO).

(f) Ruling out interference with potential co-administration with already established vaccines. As children already receive at scheduled visits a number of recommended vaccines it is necessary to make sure that the addition of the new vaccine during the same vaccination visit does not adversely affect the immunogenicity of routine vaccinations nor increase their reactogenicity.

*Phase III*

At this stage of development vaccine testing should be normally performed with the final vaccine formulation, produced at production scale in the final manufacturing facility, and using the proposed immunization schedule in order to produce, in large randomized and controlled clinical trials, pivotal data for registration on the safety of the vaccine, the efficacy in the prevention of the disease and the clinical consistency of vaccine manufacturing.

Efficacy

The objective of these trials is to evaluate vaccine protection by measuring the reduction in the incidence of the disease among individuals who have received the test vaccine compared to the incidence in unvaccinated individuals. These trials are normally very large and may require, depending on the background incidence rate of the disease, tens of thousands of subjects: an example is the efficacy trial of the first licensed heptavalent pneumococcal conjugate vaccine, conducted in approximately 38,000 infants. The primary endpoint of that large efficacy trial was prevention of invasive pneumococcal disease [1]. These field trials should also look at the possibility to define immunological correlates of protection (i.e. the identification of the threshold of an immunological response, normally an antibody titer, which is associated to protection from the disease). According to CHMP (EWP/463/97), *for vaccines (antigens) for which the protective antibody level is established, immunogenicity studies may be more suitable in establishing efficacy.* Therefore, once correlates of protection are defined and accepted by the scientific community and regulators, they can be used as trial endpoints to assess the efficacy of the vaccine in an immunogenicity trial and for subsequent investigational vaccines. Licensure of vaccines based on immunological data in comparison with a licensed vaccine (non-inferiority) have occurred so far for vaccines like the Hib and meningococcal conjugate vaccines

and most recently for new pneumococcal conjugate vaccines.

The feasibility of efficacy trials depends largely on the incidence of the disease in the target population. In case the incidence of the disease is so low that a huge number of subjects would be required for demonstration of efficacy and in case immunological correlates of protection are not available, the only other theoretical approach potentially available, with concurrence by regulators, for producing the efficacy data needed for registration of the vaccine is the so called 'animal rule'. Based on the animal rule, efficacy data obtained from animal studies may be extrapolated to humans. Although this approach has been discussed mostly to allow registration of antibioterrorism vaccines (e.g. anthrax vaccine), it remains the only other possibility in case the epidemiology of the disease would not allow an efficacy trial in humans to be conducted, ethical considerations would not allow a challenge trial and immunological correlates of protection would not be available. Should this approach be viable, a post-licensure trial would be needed to verify the product's clinical benefit should feasibility conditions be satisfied.

Sometimes, the expected benefit of certain vaccines may not be the reduction of the incidence of disease but rather the demonstration of an impact on disease complications (e.g. hospitalization, severity of disease). When a clinical endpoint cannot be measured for ethical reasons (e.g. reduction in occurrence of cervical cancer in women with HPV infection), or when the expected benefit is delayed over time (reduction in occurrence of cervical cancer), a valid alternative clinical surrogate needs to be established (e.g. reduction of pre-cancerous lesions; CIN 1, 2 and 3).

Safety

According to the type of vaccine (novelty of the vaccine, inclusion of a new adjuvant, etc.) additional safety data may be required to support registration of the vaccine in children. Ellenberg [2,

3] examined, based on the expected rate of certain adverse events, the number of subjects needed in a trial to detect such events and, in addition, the number of subjects needed to demonstrate that the investigational vaccine is responsible for an increased rate of these events. The number of subjects needed to detect a twofold increase in the rate of an event expected to occur in 0.1% of vaccines is approximately 50,000 while to detect a threefold increase in the rate of an event expected to occur in 0.01% of vaccines at least 175,000 vaccinees would be required. Recently, large-scale safety trials were conducted with new candidate live oral rotavirus vaccines in over 60,000 infants each, to rule out the risk of intussusceptions at a rate of 1 in 10,000 vaccine recipients. That was the estimated risk associated with a previously licensed but subsequently withdrawn rotavirus vaccine [4, 5].

Most Phase III vaccine trials are based on much smaller cohorts of vaccinees, typically in the range of 5,000–20,000 individuals, when the objective of the safety analysis is to rule out a two fold increase of adverse events expected to occur at a somewhat higher incidence (i.e. 1–0.5%). Reliance on the phase IV post-licensure experience and the reporting of adverse events is regarded as the most efficient way of bringing a vaccine into use.

## Special Considerations in Paediatric Vaccines Clinical Development

### Use of Placebo in Paediatric Randomized Controlled Trials

According to article II.3 of the Declaration of Helsinki: 'In any medical study, every patient – including those of a control group, if any – should be assured of the best proven diagnostic and therapeutic methods'.

The general rule for use of placebo in paediatric vaccine trials holds that placebo vaccination is allowed if no licensed vaccine against the target disease exists. The use of placebo arms in phase III pivotal clinical trials allows to conclude on absolute efficacy of the vaccine rather than relative efficacy compared to an older effective and available vaccine.

Vaccine placebo ratio of 1:1 generally gives the best opportunity to evaluate safety for rate adverse events. For efficacy, a smaller placebo group, for example, in randomization ratio 2:1 may be sufficient. Vaccines to vaccine (new vs. old) comparisons are generally done at 1:1 ratio and will require a larger sample size than placebo-controlled trials.

Although the type of placebo used in clinical trials may vary, i.e. true placebo control (e.g. saline, alum adjuvants) or non-true placebo control (e.g. a different vaccine) in either case subjects, and especially children in the placebo arm, should be offered to receive a dose of the investigational vaccine (cross-vaccination) within the scope of the study or of a similar licensed vaccine at the study end (outside the scope of the study).

### Paediatric Vaccine Trials in Developing Countries

The clinical profile of the candidate new vaccines may be different in developing countries. Typically vaccines may show lower immunogenicity and/or efficacy in developing country populations. Therefore, in order to achieve a global recommendation by the WHO, demonstration of clinical efficacy in developing countries is required. Similarly or even more importantly, testing in developing countries is necessary for vaccines that are indicated to prevent diseases which primarily affect developing countries.

Normally, the safety and immunogenicity of the candidate vaccines are first evaluated in young healthy volunteers in other settings, e.g., where the vaccines are produced. Following satisfactory results of the phase I trials conducted in Western countries, the phase II age de-escalation trials (from adults to adolescents, older children and infants) to reach the targeted age group for immunization (e.g. infants) may be done directly in developing countries.

Practical complexities of performing clinical studies in less developed clinical settings require a lot of efforts and commitment in capacity building, including staff education, training and facility upgrade.

The ethical aspects of clinical research in developing countries require that the proposed study is epidemiologically relevant and suitable from a country public health perspective, and that the study is well designed and aimed to achieve results that are important to the country where the trial will be conducted, including the accessibility to the new vaccine once the trial is over and the value to the local population has been demonstrated.

Additionally, the good clinical research practices should be applied in the developing countries, making sure that the rights of trial subjects and the integrity of the clinical data are not jeopardized. Review by local ethics committees may be supplemented with independent ethical review by western ethical bodies to assure that ethical guidelines are fully respected and to mentor less-experienced local review committees.

## References


1 Black S, et al: Efficacy, safety and immunogenicity of heptavalent pneumococcal conjugate vaccine in children. Pediatr Infect Dis J 2000;19:187–195.
2 Ellenberg SS: Evaluating the safety of combination vaccines. Clin Infect Dis 2001;33(suppl 4):3919–3922.
3 Ellenberg SS: Safety considerations for a new vaccine development. Pharmacoepidemiol Drug Safety 2001;10:411–415.
4 Ruiz-Palacios GM, Perez-Schael I, Velazquez FR, et al: Safety and efficacy of an attenuated vaccine against severe rotavirus gastroenteritis. N Engl J Med 2006;354:11–22.
5 Vesikari T, Matson DO, Dennehy P, et al: Safety and efficacy of a pentavalent human-bovine (WC3) reassortant rotavirus vaccine. N Engl J Med 2006;354: 23–33.



Francesca Ceddia, MD
Vice President and Head, Global Clinical Development
GlaxoSmithKline Biologicals, Wavre, Belgium
Avenue Fleming, 20 (W23), BE–1300 Wavre (Belgium)
Tel. +32 10 85 94 10, Fax +32 10 85 33 63, E-Mail francesca.x.ceddia@gskbio.com

Rose K, van den Anker JN (eds): Guide to Paediatric Drug Development and Clinical Research.
Basel, Karger, 2010, pp 212–214

# Future of the Paediatric Pharmaceutical Market

Vincent Grek[a] · Klaus Rose[b]

[a]Only for Children Pharmaceuticals (O4CP), Paris, France, [b]Granzer Regulatory Consulting and Services, Munich, Germany

The provision of pharmaceutical treatment to children is extremely complex and will become more complex in the near future. As explained in previous chapters in this book, there are multiple challenges, which include segmentation of the paediatric market into different age groups, communication challenges and sometimes insufficient collaboration between treating medical doctors and regulatory authorities, technical challenges, and many more. There are many disconnects, e.g. between public statements of all political parties that children are our future and deserve the best treatment, etc., and the reality where pressure for low pricing is quite often a strong factor. However, medicines for children are in the focus of regulatory authorities, paediatricians, paediatric pharmacologists and other stakeholders. Both US and EU governmental agencies have initiated large programs to make appropriate pharmaceutical treatment available to more and more specific paediatric needs. There is an illusion that good drug treatment can come cheap. The more the children will be included into systematic development of new and better drugs and appropriate use of existing drugs, the more the treatment patterns and attitudes will be challenged among key stakeholders and in the public opinion.

The private sector has so far been predominantly reactive to initiatives made by regulatory authorities and local governments. In the following, we give a few postulates on how key patterns in the provision of medicines for children might evolve in the near future, followed by some explanations.

1 The paediatric drug market will expand and will change its structure.
2 New specialized companies will emerge.
3 Research-based companies will include increased costs of paediatric drug development into their pricing calculations.
4 Pressure on regulatory authorities, available grants, and competition will lead to the rapid availability of new drugs and adapted treatment of older drugs for children. New technologies will emerge.
5 Pricing of paediatric medicines will shift from a multiple/fraction of the price of reference adult treatment to a true evaluation of innovation for children without reference to the adult treatment. It will induce an increased price of pharmaceutical treatment of the respective paediatric disease.
6 Society and parent will welcome companies making a profit provided they offer value for money in terms of efficacy, safety, availability, innovation and service.
7 Society's obligation to provide treatment for all treatable rare diseases will be discussed more intensively.

8   The rising costs for children's pharmaceutical treatment will be debated. The positions of different key stake holders, i.e. parents, pharmaceutical companies, reimbursement institutions, will differ.

Health and well-being of children is not only a question of availability of good medicines. It is in general terms a question of healthcare, education together with drug availability, economic prosperity, and many other factors. Furthermore, with the new communication technologies, integrated services will arise around disease management. Children in developed countries will probably profit first from this new drive in better medicines for children, but the children in the developing world will certainly also benefit in the long term.

Advances in treatment of cancer in children is one of the main success stories in medical research of the last century [see chapter by Vassal et al., this vol.]. Nevertheless, the majority of medications used in the treatment of child cancer are not registered for this specific purpose. Many of them are registered for adult use only. Most cytotoxic substances that still constitute the fundament of modern cancer treatment have been developed decades ago. In other words, they are generic today and relatively cheap. In consequence, one paradigm of the treatment of child cancer is so far that the costs of medications are comparatively low. The increasing pressure to use more drugs registered for use in children will lead to the establishment of specialized companies. These will deliver the necessary clinical and other data to register medicines for the different child age groups. Clinical trials, however, and drug development measures in general are expensive. One consequence of the current movement towards more evidence-based pharmaceutical treatment in children will be that the price of off-label substances used so far in children will increase substantially or even dramatically. Patent ductus arteriosus Botalli is a condition that predominantly affects preterm newborns. It can be treated surgically, which is very expensive and bears all the risks that come with it, or pharmaceutically by nonsteroidal anti-inflammatory substances, e.g. ibuprofen. Medication costs to apply one or a few unlicensed suppositories to a newborn are a few USD or EUR. The i.v. application of the same substance today costs several hundred USD or EUR because the new dosing has been tested clinically, expensive manufacturing insures that the highest quality has been developed and maintained for a small population, and the new indication is fully registered.

Examples where child-adapted doses or formulations have increased the price of pharmaceutical treatment are still comparatively few. With more medicines registered specifically for child use this will change considerably, which will have several consequences.

At present, the number of companies that specifically focus on the pharmaceutical treatment of children is very limited. Large pharmaceutical companies focus on adult blockbusters. However, the visible profitability of child medication will attract more companies. New companies will be established, and areas may develop where the paediatric markets reveal themselves to be profitable enough even for large companies.

The combined size of the paediatric pharmaceutical markets will grow exponentially over the coming years. Somebody will have to cover these increased treatment costs. This could be achieved by just increasing the general pharmaceutical treatment budgets (not probable in the current situation of world economy), or by shifting more money within in the overall budgets of pharmaceutical treatment. One way would be to reduce the reimbursement of treating trivial adult conditions.

People that advocate more rational pharmaceutical treatment of children might be shocked about the size of the paediatric markets in a few years time. But 'rational' should not mean 'cheap'. We are still used to relatively low pharmaceutical treatment costs in children. Paediatricians' prescriptions will increase substantially well beyond the growth rates of the current economy. Innovative new drugs for adults will probably cost more from the beginning as companies have to include the costs of paediatric drug development into their cost calculations. Once this development reaches dimensions that seriously affect the calculation of reimbursement institutions and insurance companies, the current debate on medicines for children will certainly become more intense and will reach beyond the still limited circle of people involved so far.

Children cannot vote. Their voice is not part of the public decision-making machinery. In health care, as in many other areas, many things are desirable as long as somebody else pays the bill. The consequence for children so far was that their share of the medication costs was comparatively low. This is changing now. The budgetary consequences of this change, however, have not even made it into public debate. Once this level of attention has been reached, we will face new interesting debates.

Klaus Rose, MD, MS
Principal Consultant
Granzer Regulatory Consulting & Services, Zielstattstrasse 44
DE–81379 Munich (Germany)
Tel. +49 89 780 68 98 29, Fax +49 89 780 68 98 15, E-Mail rose@granzer.biz

# Author Index

# Subject Index